Working with Homeless and Vulnerable People

Advisory Editor
Thomas M. Meenaghan, *New York University*

Related Books of Interest

New Perspectives on Poverty: Policies, Programs, and Practice
Elissa D. Giffords and Karen R. Garber

Social Work with HIV and AIDS: A Case-Based Guide
Diana Rowan

The Costs of Courage: Combat Stress, Warriors, and Family Survival
Josephine G. Pryce, Col. David H. Pryce, and Kimberly K. Shackelford

Best Practices in Community Mental Health: A Pocket Guide
Vikki L. Vandiver

Social Work in a Sustainable World
Nancy L. Mary

Case Management: An Introduction to Concepts and Skills, Third Edition
Arthur J. Frankel and Sheldon R. Gelman

Evidence-Based Practices for Social Workers, Second Edition
Thomas O'Hare

Working with Homeless and Vulnerable People

Basic Skills and Practices

Jeannette Waegemakers Schiff
University of Calgary

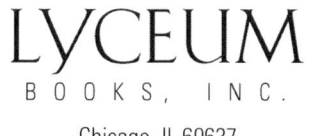

BOOKS, INC.
Chicago, IL 60637

© 2015 by Lyceum Books, Inc.

Published by
LYCEUM BOOKS, INC.
5758 S. Blackstone Avenue
Chicago, Illinois 60637
773-643-1903 fax
773-643-1902 phone
lyceum@lyceumbooks.com
www.lyceumbooks.com

All rights reserved under International and Pan-American Copyright Conventions. No part of this publication may be reproduced, stored in a retrieval system, copied, or transmitted, in any form or by any means without written permission from the publisher.

6 5 4 3 2 1   14 15 16 17 18

ISBN 978-1-935871-62-0

Printed in the United States of America.

Library of Congress Cataloging-in-Publication Data

Schiff, Jeannette.
   Working with homeless and vulnerable people : basic skills and practices / Jeannette Waegemakers Schiff, University of Calgary.
      pages cm
   Includes bibliographical references and index.
   ISBN 978-1-935871-62-0
   1. Social work with the homeless.   2. Social work with people with social disabilities.   3. Homeless persons—Services for.   4. People with social disabilities—Services for.   I. Title.
HV4493.S35   2015
362.5'53—dc23

2014016133

Contents

Acknowledgments ix

Permissions xi

Introduction and Overview xiii

    Basic Premises xv
    Aims xvi
    The Content xix
    The Journal: Integrating Learning and the World of Working with
        Homeless People xx
    A Note about Terminology xxi

Chapter 1. Who Are the Homeless and What Is Life on the Streets? 1

    Overview 1
    What Is Homelessness? 3
    Homelessness Then and Now 4
    How Many Homeless Are There? Canada and the United States 6
    Life on the Streets 8

Chapter 2. Outreach and Engagement 23

    Overview 23
    Outreach and Engagement: What Are They All About? 24
    Worker Behaviors Viewed as Valid and Invalid 26
    Intervention Skills 34
    Communication and Nonverbal Behaviors 37
    Engaging the Client 41
    Exercises 45
    Journaling 47

Chapter 3. Homelessness and Health 48

    Overview 49

vi   CONTENTS

    The Psychosocial Determinants of Housing and Health   52
    Physical Health   54
    Common Medical Conditions   56
    Health Recovery Related Needs   67
    Provider Health: Self-Care, Compassion Fatigue, and Burnout   74
    Exercises   86
    Journaling   89

Chapter 4. Interprofessional Practice   91
    Overview   91
    What Is Interprofessional Practice?   92
    Exercises   116
    Journaling   122

Chapter 5. Case Management and System Navigation   123
    Overview   123
    Publicly Administered Programs   125
    Services and Responsible Organizations   130
    Case Management: Service Coordination and Service Brokering   139
    Exercises   157
    Journaling   157

Chapter 6. *Housing First* Approaches and Housing First Programs   158
    Overview   158
    Background: Housing the Poor   159
    Housing First: A Housing Philosophy and a Program Model   175
    What about Landlords?   187
    Retaining Housing   189
    Exercises   195
    Journaling   197

Chapter 7. Mental Health and Mental Disorders (Illness)   198
    Overview   198
    Stigma   205
    Identifying Mental Health Disorders   208
    What Causes Mental Disorders and What Are Common Treatments?   223
    Basic Intervention Strategies in Unfamiliar Situations   227
    Exercises   230
    Journaling   234

Contents   **vii**

Chapter 8. Addictions: Mind- and Mood-Altering Substances and Behaviors   235
Overview   235
Substance Use Worldwide   237
Mood- and Mind-Altering Drugs: A Brief History   239
Use, Intoxication, Abuse, and Dependency   246
Drug Pathways and Body Reactions   247
Other Common Types of Mind- and Mood-Altering Drugs   252
Addictive Mechanisms and Pathways   255
Substance-Abuse Treatment   260
Motivational Interviewing and the Need for Change   266
Relapse and Relapse Prevention   268
Harm Reduction   269
Exercises   270
Journaling   270

Chapter 9. Co-occurring Disorders and Trauma-Informed Care   271
Overview   271
Co-occurring Disorders   272
Treatment of Those with Co-Occurring Disorders   278
Trauma and Trauma-Informed Care   279
Trauma and Homelessness: What Is the Connection?   281
Misidentification and Misdiagnosis   286
Worker Reactions and Interventions   290
Traumatic Brain Injury: Behavioral and Psychosocial Implications   294
Fetal Alcohol Spectrum Disorders (FASDs)   297
Exercises   298
Journaling   300

Chapter 10. Cultural Competence with Diverse People   301
Overview   301
What Does Culture Include?   302
Cultural Sensitivity and Cultural Competence   303
Personal Cultural Awareness: Who Are You?   308
Cultures, Subcultures, and Mingling of Cultures   311
Further Cultural Differences   316
Culture and Oppression   318
The Culture of Homelessness   320
Organizational Culture   322
Exercises   323
Journaling   324

Chapter 11. Ethics in Practice   325
    Overview   325
    What Are Some Ethical Issues in Working with Homeless Persons?   326
    Basic Ethical Principles   330
    Ways of Applying Ethical Principles   336
    Ethical Boundaries   341
    Ethical Decision-Making Map   343
    Boundary Crossing or Violation   345
    Boundaries in Rural and Remote Areas   347
    Ethics in the Workplace   348
    Record-Keeping and Confidentiality   352
    Code of Ethics for Frontline Workers   355
    Exercises   357
    Journaling   361

Chapter 12. Legal Issues in the Homeless Sector   362
    Overview   362
    Rights of the Homeless   363
    Victimization of the Homeless   364
    Incarceration and Homelessness   371
    Civil Law and Civil Rights   373
    Child Welfare   377
    Roles for the Worker in Legal Issues   379
    Confidentiality   380
    Exercises   387
    Journaling   388

Appendix 1. Canadian Definition and Topology of Homelessness
    (Canadian Homelessness Research Network, 2012)   389

Appendix 2. Professional Quality of Life Scale (ProQOL)   397

Appendix 3. Addiction Abstinence Self-Efficacy Scale   403

Appendix 4. Trauma Self-Assessment   405

Appendix 5. Alcohol and Other Drugs: Intoxication and Withdrawal   407

References   411

Index   431

Acknowledgments

It takes a community to raise a child, and a network of colleagues, friends, and family to support the genesis and development of a book. Without the many people who have provided inspiration, guidance, and important suggestions, this project would not have come to fruition.

The idea for this book was born out of the process of developing a course aimed to prepare frontline workers in the homeless sector in Calgary for the complex requirements of this demanding work. With the support of Tim Richter and the Calgary Homeless Foundation, and the team of Kim Ruse, Jeff St. John, Marina Giacomin, Andrea Silverstone, Timothy Wild, and John Schutte, we developed a comprehensive curriculum that became the basis for the present book. To Richard Wagamese, whose book *Ragged Company* offered much clarity for the early chapters, and with whose kind permission some excerpts are quoted, my appreciation. Steve Gaetz and the members of the Canadian Homeless Research Network have provided inspiration along the way. David Follmer, my publisher, was invaluable in providing the encouragement to broaden the scope and make this book of interest in both Canada and the United States. I am grateful for his encouragement and for his efforts to seek reviewers who were able to give sage advice in the early drafts. To Tom Meenaghan who reviewed and provided much valuable advice and support as the final draft unfolded, "merci." I am extremely appreciative of the efforts of those who read preliminary drafts and offered critical feedback: George Neffinger and Rebecca Schiff. I am especially indebted to my friend and colleague Dianne Gray for her sage advice and countless examples of sensitive and respectful interventions on the frontlines, the critical aspects of good case management skills, and for her work on a number of the illustrations that have found a home in this book. The support of my colleagues and friends has been enormous, and has provided incentive when the dark days of a late January afternoon crept across my windowsill. Those to whom I am most grateful for keeping the support and encouragement going during this journey are my family: my mother Anne; my children Daniel, Rebecca, and Sarah; their spouses Robert and David; and my husband Gordon who has witnessed and encouraged my professional life from its beginnings, as they accompanied me in the process of this book creation.

Permissions

The following individuals and organizations have provided permission to use their material.

Sullivan County Historical Society, Sullivan County, Indiana. Picture of the Sullivan County Poor House.

Bryan Passifiume. Picture of the King Edward Hotel, Pincher Creek, Alberta.

Willard Library Archives, Evansville, Indiana. Picture of the Evansville County Poor House.

Dianne Gray. Picture of the Calgary Drop-In Centre.

Barbara Campagna. Picture of the Richardson Complex, the former Buffalo (New York) State Asylum for the Insane.

Patrick Corrigan, Illinois Institute of Technology. The Attribution Questionnaire (AQ-27).

Barbara Stamm. For use of the Compassion Satisfaction and Compassion Fatigue (ProQOL) V. 5.

Patrick McKiernan. The Alcohol Abstinence Self-Efficacy Scale.

Introduction and Overview

This book is written with the frontline worker in mind. Some practitioners have come to work with homeless persons because of a personal or professional desire to help others, and some have lived experiences of homelessness and housing crises themselves. Whatever path has led to a desire to help those who are having problems getting and maintaining a foothold on permanent residence and stable lifestyle, working with those who face homelessness requires knowledge and skills in many areas of living and navigating in modern society. Working with homeless persons also cuts across the traditional boundaries of professional disciplines, as helpers assume closely related roles in counseling, advocacy, and case management. Individual chapters in this book address a broad range of knowledge and practice skills in mental health, addictions, health care, assessment and interviewing, housing strategies including *housing first*, and intervention strategies such as case management and teaching essential housing skills. (We have chosen to denote the approach with *housing first*, and the program model with Housing First, and hope that this distinction will avoid confusion as to what is being discussed.) We will also touch on additional topics that frequently arise: child welfare and legal issues are the most common. Overarching all of these is the need to be sensitive to the ethical issues that arise as we try to work respectfully with vulnerable persons.

When we talk about homelessness we are referring to a range of situations where a person lacks a safe, secure, and permanent place to live. Within this broad definition, we are concerned with those who sleep rough—that is, on the streets and in places not fit for human habitation; those who must sleep in overnight shelters for the homeless and for persons affected by domestic violence; those provisionally accommodated in temporary accommodation and those whose present economic circumstances or housing arrangements are precarious. We include in this description those who are "doubled up" in living spaces intended for fewer than the number of people actually present, and those who are "couch surfing," moving from the bed of one friend or family member to the bed of another on a frequent basis. We recognize that people who are presently in institutions, primarily hospitals and prisons, who have no place to live on discharge, are among the homeless. Homeless people can range in age from one day to over eighty years. They can be single, in relationships, or consist of entire families. For a complete definition and description of those we include among the homeless, please see appendix 1.

Fundamental to working with homeless persons is the need to understand the complexities of working with diverse persons from different backgrounds, worldviews, and value systems and priorities. We call this interdisciplinary or interprofessional practice. Homeless persons have many needs that involve various professions involved with health, psychological well-being, child welfare, legal issues, and housing issues. Workers find themselves in daily contact with social workers, police, doctors, nurses, mental health workers, and child-care specialists who come from a variety of educational and professional backgrounds. Some may have specialized professional education and experience, but many have a generalist training in basic human services. Some have no training except the most important— the reality of life on the streets. We keep all of these nuances in mind as we present material that recognizes the many backgrounds and professions in the field and the rich opportunities available when persons from multiple professions and disciplines work together.

Working with the homeless is a specialized field of practice that is beyond the scope of general professional programs. Addictions, chronic health and mental health issues, poverty and housing issues, assessment, case management, and interviewing skills are taught in disparate courses. Students rarely have an opportunity to both take all of the courses required for full understanding of the complexities in working with impoverished people, or to integrate material from these different sources to address specific issues in the homeless sector. In addition, there are few opportunities to examine the demands of a multicultural and multiethnic society. Yet many homeless persons come from diverse backgrounds and minorities are overrepresented among the homeless. All of these issues are complicated by the fact that many courses are taught from an academic stance with insufficient attention to the important experiential and practice-oriented elements needed to understand frontline work.

We want to give readers an understanding of what it means to work with persons from many different backgrounds in the context of helping a single individual or family.

Introduction and Overview   XV

We include the backgrounds of both clients and workers. When looking at frontline workers we examine both the priorities that different professionals have on the care provided and the importance of the professional ethics of each discipline. We interweave these with a look at the ethical dilemmas that are encountered in everyday work by those who see and experience skirmishes with the law, and survival skills that may skirt legal boundaries. In this process we make no effort to comment on any behavior other than to recognize that those who are desperate for food and shelter may be forced into coping behavior that is not universally respected, including dumpster diving and sexual bartering.

Working with homeless persons is based on learning skills in respectful interaction, awareness of differences, the need to empower people, and the need to let the client set the pace of the agreed-on change plan. Learned skills also include those involved in working in groups, as often the worker finds him- or herself in a team either within the employing agency or in the community with various other persons also involved in a homeless person's life. Thus, respectful team work is essential.

There are additional topics that are not covered in this introductory text. In recognizing the importance of getting a basic text and reference book into the hands of providers and would-be providers, we have chosen to limit this volume to essential knowledge and skills. In future work we aim to delve further into practice topics that involve the challenges and problems of persons fleeing domestic violence, homeless youths and seniors, immigrants and refugees, homeless families with two or more adults in the family unit, and further complexities in mental health and addictions beyond the basics in this book.

The following section begins with a brief overview of some of the organizational features of this book, the basic premises from which we offer information, the aims of the book, the inclusion of journaling as an important learning tool, and how the content is presented. We also include a note about the careful use of the language that we have elected to frame these discussions.

BASIC PREMISES

Everyone has the right to a standard of living adequate for the health and well-being of himself and of his family, including food, clothing, housing, medical care, and necessary social services; everyone also has the right to security in the event of unemployment, sickness, disability, widowhood, old age, or other lack of livelihood in circumstances beyond his control (United Nations, 1948).

More than sixty years ago the United Nations adopted a statement of the right to housing for all peoples. Basics of food, clothing, shelter, and potable water are fundamental to life. In providing for the welfare of all, we recognize the importance of the principles and priorities laid down in Maslow's hierarchy of needs (figure i.1) (Maslow, 1954).

Historically, poverty is the single largest contributor to lack of appropriate shelter and nutrition, although natural disasters such as floods and famine, as well as human disasters created by war, have become major contributors in many countries. Governments have moral and ethical responsibilities to ensure the welfare of their citizens. Thus homelessness, where it exists at all, should be an individual choice, and should not be the result of lack of resources. These statements are embedded in the United Nations Declaration of Human Rights and in the personal freedoms and protections of the Canadian Charter of Freedoms and US civil rights legislation. We would add that access to equal opportunities in education and affordable health care are additional rights that further the assurance of a healthy civil society. Working with homeless persons involves recognition that, for many, daily living is consumed by meeting basic biological and safety needs. As those are more easily met, there is room for addressing other, psychological, social, relational, and self-development needs. The growth that results when these latter needs are met can often be astounding.

AIMS

The main aim of this book is to provide frontline social service workers, and those who are beginning work in this area, with the fundamental information to provide competent and consumer-driven help to persons who are homeless or at imminent risk of losing housing. To this end, we provide an examination of the multiple personal and social service components required to adequately address their needs. We aim to do the following:

- Provide an understanding of the lived experiences of those who have faced homelessness and of their vulnerabilities in various areas so that

Figure i.1. Maslow's Hierarchy of Needs

Self-Actualization Needs: Realizing personal potential and self-fulfillment; seeking personal growth and peak experiences

Esteem needs: Achievement, mastery, independence, status, dominance, prestige, self-respect, and respect from others

Social Needs: Belongingness, affection and love, from work group, family, friends, romantic relationships

Safety needs: Protection from elements, security, order, law, limits, stability, freedom from fear

Biological and Physiological Needs: Air, food, clean water, shelter, warmth, sex, sleep

Growth Needs

Foundational Needs

- workers may appreciate those struggles as voiced by homeless people.
- Help service providers to understand the multiple systems involved in homeless services provision: individual, family, small group, agency, and government.
- Provide an understanding of how the multiple service systems interact with each other in housing and support services.
- Help service providers understand and be able to work with diverse professionals.
- Examine the individual challenges faced by vulnerable persons: lack of education, job skills, mental health, and physical health; and addiction issues.
- Provide basic training in interviewing and group process skills.
- Explore the challenges of frontline work, including the professional use of the self in engagement of clients in the helping relationship, self-care, and dangers of burn-out.
- Provide training on the importance of case management, its components, and its effective utilization.
- Help providers to understand the philosophy of *housing first* approaches and the specific components that allow for their effective use with different groups of people.
- Explore the multiple legal and ethical challenges faced by vulnerable individuals, service providers, and service agencies.

The aim of this book is to unite all of the basic information and skills for frontline workers in a single volume that can be used both as a college- or university-based text on working with homeless persons, as well as a reference for those who are looking for information useful to job-based training. Because many frontline workers may not have educational experiences beyond high school or junior level college, the material has been presented in ways that are user friendly. The references provided are meant to support this information and often direct the reader to professional Internet resources (not to for-profit or commercial organizations) and to government sources that update statistics and other data more frequently than is possible in a printed book.

THE CONTENT

We stress the concept of interprofessional work because the homeless services sector includes representatives from multiple backgrounds who need to recognize each other's competence and develop effective ways of working together. This recognition prepares frontline practitioners to work with the complex array of personal and interpersonal problems that are common to those experiencing homelessness: mental health, substance abuse, concurrent disorders, complex health issues, access to necessary and eligible social services and employment rehabilitation program, and ongoing supports to prevent another housing loss. At the same time, understanding the complexities of working with different disciplines orients practitioners on how to navigate a complex system comprising government, mental health, medical, legal, and social service agencies; how to effectively manage client caseloads; how to provide linkage to best serve the client's needs; and how to develop skills working with service workers and professionals from multiple viewpoints to effectively communicate and advocate for the client. Finally, we hope that it provides a greater awareness of diversity and culture, proper professional conduct, the importance of self-care for practitioners, and the complexities of ethical behavior and decision making.

We hope that the use of this as a textbook or an in-service training guide will provide a common foundation for training practitioners working with the homeless population. The content for this book has been developed using evidence-based practices that have been shown to be effective in treating the homeless population and are accepted interventions within the field. We anticipate that it can be used to train practitioners in interprofessional and cross-disciplinary practices so that they will be able to competently respond in a variety of situations and contexts. In this text, we strongly emphasize the understanding and implementation of a *housing first* philosophy that has rapidly come to be adopted in many areas, because it affirms the unconditional right to housing. To that end, we differentiate the *housing first* philosophy from the program model by the same name (Housing First), which is currently considered a best practices for homeless mentally ill and substance-abusing (co-occurring disorders) persons. Finally, we focus on developing cultural competency and ethical practices because these aspects of services delivery are essential components of respectful and competent practice in a multicultural society.

THE JOURNAL: INTEGRATING LEARNING AND THE WORLD OF WORKING WITH HOMELESS PEOPLE

At the end of chapters 2–12 are exercises that can help to integrate the material in that section and suggestions for journaling. Learning is also the integration of content and experience, and the use of critical thinking in melding these two. It is insufficient to be exposed to information; a worker must learn how to filter it for relevance, critically evaluate its appropriateness, and apply it in a meaningful way in real life. One highly effective way to develop this integration is through the use of a journal to focus reflection between the written word and the world of work. Journaling is an important part of self-reflective learning and skill development. It is an opportunity for a new worker to become aware of the connections between what she learns in the classroom and the realities of her work environment. Journaling is an excellent way to become increasingly aware of your feelings, roles, and actions working with others, which also allows you to reflect on the process of developing effective helping skills.

The format of these journal entries is set up to parallel that of record-keeping—stating facts separately from reflecting on feelings—and will reinforce your ability to write concise, focused entries required for work. Thus it is important for you to consider the journal as an active part of this learning experience and one that you will attend to regularly. There is no single specific topic that is relevant or appropriate for your journal entry because what you experience on the job will determine what connections you make with the text material. Each journal entry should focus on an interaction or event that happened during your work week. It should relate to material that you have learned in the previous chapter, but over time may be relevant to more than one module. For effective journaling, each entry should

- start with what has happened;
- include your actions (behaviors) and personal reactions (thoughts and feelings);
- reflect on how this is relevant to what you have learned in previous chapters; and
- offer any conclusions, if that is appropriate.

If you are reading this book as part of a course, you should make at least one entry per week. This allows you to develop a regular habit of self-reflective learning and to monitor your growth in knowledge and understanding of the material. It will ensure that you recall significant classroom information while you work. It will also allow you to appreciate the development of your own personal reflections over time. You may make more entries if you so choose. The journal becomes another learning opportunity for you. When the journal is part of a course requirement, you should be evaluated on whether you have included all of the above components in your reflection and *not* on the nature of the experience or what conclusions you draw from it (unless they violate ethical, legal, or moral norms). Your reflections may include

- specific incidents working with homeless persons;
- issues of practice and ethics that arise in your workplace;
- challenges in working with colleagues in your agency and in other agencies; and
- observations on what obstacles there are in trying to help homeless people.

We hope that as you journal you allow yourself to become a self-aware individual who continuously engages in reflective practice.

A NOTE ABOUT TERMINOLOGY

In the human services field, as in others, the words that we use to describe people and their situations often change as we become more sensitive to the various aspects of a social issue or a specific group of persons. The first challenge has been around gender-related words. We interchangeably use either "he" or "she" when speaking of individuals, and do not intend to suggest a sexual bias. A second challenge is that over the past fifty years we have witnessed many changes in word usage and connotations, and we are aware of, and sensitive to, their implications. For correct descriptions when examining historical antecedents to the current issues, we have chosen to use the terminology in prevalent use during the period mentioned. Thus the reader may encounter words such as addict, drug user, substance abuser, battered women's shelter, asylum, insane, the chronic mentally ill, and others. Where these may be offensive to modern readers we have placed them in quotation marks to indicate a word or term that is no longer acceptable or in popular use, but that is historically accurate. This will also help those who may seek further information by providing the search words likely to target historical material.

In the first couple of chapters, where we focus more on the absolutely homeless, we have used some terminology to differentiate those who are housed and not housing insecure as coming from Main Street, and those who live in shelters, and outside of shelters (sleeping rough) as living on the streets and living rough. We also refer to those who are in marginal accommodations or on the verge of losing housing as fragilely housed. This has slightly different connotations than the term "marginally housed," as the latter can more accurately speak to deficits in the physical shelter while the term "fragilely housed" connotes a person whose housing security is very tentative. We have not chosen to use street lingo because it frequently varies with geographic location. However, where used, it is meant to convey some of the culture of those who have no home of their own (Schutt, 2011). At the same time, we encourage practitioners to become aware of local street language in order to be aware of the local culture and its variations.

Throughout this book we have made a deliberate effort to respect the worldview of those who are housing vulnerable. Often words acquire a negative meaning that can act as a stigma. Thus we avoid constantly referring to people as "the homeless." One option, which may not be acceptable to everyone, is to use the term "vulnerable" or "housing vulnerable" to refer to those who have no stable dwelling place of their own. These terms include those who are without shelter as well as those who are temporarily housed; they refer to the housing (shelter) vulnerability and not to personal vulnerabilities. Indeed, it has been noted by others that those who sleep rough have impressive resiliency and coping skills (Smith, 2010).

We have chosen the term "working with homeless persons" to denote the partnership of helping alongside rather than putting ourselves in a one-up position. This term is long and may not fit agency vocabulary that more frequently uses terms such as "client" or "patient." However, we have been careful not to use the word "client" to refer to anyone unless a formal relationship has been established. There are many places that use the word "client" to denote a person who seeks shelter in an emergency hostel for one or many nights. Is the recipient of relief services really a client? It is more appropriate to denote as clients those who have agreed to a service relationship in which there is at least one goal or action plan and an agreement to work with staff in a designated agency. Thus, in the section on engagement (chapter 2) you will note that there is no mention of a client until there is at least a tentative and implicitly agreed-on goal or action plan to which the worker is a facilitator. Where appropriate we use the above terms, but that should not be taken by the reader as a statement of preference. Rather it is one of reality that different service and health organizations have their own preferred terminology. In all of our usage we aim to be accurate but not offensive. This sensitivity to language, we suggest, is extremely important in working with people who have been disadvantaged.

CHAPTER 1

WHO ARE THE HOMELESS AND WHAT IS LIFE ON THE STREETS?

How do you feel...
When you have no home...
When you have no place to eat, sleep, or feel safe...
When you have no place to belong...
When you know no one who will take you in...
When you have no hope...
When you are all alone...

KEY ISSUES

Description and definition of the homeless

Universal features of homelessness and some country-specific issues: Canada and the United States

Overview of the subcultures of the streets and shelters

Specific needs of clients who are currently homeless or have a history of homelessness

Building rapport and a therapeutic alliance with clients who distrust treatment providers and agencies

Providing practical assistance to clients to meet their basic needs

Safety on the streets for community providers

Understanding street crime, drug trafficking, and gangs

OVERVIEW

This book is about reaching with a hand out to give someone a hand up. It is about understanding that the most important thing is to always be aware of how it feels to "walk in someone else's moccasins." The most important thing for a worker is to be sensitive to the many challenges posed by a life in severe poverty with few resources that is the mainstay of existence on the edge. In the following pages we introduce a frontline view of life on and the culture of the streets, and of those who are without a fixed address, such as couch surfers. Then we turn to an overview of specific needs of people who are absolutely homeless or among the hidden homeless, with a temporary roof offered by family, friends, or kind strangers. We begin here because in order to work with people it is essential that you recognize and accept "where each person is at"—that is, what the individual's current state is, physically, mentally, emotionally, and spiritually. That means understanding the fundamental issues that face those whose worldly possessions may well be what is in their backpack or a wheeled laundry cart. A respectful acknowledgment of these life circumstances will contribute to building a connection and eventually, hopefully, a pact built on trust. Without understandings at the beginning, no effective helping strategy is possible.

The aim of this first chapter is to provide you with an appreciation of the many challenges that confront a person who is in extreme poverty and who has few resources. To do so, we explore street culture and how survival depends on learning and using skills in dealing with various people, both those in similar circumstances and those on the other side: those in authority, with power, money, and the privileges that stable housing provides. This includes recognizing that lived experiences impact people differently: the issues and struggles in southern towns are different from those in northern cities; those in warm, dry climates are different from those in climates with snow or rain; those in rural areas are different from those in congested cities. The issues and struggles vary depending on an individual's age, sex, ethnicity, and other personal characteristics. These lived experiences are impacted by what led to the houseless circumstances: be it domestic violence, alcohol and drugs, a mental illness disability, or evictions due to financial crises brought on by high rents, low wages, or immense debt. They are also influenced by what we think of when we think of home—a place to live, a place to belong, a place where we have or can put down roots, and a sanctuary from life's hardships and challenges.

Having some understanding of the streets sets the stage for us to suggest how you as a frontline worker may acquaint yourself with the local street culture of your community and what local homeless people experience. We also take a look at life on the edge—what the imminent threat of losing housing does to a person's sense of security and ability to plan for tomorrow—even if "tomorrow" is just the next few days. When more than one person is involved, this insecurity extends to everyone in the household and is especially critical for children whose insecurity is fueled by adults unable to predict what tomorrow may bring.

WHAT IS HOMELESSNESS?

Home is a special place. It reaches inside us and awakens feelings of belonging, comfort, and shelter. For some it arouses painful memories of places that should be comforting but are not. For many others home arouses reminders of what is lacking in their lives: a place to be welcome, to call your own, to be able to close a door and leave your public faces outside. Home is a place to relax and be in control of who walks through the door and who leaves. Home, for many of us, is the place where we can be who we want to be. For some people home is a place to hang a hat but lacks the emotional safety that it should provide. That kind of safety comes from feelings that this place of shelter is secure and conveys a sense of belonging, as well as from the knowledge that this home is not a makeshift or temporary accommodation that can be removed because it was an expedient for protection from the elements without promises of permanency.

Most of us have a home to turn to—even if where we currently live is a stop along life's road, such as it is with college-bound students who still consider the parental house as home, extended travelers on a long road trip, or those young adults seeking their own place to live. These young people do not worry about home because there is a place of safety they can still return to. They are transitioning from what was the childhood home to one they will establish as adults. But for an alarming number of people, from children and youths to seniors, home is a dream of something not currently available and perhaps, they fear, never achievable. These people are the dispossessed of the twenty-first century, those who have no abode that is permanent or secure, that is a shelter that keeps out the elements, provides essential electricity, heat, and running water, and is not in imminent danger of being lost for a variety of reasons. These are the people we refer to in this book as the homeless. For many, the first challenge is obtaining housing, before even attending to the other aspects of creating a home. Getting and maintaining housing is not easy; there are many complex factors that contribute to this dilemma. For a complete description and definition of homelessness that is the basis of our understanding of this complex phenomenon, please read the definition of homelessness in appendix 1.

Homelessness is about many "nots": *not* having a safe and adequate shelter from the elements, *not* having a voice in who shares a shelter or how long one can stay in that place, *not* determining the rules of how one lives in a shelter, and *not* having a feeling of belonging in that shelter. While a tent may be a regal home for a Bedouin prince, it is a precarious place to live in the Yukon or Alaska. What is adequate shelter will always have some regional variations. What is an emotionally and psychologically safe place has universal elements. A shelter that is not safe and has no promises of permanency is not a home. Staying in a large urban shelter that houses hundreds of people may be less safe than sleeping under a bridge, as the chance of having personal possessions stolen is less out in the open than it is when a cot with a stranger is thirty inches from your own.

HOMELESSNESS THEN AND NOW

Homelessness is not a new phenomenon. There have been homeless and displaced persons in all societies for thousands of years. The majority were poor and disabled. But homelessness in the twenty-first century is a problem within an industrialized society that has new features not encountered before. Poverty, rising costs of housing not in keeping with low-income wages, lack of housing subsidies, and the complications of those disabled by physical and mental illnesses as well as addictions have created a new profile of those who are homeless. A hundred years ago asylums and poorhouses sheltered the most destitute. Some slept rough and in hovels unfit for human habitation. These have been demolished but nothing has been substituted to shelter the most needy of society. The demolition of marginal housing and asylums was coupled with a rise in the standard of living in urban North America. Low-cost cold water flats with a single toilet on each floor, which were found in tenements in major cities, were replaced by apartments featuring indoor plumbing and central heating in each housing unit. Large boarding houses for the urban poor disappeared. At the same time, many cities and towns demolished shanty towns and other poor housing that was seen as an urban blight (Jencks, 1995). The result of these events was that a great deal of affordable housing for the poor disappeared. In figures 1.1 and 1.2 you can see how this accommodation was handled in poorhouses; present-day variations continue to be found in rural communities. A "King Edward Hotel" is found in many small towns throughout English-speaking Canada. It is frequently the only low-cost accommodation available and is often used for emergency shelter in rural areas.

The closure of many psychiatric hospitals in the 1960s and 1970s forced those disabled by mental illness into inadequate housing, competing for scarce space with the poor who had also been dispossessed (Grob, 1994). Currently, persons with a mental illness, single parents with children, and those with physical disabilities, all formerly cared for by the state, now live in the community with inadequate financial and social housing supports to manage even a marginal existence. These groups of housing poor are joined by many people whose education and job skills make them eligible for only minimum wage jobs, which, as we will explore later, is not enough to shelter, feed, and clothe an individual (Burt, 2001). Those with an alcohol addiction, who were among the homeless hobos of the Great Depression, have

Figure 1.1. Sullivan County Poor House, Sullivan, Indiana

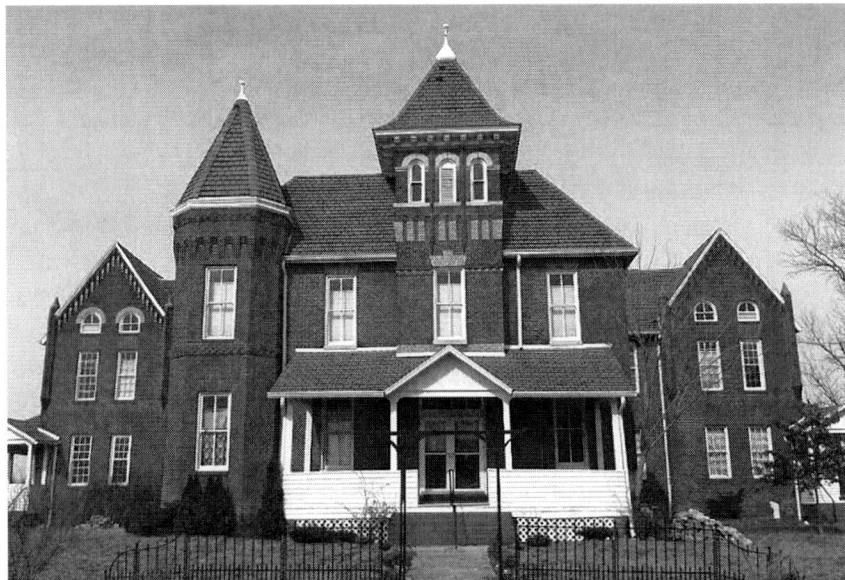

Source: From the archives of the Sullivan County Historical Society. Used with permission.

Figure 1.2. The King Edward Hotel: Low-Cost Accommodation in Rural Canada

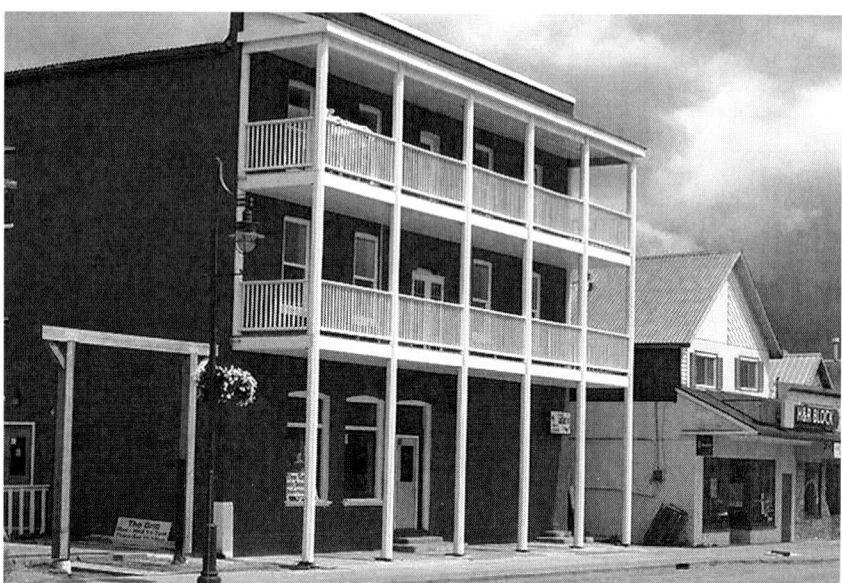

Source: Used with permission from Bryan Passifiume.

been joined by many with serious drug addictions that rob individuals of the ability to hold on to housing and stay out of jails. In the past two decades prisons have only too often become alternative institutions for those with mental health and addiction issues who fall outside the law (Fitzpatrick & Myrstol, 2011). Local jails have also become a shelter from the cold for those who are publicly intoxicated or who commit minor infractions of the law, with a return to street life when the sun rises.

HOW MANY HOMELESS ARE THERE? CANADA AND THE UNITED STATES

In Anglo-Franco North America homelessness is a major issue; many of the issues encountered are similar in Canada and the United States. Because the definition of who is homeless differs, and thus who are counted as homeless are not the same in both countries, the comparisons between the homeless populations in Canada and the United States are not always exact. The history of government supports for those who lack proper housing is also different in the two countries. Nonetheless, on both sides of the border there is a similar picture of those who are most vulnerable to homelessness: victims of poverty, disability, unemployment, educational disadvantage, racial and ethnic differences, economic circumstances, and foreign wars. In the United States a biennial count of those who are homeless includes those sleeping rough (unsheltered) and in shelters; these numbers are reported as over 636,000 (National Alliance to End Homelessness, 2013) and do not include those in prison or other institutions such as a hospital with no place to return after discharge. When those who are doubled up (individuals couch surfing or multiple families sharing one dwelling unit) are included in the tally, an additional 6.8 million persons are estimated to be without a home, which represents a 50 percent increase since 2005 (Sermons & Witte, 2011). In Canada there is no official national count of homeless persons. Data on shelter use includes congregate care, hospitals, and religiously based communities as well as shelters, and thus do not offer any accurate measure. Nonetheless, there is broad consensus that the homeless, not counting those marginally sheltered on reservations, ranges between 200,000 and 300,000. While some large cities such as Toronto, Vancouver, Calgary, and Edmonton conduct regular counts of homeless people and thus have a breakdown by age, ethnicity, sex, and family status, there are regional variations (as there are in the United States) that make it impossible to generalize to all areas of the country.

The United States and Canada have vastly different populations, with the United States having ten times the total population of its northern neighbor, and centers of population are grouped in different ways in each country. In Canada, most of the population is along the southern border and concentrated on the shores of the southern Great Lakes, Erie and Ontario, along the banks of the St. Lawrence River, and along the west coast of British Columbia near Vancouver. In the United States, population density follows historical paths of immigration and settlement, especially along the coastal areas and major rivers. The greatest population concentration is in the eastern half of the country, in California, and in a portion of southern Arizona. What is equally important is that the average population density in the United States is 34.06 persons per square kilometer, while it is a mere 3.79 in Canada. These comparisons are useful for understanding the locations of major centers that have large concentrations of homeless individuals and the vast regions where rural homelessness is likely to exist. The places most likely to have major concentrations of homeless persons include older industrial cities, but in both countries they are especially prevalent near coastal cities and in warmer climates.

We continue our comparison of the two countries with some further details. Homeless people are a heterogeneous group whose present housing dilemmas come from multiple causes. The diversity in the homeless population varies by country, and reflects a picture of the nations' poor and oppressed. There are many similarities in North America as Canada and the United States share many demographic features as well as similarities in poor persons. Tables 1.1, 1.2, and 1.3 compare some of these differences.

LIFE ON THE STREETS

In order to understand the issues and needs of homeless persons, it is important to have an awareness of what absolute homelessness is like, as many people either experience this or fear that this will happen in their struggles to maintain stable housing. We present here a frontline view of life and culture on the streets, specific needs of clients with a history of homelessness, and the challenges of developing rapport with clients who typically distrust providers. This presentation is based on the basic premise that in order to work with people who need assistance it is essential that we start with where the person is, which includes understanding the challenges of utter destitution and lack of belonging. This understanding contributes to building a connection and eventually a pact built on trust. Without this fundamental connection no effective helping strategy is possible.

> **Textbox 1.1. Emotional Burden of Homelessness**
>
> In *Ragged Company* the sole woman of the group, thinking about the realization that she has the chance to move to and stay on Main Street reflects, "Digger carried the street in his chest. Timber and Dick carried the street on their shoulders. They carried the story of their street life, the story of how they got there, the story of how they had survived. Even though that splendid old bear of a house we lived in bore no weight of loss, no burden of sorrow, no hauntings, it didn't need to. Some of us brought our own."
>
> (Wagamese, 2008, p. 192)

Life on the streets is also about experiences that leave people traumatized, as they witness human suffering, brutality, and violence. It includes the stigmatizing behaviors of the privileged who are housed and who ignore,

Table 1.1. The United States and Canada: A Comparison of Homelessness

United States	Canada
The composition of the homeless population, meaning those unsheltered and/or living in temporary shelters, is well documented in the United States. A comprehensive report by the National Alliance to End Homelessness presented the following description of the American homeless population (Witte, 2012). Single persons account for 63% of the total and persons living in families account for 37%. The number of families and family members has risen significantly in the past eight years, driven to a large extent by the economic downturn and the mortgage crisis that saw many people evicted from their homes. Homeless people are a heterogeneous group whose present housing dilemmas come from multiple causes. Homeless counts do not always categorize people by ethnicity or race and thus these national profiles are missing some details, but local reports indicate that African American and Spanish-speaking people are overrepresented. Poverty and low income are significant contributing factors to homelessness. The very poor in any given sector of the country are the most frequently unhoused or living in substandard conditions.	In Canada the larger cities that complete a homeless count periodically report on demographics such as Aboriginal origin, immigrant status, youths, adults, families, and seniors who are homeless and the length of time they report being without housing. Both sheltered and unsheltered people are included in these point-in-time counts, but those who are doubled up or couch surfing are not usually part of the overall totals. The rate of homelessness varies by city and region of the country, but also by size of the city: large urban areas are more likely to have shelter beds. Rural homelessness has recently begun to receive more attention in both countries. While the number of homeless families has reportedly grown somewhat in some cities such as Calgary where the economy is strong, affordable housing for low-income families is scarce and family homelessness continues to be a significant problem. Canada also continues to have an economy that has withstood the extremes of economic hardship experiences in the United States and has not had the enormous burden of mortgage defaults that has impacted large numbers of Americans.

overlook, or move away from a person who appears to be homeless. Homelessness means being singled out by police and enforcement officers who are charged with reducing vagrancy, loitering, bylaw infractions, and petty crimes of turnstile hopping or riding without a ticket on public transport. In painting this picture we hope to emphasize that homeless persons may be victims of crimes and injustices, that they may also be perpetrators of immoral and evil acts, or they may be helpless bystanders. All of these experiences leave a person more vulnerable and potentially scarred. Often these

Table 1.2. Distinct Groups in the Homeless Population

United States	Canada
In the United States, demographics on five distinct groups are reported: singles (63%), families (37%), those chronically homeless (17%), youths (size of this group is unknown), and veterans (11%). The totals amount to more than 100% because some people fall into more than one category. Veterans are a sizable group of about 67,500. Their numbers are declining because of active government interventions, but they still present a large and troubled group of people with special circumstances and special needs. Homeless counts do not always categorize people by ethnicity or race and thus these national profiles are missing some details, but the National Coalition for the Homeless (2009) notes that African American and Spanish-speaking people are overrepresented. Poverty and low income are significant contributing factors. The very poor in any given sector of the country are the most frequently unhoused or living in substandard conditions.	In addition to capturing information on singles, families with children, youths who are homeless, and those who have short- and long-term issues with homelessness, some Canadian reports include those who have an observable mental illness or substance abuse. Visible minorities (self-defined) as well as those of Aboriginal, Metis, and Innu/Inuit origin are also documented. Aboriginal people are overrepresented among homeless people in major Canadian cities. In Vancouver they account for 2% of the overall population but 13% of the homeless population (unsheltered and living in shelters). In Calgary the numbers are 2% and 18%, respectively. In Edmonton the numbers increase to 4% and 22%, respectively (Hanselmann, 2001). Toronto has a large immigrant and refugee population that makes up a significant proportion (21%) of those who are homeless. This reduces the proportion of Aboriginal homeless to 8%, but that figure is still inordinately high as Aboriginal people make up only 0.4% of the overall population. These numbers show that in every major Canadian city Aboriginal people are significantly overrepresented in the homeless population (Hwang, 2001).

experiences will involve service providers as witnesses or inadvertent participants, leaving them all the more sensitized and ultimately desensitized to the stress of the streets. These traumatizing issues will be explored in greater depth in chapter 9 when we look at co-occurring disorders and trauma-informed care.

People do not choose to be homeless. Homelessness happens because of personal circumstances and society's failure to offer basic human protections (see appendix 1 for a full description). Homelessness is the result of

Table 1.3. Counting Homeless People in Rural Areas

United States	Canada
Until US Department of Housing and Urban Development (HUD) regulations were revised recently, homeless persons in rural areas were not counted if they were doubled up or couch surfing. Recognition that lack of available shelters in rural areas meant that many people moved in with family or friends has recently emerged in a new HUD initiative that will make specific rural-oriented services available in those areas. The Homeless Emergency Assistance and Rapid Transition to Housing (HEARTH) Act of 2009 was revised in 2013 to specifically address unique rural issues. Section 1504 of the HEARTH Act directs HUD to establish regulations for this program. (See 42 U.S.C. 11301.) These regulations include a description of homelessness salient to rural areas: "housing situations of individuals and families who are homeless or in the worst housing situations in the geographic area; stabilize the housing of individuals and families who are in imminent danger of losing housing; and improve the ability of the lowest-income residents of the community to afford stable housing" (HRSP, Section 579.1 Subpart A). Funding under this assistance program may be used for items such as rent, mortgage, utility assistance; relocation assistance; short-term emergency lodging; new construction; acquisition; rehabilitation; emergency food and clothing; employment assistance and job training; health related services; housing search and counseling services; referrals to legal services; mental health services; substance-abuse treatment services; and transportation (HUD, 2013).	Canada recognizes those who are staying with friends and family on a temporary basis as homeless, but there are few rural programs to help with rapid rehousing or prevention of housing loss. Some rural areas have adopted a housing coordinator to take on a brokerage role in homeless prevention and rapid rehousing (e.g., Newfoundland and Labrador), but the singular effort of one individual to support high-needs families and individuals, even with community services in place, may be underresourcing the need. In addition to lack of available housing, in remote areas the cost of food is prohibitively high; this burden is not offset by northern food allowances for those who do not qualify. Feeding programs are infrequent and relying on traditional hunting does not provide sufficient food security, especially for a single mother or an elderly person. Rural poverty and housing insufficiency is a significant issue, even more so for the 25% of Aboriginal people who live in rural areas but not on a reserve (Waegemakers Schiff & Turner, 2014).

multiple factors, individual and societal, that result in an individual or family being unable to get or sustain independent living. Low income, unemployment, illness and disability, health, mental illness, and substance use all may be contributing factors, as may be the disadvantages created by lack of education, and experiences with the child welfare and justice system. The personal devastation of war trauma adds further risk factors of homelessness for veterans who have seen combat. Homeless persons may be single adults, youths fleeing abusive family situations, families dispossessed through economic hard times, single parents without adequate income to pay rising rental costs, and seniors whose rent has exceeded their ability to survive on a fixed and inadequate income. Social services workers who strive to help those dispossessed come from a variety of backgrounds, ranging from those with lived experience, those who find employment in low-paying shelter positions, to college and university graduate students seeking to help disadvantaged people and working toward social justice.

The lens of values and attitudes that we use to view the world around us shapes our reactions and behaviors in whatever situation we find ourselves. A man with a full backpack and a week's worth of facial hair that we encounter on a mountain trail evokes a very different reaction from the same person walking in a busy downtown area known to have a homeless shelter nearby. We associate the first picture with a healthy outdoor athlete, and the second more likely as a vagabond with no secure place to spend the night, attend to personal hygiene, or stash his belongings during the day. That scruffiness, whether it be in a man or a woman, is one common feature that most of Main Street society uses to distinguish the housed from the unhoused. Body odor, personal neglect, unkempt and uncut hair, and worn out and unwashed clothing are additional signs. While most of us travel with intent from one destination to another, those who are homeless might take a long ride to no particular place. In urban areas you can cleverly transfer on public transportation to different routes and ride out a bad snow- or rainstorm, and be going no place in particular. These behaviors are more subtle than the panhandler who sits on the sidewalk or the person sleeping by an open grate that spits hot air into a dark December night. We have all seen the homeless, and have all walked quickly and widely around those whose behavior seems odd or unpredictable, or makes us uncomfortable.

What is it about homelessness that makes most Main Street people uneasy? Are we worried about behavior that may be threatening, or do we wish to avoid those who are the victims of society's failure to provide? Is it guilt or fear of contagion—their homelessness, their despair—that makes us cross the street to avoid them? Do we think that all homeless people carry disease and may pass on the lice and bedbugs that we associate with poverty and uncleanliness? Or do we feel guilty that our fortunate lives have kept us out of the gutters of life? Do we think that "these poor unfortunates" (as some would describe those who are homeless) have no education, no sense of deportment, no understanding of Main Street society? Do we see them all as afflicted with moral deficits that lead to alcohol and drug addiction?

These fears and attitudes are central to the stigma that we associate with being homeless. Because so many of these attitudes allude to personal flaws, we assume that it is within the individual's power to change his or her circumstances. In that assumption lies the misbelief that homelessness is a personal flaw. Stigma about homeless individuals is also about how we are viewed by society, as in the adage "you are known by the company you keep." Few people want to be associated with those who are outsiders to Main Street, since we live in a world where association with money and appearance and a life filled with gadgets is a symbol of being successful and thus being wanted. No one wants the baggage associated with being homeless. As we try to shift our attitudes we must first look through the eyes and walk in the shoes of those who live on the streets.

Some Typical Scenarios

Why begin with an exploration of personal experiences of homelessness? Many years ago the helping process was described in basic and simple terms that began with identifying and starting where the client was at (Perlman, 1957). This simplicity hides its importance. It is this principle that is foremost in reaching out to work with a homeless person. In recent years we have come to realize and accept that help, if it is to be acceptable and effective, must begin with whatever issue, concern, or problem a person identifies as one she will accept help with. While there was a time when helpful good Samaritans distributed aid that they presumed those in need wanted, these efforts frequently missed the mark or failed to deal with the most primary issues, as identified by the person being helped. The result was that recipients of those good deeds felt humiliated and demeaned as others, in better circumstances, would try to dictate how they should live their lives and overcome their problems. For example, no one wants to be told with whom to live, and many choose to opt out of various housing and other options if treatment interventions for various psychosocial, behavioral, and substance-using behaviors are mandated by service providers (Tanzman, 1993).

Experiences of homelessness are manifold, as diverse as the lives of those who find themselves on the edge or without a stable place to live. They vary from the teenager who has left an abusive household, to the young adult who traveled a thousand miles in search of work only to find that the job didn't pay enough to cover housing and food costs. It might be the young family dependent on two incomes who finds itself with the primary wage earner sick, unable to work; the family has no health benefits, and is suddenly less than a paycheck away from eviction. The faces of the homeless are as varied as the rest of society. Homelessness is the soldier returning from combat duty in the throes of anxiety, nightmares, and an inability to concentrate, who is frequently intoxicated to relieve these distressing symptoms, and who has no emotional resources left to find and keep work. After alienating family and friends, he finds little solace in an emergency shelter. It is the single mother with a couple of small children who struggles to pay for babysitters, travels across town to a menial, low-paying job, and then is laid off because of lack of business. It is the downtown career woman who worked her way through business school, rose to top of the class, began a promising position, and is then laid off because of the struggling economy. Faced with debts of over $100,000, she has few options as she can't afford to pay her rent, can't return home, and is couch surfing with friends. Or it is the bus driver who served the route you rode who has been let go, the bus route eliminated. She has three dependents, including an ailing husband, no means of support; her house is almost paid off, but she must refinance it and can't, because she has no income. Selling it in a down market will be difficult and without substantial help she will lose her house and be on the streets.

On the other side of town live a group of people who prefer to call cardboard boxes, salvaged boards, and blankets cobbled together, home. Near them is another assortment of people who have found an abandoned street tunnel for sheltered sleep. Booze and drugs are for many of them, but not all, a fact of life. Some choose to remain clean and sober and help those who have fallen off the wagon. Meanwhile, in the Latino quarter families double up and share living and sleeping spaces, taking turns while others work evening and night shifts. The same scenario of overcrowded housing is found in many immigrant homes, especially those with single men seeking a foothold in Western society. Tempers flare in hot humid weather and teens stay out till all hours, preferring the streets to the crowding tensions of home.

After eight years of violence and spousal abuse a woman leaves her home. Lacking job skills and married at the age of eighteen to a man who could find employment only in low-wage jobs because he too lacked technical skills, she has no savings and must rely on the local domestic violence shelter to provide a safe haven. She takes her children with her, but then worries about the ever-vigilant child welfare authorities and their powers to take the kids away. Meanwhile she wonders how she will pay for food and necessities, including the endless diapers that the two-year-old still needs.

Across town is a man, age twenty-four, who was hospitalized for the third time this year and now faces a diagnosis of schizophrenia. He does not yet qualify for disability income because he struggled to work in a warehouse until his last episode resulted in his being fired. His family lives 1,500 miles away and does not have the money to bring him home. Besides, he refuses to return home. His latest psychotic episode led to him trashing his apartment, so he has been evicted and no one knows what has happened to his belongings. He has the clothes on his back and no place to go when he is discharged from the hospital. He also has celiac disease and must have a special gluten-free diet. Any food made from wheat, such as bread, will make him sick. He does not know how he will manage this. These are but a few scenarios. One could easily find examples from every age group and social class as economic hardships are faced by those who have lived a paycheck away from losing housing.

What is common to all of them is the fear and anxiety that pervades the life of a person caught on the edge. With housing loss you lose more than the roof over your head: you lose your privacy, your independence, your right to choose where and when you will do basic activities of daily living such as when you eat, sleep, and even use the washroom. Your access to washing facilities for showers and cleaning clothing is limited to those few places that provide shelter to the public. You no longer can determine what bed you will sleep in each night and who has used the pillow the previous night. There is no place you can call your own, no private nook to cuddle in, no haven for a bit of relief from public noises. The possessions that you have you must carry with you, unless you are fortunate enough to find and to be able to afford a public locker to store your worldly possessions. But that last resort is only good as long as you can pay the rent for it.

How Does It Feel to Be Homeless?

So how does all of this make you feel? Fear and panic at the possibility of becoming homeless quickly turns to depression, sadness, and despair as you see your world collapse around you. Without a place to call yours, no matter how humble, you have lost status in the eyes of society. You feel marked as a failure, even if the circumstances were entirely beyond your control. Provision of your basic needs for food and shelter is now in the hands of others, and your struggles for independence and self-sufficiency are battered by those who hold the power of providing them. The longer this situation continues, the more likely you are to lose hope of having things change, the more likely you are to acquiesce to demands from others. This may mean bartering your body for shelter, more prevalent for women but also a threat for men and especially for teenage boys. You may be fearful of being out of doors in the evening, especially near the local shelter where you must sleep—if the weather is too cold for rough sleeping. We know that for homeless persons, trauma is often something they flee from and something that also confronts them on the streets (Coates & McKenzie-Mohr, 2010). Life on the streets is not easy. You feel as though you have lost your dignity and respect as a human being. People walk by you and avoid eye contact if they sense that you are in need. Your appearance is not what it would be if you had adequate access to bathing and grooming facilities. Even walking into a grocery store or deli can rouse suspicion, with people watching to see if you will steal or panhandle. Your presence at the local fast food joint is discouraged, even when you scrape up the cash for a coffee. You can feel the social scorn and avoidance from the other side of society that easily ambles into and out of these places. You are often not welcome at the library as it discourages those who are not actively reading or using its resources, which is not possible when you have lost your glasses, and so this is one fewer option for shelter on a rainy day.

Then there are the police and law enforcement officials. They turn up everywhere and seem to target the shabbiest looking to harass. They ask for ID—which you no longer have because it was lost when you were evicted, or was it when you were robbed at the shelter? In any event, you no longer have a birth certificate. Your license expired long ago and you have no money for another. Who needs a passport? You don't ever see yourself able to leave town, never mind a trip out of the country. So with no ID you are not a person. Your access to health care is limited because you don't have a health-care card (in Canada) or a U.S Medicaid/Medicare card (Hwang, 2001). You can't get a voter's card if you can't provide proof of residence, and only some jurisdictions will accept the shelter as a legal residence so you may lose your ability to vote. You are a noncitizen.

Being homeless means that you must get up when someone else tells you to—there is no sleeping in when you stay in a shelter. Nor is there a place to go and lie down if you are sick. You may be sleeping thirty inches away from someone who has a communicable disease or is carrying parasites such as bedbugs, lice, or scabies—and you may not even know it. People who are homeless have more health issues, and more-serious health issues, than those who are housed, as we discuss later. These issues exist regardless of whether you live in a place with socialized medicine services such as Canada, or in the United States where public clinics and emergency rooms treat the homeless (Hwang, 2001). You have trouble getting care, getting the prescribed medicines, diet, and rest needed for recovery. And you continue to risk increasing your health problems (Hwang, Tolomiczenko, Kouyoumdjian, & Garner, 2005).

You are constantly faced with booze and drugs. Your buddies—if you can call those you hang around with buddies—are most likely ready to toke up, get high, or get smashingly drunk the minute stuff is available. You may well join them since there is nothing else that will take away all of the bad feelings you harbor. Cops to harass you? That is probably the least of your worries, as a dirty joint or needle are even greater dangers. At least the cops would give you "three hots and a cot"—food and someplace that you could lie in all day, something much safer than what most local shelters provide. All this somehow seems better than the street, and less violent as well (some of the time).

If you are single, you may not have anyone to watch your back—or the few things you have while you take a shower in a shelter. As a woman you constantly face the dangers of predators; your risk of any kind of assault is extremely high, especially near and around shelters where predators often lurk. Your protector may be a pimp, in which case your life is controlled by another abuser. You avoid authorities because jail time does not appeal to you. But the loneliness, emotional pain, and isolation may drive you to increasingly use more drugs to dull the pain. And you find yourself in a downward spiral. If you have children, you face the additional fear that child welfare workers may appear at any time and remove your kids, your only lifeline to someone who cares.

Homeless youths face additional threats as their legal status is precarious, their income sources limited, and their support systems fragile to nonexistent. They most often rely on peers for support and assistance, but this is a two-edged sword as peers have their own set of problems. In addition, the widespread use of drugs and alcohol as a social lubricant and anxiety-reducing mechanism leads to all of the dangers that drugs pose. The banding together of youths has a dark underside for those who become involved with gangs. They are likely to become victims, fueled by peer pressure and coercion, as the pressures of gang conformity become straitjackets (Harper, Davidson, & Hosek, 2008; Yoder, Whitbeck, & Hoyt, 2003).

Life on the streets is a constant confrontation with trust—whom to trust, if anyone. It is a never-ending challenge to stay dry and warm, especially if you live in a cold climate. You face the constant warning that you should not linger any place for too long and that you are not welcome in those public places others move around in with ease. Large stores, supermarkets, libraries, public halls, and train and bus stations are all warmer than outside—or cooler in the heat of midsummer. But most cities and towns have watchful police or bylaw officers ready to pounce on any infraction, even those outdoors in public parks and streets. In some places park benches have been reconstructed to discourage sleeping. Fines are impossible to pay and result in an increasingly long record for vagrancy and bylaw violations (Sylvestre, 2010).

Faced with being one of hundreds or thousands, depending on the size of your city or town, you stand little chance of getting enough time with a frontline worker to make a solid plan as to how to get out of this mess that your life is in. Moreover, many of these workers are here today and gone tomorrow. So whom can you trust to really be of help? When you are down and out, as are your friends, your mutual support is not enough to lift you above the bottom rungs of the ladder.

When Is Help a Step Up?

Many organizations have come to realize that blankets, hot coffee, and warm socks in the winter are the first order of business for those who are out in the rough. Having a stable, safe place to sleep each night is an important step to establishing a foothold in moving forward. Thus sleeping in large-scale shelters that house hundreds each night is for many who live on the streets no safer than sleeping under a bridge. For those who try to find day labor jobs, the stability of a secure sleeping place, one that will accommodate shift work, and the opportunity to work with a counselor who helps develop a plan to finance a way out of the shelter are vital to personal progress.

For most persons, meeting the basic necessities for food, shelter, and clothing consumes most of their available physical and emotional resources. Health problems and access to health care are major issues for persons without housing, and are usually not addressed because getting food and shelter takes all the time and energy a homeless person has available. Maslow's hierarchy of needs (see figure i.1) illustrates this challenge (Maslow, 1954).

Seeking medical attention for all but the most painful and distressing symptoms becomes a secondary matter. Emergency rooms are often uncomfortable places, and waiting for services often takes hours. This assumes that a person can get help without being able to show proof of ability to pay either through insurance or a Medicaid/Medicare card (United States) or health-care card (Canada). In addition, those who obviously are homeless are often accorded less priority in treatment and are assumed to not follow through on recommended care. Thus basic medical issues are generally neglected until an emergency arises (Hwang, 2001). Even in the event of medical treatment, follow-up care frequently requires access to medication, perhaps a special diet, and plenty of rest. These services are usually not made available in first-stage shelters (basic, straight from the streets). In secondary, transitional shelters where families and women with dependent children, or those fleeing domestic violence, may stay for a longer period, permission to stay in bed, to have a special diet, and so on may still not always be forthcoming. It is a vicious cycle, because without good health the opportunities to seek and obtain housing are greatly diminished.

While research reports on the precarious health of those who are homeless, most studies and commentaries focus on physical health problems but neglect to include oral health. We know that poor oral health—gum disease, abscesses, cavities, and missing teeth—contribute to poor nutritional intake and general ill health. In addition, poor teeth disfigure the face, marking a person as poor, lacking resources for self-care, and socially less acceptable. Other than pulling abscessed teeth, which can result in systemic poisoning, there are few if any opportunities for housing-insecure and homeless people to get dental care, and almost never to get replacements such as crowns, bridges, and dentures. Yet without this basic remediation people with major dental problems continue to face disfigurement as part of the stigma of homelessness, further lowering their self-esteem.

Some cities and town have developed programs that provide help beyond the basics of food, and a place to sleep and tend to basic hygiene. These programs often consist of a day during which multiple local service providers and support persons set up booths, much as at a convention, in a large public space such as a town hall, arena, or other building with open areas, for the purpose of providing immediate, free, services to those who need them. As grooming and personal appearance is always a primary issue for homeless persons, barbers and hair stylists offer complimentary haircuts and beard trims or shaves. In some places dentists provide oral care and public health nurses attend to minor ailments. Some have added opportunities for those without basic ID to complete applications for birth certificates, and residency and other ID cards, with application costs covered by government grants. Shoes and clothing appropriate for workplaces may also be available. In many localities these services exist in disparate locations that may be difficult for a homeless person to access and are often at a cost that most people on the edge can't afford. These service fairs are a tremendous asset for those who seek to improve their physical well-being, which also results in improved mental well-being.

There is no way to adequately capture the experiences and emotions of those who face life on the precipice of homelessness, or who are truly without an adequate place to sleep at night. Yes, there are a few stalwart individuals who prefer this lifestyle, but the overwhelming majority of persons with housing problems want a place of their own, without a stranger dictating how they should live in that shelter, and with whom. In a society that has too often depicted those who are homeless as antisocial street vagrants, with drug and addiction issues, it is important to remember that many homeless persons do not fit this stereotype. In order to provide meaningful, respectful help, we must remember that in many cases it is fate, circumstances of birth, and life events that place some people in safe homes and others on the street. With this in mind, walking in another's shoes, rather than presenting as critical interlopers, we can be respectful and effective helpers.

Doubling Up and Couch Surfing

Many people do not go straight from housing to a shelter. They often move in to a friend's spare room, or sleep on a friend's couch. For some youths, couch surfing is a popular way of meeting people while traveling, absorbing the local culture, and living inexpensively. Accommodation, while sparse, is free. For those who are homeless, couch surfing does not entail such idyllic adventures, but is a means of surviving at the edge—close to, but not in, a public shelter. Also called doubling up, it may be with family, close friends, or acquaintances. It may be freely offered, or come with expectations: child care of others' dependents, cooking, cleaning, or other duties in exchange for a place to sleep. In rural areas, doubling up is frequently the place where one finds homeless people, as shelters are few and far away.

Doubling up is not intended as a permanent solution to housing but often goes on far longer than anyone involved had intended. Along with expected chores comes the need to pay for food and other household necessities. Many persons who double up fall into the trap of thinking that this is a free holiday and forget the burden placed on the host(ess). Lack of reciprocation is one of the frequent stressors that results in this type of arrangement breaking apart. The stress of lack of privacy, and neglect of emotional and physical boundaries also contribute to the short-term nature of many of these arrangements. In rural areas doubling up may be an accommodation to harsh weather conditions. When the cold eases up, many, especially single men, will seek shelter in unused cabins, tents, unheated trailers, abandoned cars, and even sweat lodges (on and around reserves). The following present some pictures of where persons who do not want to stay in a shelter, or have no shelter available, double up.

Frequently, doubling up is a final step between being domiciled and homeless. Domestic violence is a precipitant for women who choose to live with friends or family rather than continue to live in an abusive situation. Many women, youths of either sex, and some men find that sexual favors are often expected in exchange for a place to stay. In some cultures, sharing a dwelling with extended family members is a norm. Those who come from "away" will generally find a place to stay with kin, no matter how remote the relationship. However, even kinship accommodations have their limits of tolerance, especially if the guest's behavior challenges or violates the house norms. Those who double up encounter many of the emotional challenges of those who are in shelters—depression, a lack of hope, an inability to see a brighter future, and a feeling of lack of empowerment.

Somehow life on the streets in the twenty-first century has many echoes of the streets of London in the nineteenth century that Charles Dickens wrote about. Our shelters are the modern replacement for poorhouses, but not much better when it comes to personal safety and security. Many people still sleep with their shoes around their necks for fear of theft of their transportation. We do differ in one way—our homeless have access to potent drugs that were not known in Dickens's time, and we will look at the issue of addictive substances in chapter 8. These substances alone have added a measure of violence and insecurity to the streets that were not seen a century ago. For now it suffices to say that the streets are dangerous places to be and no place for the poor, weak, helpless, sick, and disabled of all ages and lifestyles.

CHAPTER 2

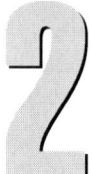

OUTREACH AND ENGAGEMENT

KEY ISSUES
- The structure and goal of outreach activities
- Importance of engagement and rapport
- Common mistakes and errors in engagement
- Introduction to basic counseling techniques and styles
- Introduction to motivational interviewing
- Challenges when working with a guarded or hostile client
- Finding common ground and goals with the client
- Professionalism in the workplace including language, mannerism, documentation, and interacting with coworkers
- Worker self-care and protection

OVERVIEW

In this chapter we focus on the basic skills necessary to provide outreach services and engage homeless persons in the service networks. We examine ways to develop therapeutic rapport and a helping alliance with homeless persons. Various aspects of outreach focus on means to provide respectful, empowering assistance. We also explore issues of the professional self and the need for workers to ensure personal physical and psychological safety for themselves and those with whom they work.

This chapter covers basic interviewing and outreach skills. Although this is familiar content to students from a variety of disciplines that use motivational interviewing in helping others, the focus here is on how to best implement these skills with the housing vulnerable and those living rough. The content flows directly from an understanding of the life experiences of potential clients. It emphasizes a low-key, down-to-earth approach that aims to minimize the existing status disparities. The language that we use shifts from "homeless person" to "potential client" and on to "client" gradually, in keeping with the process that evolves gradually on the street. Until a person has agreed to accept some form of help from a worker, she is not a client; we must be careful not to assume a relationship that has not been mutually agreed on.

Working with homeless persons requires an individual to be real—to offer genuine conversation and to recognize but not emphasize apparent differences. It requires use of language that is not technical or complicated, and can include street language where necessary. It challenges the worker to remain in the role of "helper" while not emphasizing the negative aspects of professionalism, power, and authority that are often perceived as part of service provision—and then create unwanted and unnecessary boundaries that impede the helping process.

OUTREACH AND ENGAGEMENT: WHAT ARE THEY ALL ABOUT?

Long before a person becomes homeless he has had one or more instances where service providers, who were in positions to help, failed to do so (Kryda & Compton, 2009). Distrust of those who present themselves as helpers is thus real and bitter. As a result, changing attitudes and perceptions about potential helpers (outreach workers) can be a slow and tentative process. The goal of outreach is to establish a tentative acceptance of instrumental help with the issues or problems that are most important and immediate for the homeless person. That may be a meal, a sleeping bag, connection with a street health service, or just about anything within legal limits that the worker may have access to. It may come as an invitation to a homelessness services fair where food, clothing, haircuts, and dental services are available at no cost. It may start over a cup of coffee or after weeks of passing the homeless person on the streets and giving a respectful nod. Whatever it takes, the person's tentative willingness to talk to a worker, to hear what may be available as help, is a beginning.

We speak of engagement when a person is willing to talk with a worker and accept some preliminary help—based on her needs and not that of the worker or agency the worker represents. This engagement depends on the ability of two people to build a preliminary relationship based on truth and trust. Although the homeless person may test this relationship, it is fundamental that assurances of a valid connection are established before a worker begins any more-serious conversation about lifestyle change.

> **Textbox 2.1. The Importance of Flexibility**
>
> Many homeless persons may change the priority of their needs from one day to the next. It may not be that their overall priorities have changed, but that circumstances have thrust a new wrinkle into their lives.
>
> Being flexible, having no hidden or predetermined agenda, and knowing your audience are key aspects of establishing rapport.
>
> Remembering other aspects of personal and family needs, such as helping to get some pet food or having a toy for a child, is also important.

This recognition needs to come from the other person and not from the worker. It is another form of accepting that the homeless person must be in charge of what courses of action will be tried. In this chapter we take the insights developed previously in order to explore the respectful and effective ways in which a practitioner may begin to engage a homeless person in a conversation that eventually may lead to a plan for change. In the rough-and-tumble world of those who live on the streets and in emergency shelters, words such as "respectful" and "effective" are important because they establish the equality between two humans and the mutual regard they have for each other as individuals. The tentative words of "may begin to engage" and "eventually may lead" have been carefully chosen to reflect the reality that engagement rarely occurs at the first meeting and that it will always be dependent on the free choice of the other person to accept or reject offers of help.

In the worlds of those who live in temporary shelters and transitional accommodation, a preliminary engagement has already occurred by virtue of the fact that those vulnerable persons agree to the exchange of cooperation and adherence to rules for the opportunity to remain in a consistent place that provides food and sleeping accommodation. In each case, the persons who the shelter provides with basic life necessities recognize that they are required to forgo to some extent their rights to independent choices and freedoms (such as how late to stay out, when to eat, what time to get up in the morning), for the food, shelter, and other assistance being offered.

Those who choose to leave the rough housing of the streets must accept similar restrictions: all temporary shelters have rules about these basic activities.

Practitioner Attitudes and Values

Our fundamental attitudes toward the actions of helping shape our behaviors and thus the ways in which we try to reach out. Before looking at how to engage with vulnerable persons, we need to take a look at what our attitudes and objectives are: Do we want to help because it makes us feel good? Because we feel more powerful when we help? Because we feel in control? Do we feel superior because we are better off, or have risen above our own housing instabilities and human weaknesses such as addictions? Competent because we have knowledge and access to resources? Does helping make us feel more accomplished? Does it take away the feelings of guilt over not having done more with our lives? Do we feel better when we give than when we receive? In order to examine your own motivations for helping, we suggest that you take the time to complete the exercise at the end of this chapter that addresses your values about helping.

The most fundamental attitude that practitioners need to have and maintain is that of respect for the dignity and self-worth of each individual that one works with. Those who have ever spent time in a hospital, unable to take care of their basic needs without help, will quickly understand the heightened sensitivity that one acquires in helpless situations. For example, the small but perceptible differences between valid and invalid attitudes are illustrated in table 2.1.

WORKER BEHAVIORS VIEWED AS VALID AND INVALID

Persons who are vulnerable, regardless of age, social class, life circumstance, and degree of independence, are acutely sensitive to being treated respectfully and as equals. They are the first to note the false assurances, insincerities, and other behaviors that place those who are vulnerable in positions of less respect. This need for positive regard is emphasized because those who want to help but who have an attitude of superiority or greater competence will be largely ineffective and will only be able to exert influence through

Table 2.1. Valid and Invalid Attitudes

Valid	Invalid
Empathy	Claiming to understand something that can't be easily comprehended
Concern	Superficial remark with no sincere follow up
Sincerity	Hollow and patronizing remark
Interest	Lack of acknowledgment of a response—or moving on to another issue without acknowledging what someone has said
Care	Not asking what the other persons needs
Truthfulness	Promising what you can't deliver
Respect	Not allowing for personal boundaries, space, privacy

rule enforcement. Rule enforcement may provide temporary acquiescence but never cooperation and engagement.

The issue of trust is intentionally not listed in table 2.1. Trust is not a single entity but develops from attitudes and behaviors that emerge from a host of activities and is the basis on which a helping relationship forms. It depends on the interactions between two persons in which, over a period of time, each person builds reliance on the sincerity, honesty, truthfulness, reliability, dependability, and integrity of the other. It is iterative, in that each small step in trust leads to the next and is essential in building the bonds that will allow for an open helping relationship. Practitioners must remember that vulnerable, homeless people have had their trust destroyed by others, usually numerous times, and find it difficult to rely on anyone, especially those from Main Street, to walk the talk. For workers this entails two fundamental rules: (1) Do not promise anything that is not within your power to deliver. (2) Expect that trust will build slowly, over time, and according to your integrity. Accept the fact that you will be tested as those you seek to help have experienced many disappointments in the past. This testing will occur daily, and will lessen only over time. It will include storytelling, sometimes lies, and checking on your reputation with others. This is a normal process and should not be considered as focused on you, the worker, alone.

Another challenge to building trust is the reality that many people do not work in frontline positions for long periods. The jobs are demanding, often have elements of danger, do not pay well, and tend to attract those with minimal formal training. Those who are new to the field, often lacking formal preparation, are prone to becoming overinvolved and to lacking the supervisory guidance to strike a balance between empathy and overengagement. The result is often the danger of burnout—as we will discuss in the next chapter. Supervision is often provided by those who have graduated from the frontlines or by those who have never experienced the immediacy of this kind of work. The learning available through supervision is often a combination of self-taught practices and suggestions from those who do not understand the details of this type of work. So what does this have to do with trust? The primary issue is that many people move on to take other, more financially rewarding jobs, thus those on the streets are constantly expected to form new relationships with those who would help. A second challenge comes from the mix of supervisory suggestions based on personal experience or, alternatively, lack of frontline experience. Conflicting and mixed messages can place the worker at risk since there is no clear understanding and "go forward" message. In either case the input may be well intentioned but not helpful because it continues a system of biased and only partially effective interventions. These scenarios continue the skepticism about trusting helpers.

Challenges for Frontline Workers

People who work with those who are homeless and near homeless are challenged on a daily basis with the physical and psychological dangers on the streets. They recognize that the streets are often violent places, where persons who have limited ability to control anger and impulses reside. Dangers from assault and robbery are everywhere, but so is dirt and its attendant diseases. The challenge is to be able to reach out without reaching into personal fear, and to be able to have a stance of attentive calmness, even when surrounded by noise and seeming chaos. The attentiveness is critical because the environment is a shifting scenario and danger can appear rapidly. On the other hand, overvigilance is also a barrier, both to engaging clients and to keeping a balanced perspective. The turmoil of the streets also contributes to worker burnout if the worker is unable to leave this at work. The challenge is to have a set of protective actions available as needed, and a street presence that does not indicate hesitation or fear. Homeless people are acutely sensitive to the vulnerabilities of others, and may not hesitate to take advantage of them if necessary or opportune.

One of the important considerations for frontline workers is how to handle the boundaries between personal and professional practice. This is especially challenging when the customary boundaries and structures of an office, with chairs and desks, are not present. On the streets, delicate conversations may be held curbside. This raises the question of whether confidentiality may be breached in a public location. The rest of the world need not be informed that the conversation taking place is between a worker and a (potential) client. Workers in the community need to blend in. Thus, casual, nondescript layered dress is important. Likewise, it is important to not give incorrect impressions in what one wears: no T-shirts with drug or violence or value judgment–related slogans, tight-fitting and overly revealing clothing, or skirts that are too short and pants that are too tight. At the same time, the worker should be both casual and not so informal as to challenge boundaries between professional helping and social or romantic relationships.

How you dress and how you behave convey important information about your level of confidence and competence, and your understanding of the need to not give the wrong message. The necessary street skills, especially for women, for when you are out in the community, even when working with those who are marginally housed, include the following:

- Wear loose, comfortable clothing that does not reveal too much skin. This is especially important for women who may be mistaken for sex objects.
- Wear flat or almost flat-heeled shoes. They are essential for mobility—for speed if you need to make a fast exit. They are also less likely to be misperceived as sexualized foot wear.
- Keep makeup to a very modest, understated level, as to be almost unnoticeable. Makeup is expensive. It is preferable to wear no makeup as this luxury is often out of the lifestyle of those who are homeless.
- Depending on the people you are with, or on the area or environment you are in, stand sideways to those you are interacting with to avoid any sudden hits or jabs or even spitting. This also avoids head-on confrontation and provides an easier escape if necessary.

Goals of Engagement

Engagement refers to a stage in the helping relationship when a preliminary agreement between a worker and an individual (sometimes a couple or a family) has been reached such that they will work together toward an agreed-on goal. Make sure that this goal is easily attainable, within the control of the individual, and not dependent on the behavior or decision of others. The goal should be singular or have few components so that is easy to understand, perform, and complete in a short period of time. The goal, then, is to establish self-efficacy, empowerment, and success. This goal may be the first step to obtaining secure housing or it may be the first of multiple steps along this path. The agreement is based on the willingness of a vulnerable person to commit to a course of action in return for some instrumental help in that action plan. As many people can easily feel coerced into accepting help, at least superficially, engagement has not occurred if the plan is primarily that created by the worker or if the person has only reluctantly agreed to it. Preliminary plans to engagement may be as simple as an agreement to meet again and continue to discuss possibilities. A final word of advice: keep your emotions as a worker muted. Appearing too enthusiastic or too negative may send warning signs of distrust to the potential client. Most of those who have been on the streets are accustomed to keeping a close check on their feelings and allow little public display.

In these initial encounters is the first opportunity for the worker to recognize that help is only effective if you begin where the potential client is at, psychologically, socially, emotionally, and physically. This is a fundamental tenet of good practice. Clients will not respond to an agenda of action and change that is imposed on them (Miley, O'Melia, & DuBois, 2012). Much has been written about the need to start with an understanding of the needs and priorities as seen by the homeless person, and not as assessed by the worker. Too often people fail to keep appointments or follow through with an action plan because it was not what they wanted, but was what they perceived that the worker wanted. A second aspect is that almost all housing vulnerable people are dealing with present-day, immediate issues, and have few resources for broader or long-range problems.

From the pyramid of Maslow's (1954) hierarchy of needs in the introductory section, it becomes apparent that when there is no food and housing security there are few personal resources to deal with other issues. As frontline workers you need to do your homework. If a client is known to your organization, and there are contact or progress notes, then it is important that you let the client know that you have taken some time to understand her issues. The important component is to convey this without showing that you have any preconceived ideas about the client or her situation. Finally, it is important to include an assessment of strengths and resources that a client brings to the helping relationship (Miley et al., 2012). A strengths-based approach is not new in the field of social services and social work. It builds on fundamental values that emphasize positive and unconditional regard for the other person. It emphasizes lovingness (warmth), respect, positive regard, and a nonjudgmental attitude that includes acceptance of the other (Hepworth, Rooney, Dewberry-Rooney, Strom-Gottfried, & Larsen, 2010, p. 55).

The objectives of engagement are often dictated by the mandates of the agency that the worker represents. This is a reality that the worker must openly acknowledge so that neither the worker nor the homeless person is misled as to what can be accomplished. For example, a support counselor in a transitional housing program for women who are victims of domestic violence can't assure a client that she will retain (or regain) custody of her children: child custody is determined by child welfare authorities. Similarly, a legal aid representative can't keep someone out of jail.

A first objective for the worker is to recognize what the objectives of engagement are. If the goal is short term, then the boundaries of the helping relationship must keep in mind that the contact is time limited. No one should be asked, even implicitly, to enter into a relationship that demands more emotional commitment than is feasible. That is, as most outreach work is hopefully short term, no long-term commitments are made in a short-term situation. A corollary to this is that a worker avoids becoming involved in a relationship that encourages a person's dependency on the worker. Many vulnerable people have problems with emotional attachment because those bonds may have been broken and violated in their lives. Too much attachment produces anxiety over dependency and closeness, and too little may be safe, but not helpful, as there is little engagement. The conflicts over emotional attachment and wariness over attachment are major forces in the homeless community. They may be hidden under the guise of giving the impression that they don't matter, but they are most often real and painful.

Workers learn to manage the dance of engagement, neither too fast nor too slow, neither too close nor too distant. In this dance the worker is the facilitator, but should not lead the dance, as it is the vulnerable individual who should determine what and when a course of action is taken. This includes limiting eye contact, and making either no eye contact or not much eye contact, because eye contact can be seen as a power struggle or intrusion into personal space. The dance may be slow and there may be silences in the conversation. Accept silence, unless it has a hostile overtone, as a positive step, and accept the fact that the engagement may move in and out as part of the testing process. In the beginning, let the potential client lead the conversation, and let him do more of the talking. Listen to where the person is at and observe if there is something that you may be able to offer help with. Don't be too eager because eagerness is mistrusted on the street. The dance also has different characteristics depending on whether the outreach occurs on the streets, in primary hostels (shelters), or in transitional housing programs. In each setting the dance has some predictable stages.

1. As in many new situations or with strange people, most persons—street-wise or not—prefer to check out someone from a distance; this is called "casing." Casing is where many nonverbal aspects of communication occur. Issues of how you are dressed, how you smell, how you stand, the gestures you use in talking, perhaps the tone and inflection of your speech, if it can be heard, are all assessed. The military-style posture of a law enforcement officer will be quite different from the casual, at times slouching or defensive, stance of a dealer. Casing may change with locality, but inevitably points to what can be learned about a person from a distance.

2. Once you pass the distance test (you are neither a threat nor a danger) and enter into more-direct interaction, you will usually experience some forms of limit testing and checking for boundaries. This may include:

- Swearing. What is your tolerance for rough language? Can and/or should you use rough language in specific situations?
- Sexual comments. To what extent will you allow a remark to pass unnoticed and when do you call a halt? This is especially true for male–female interactions, but is not restricted to them.
- Personal space. We all have a personal space, usually about eighteen to twenty inches between people in most North American cultures, that provides a level of comfort. In some other cultures, specific societies, and religious groups acceptable personal space may be greater or less than this norm. The variations may also be due to gender differences as personal space between women or between men may be different from those in mixed company. Some people need and prefer larger amounts of space; on initial encounters you need to be

sensitive to what distance between the client and yourself is comfortable and acceptable to the other person. Some people will test limits with your personal space, so this is another aspect you must consider. Some reflective questions about personal space include, Do you allow people into your personal space while talking to them? Is intruding on your space threatening? You may want to do the exercises at the end of this chapter to help you understand this concept. A high five may be the most positive and closest a worker gets to positive touch—and then only when you have gotten to know the person. Hugging and positive touch should be off limits because it can send very confusing messages, especially around attachment and issues of sexuality, and make a worker or client more vulnerable. A hug may also make a client appear to be vulnerable to others on the street—something that most people try to avoid. A side hug may be a more muted and acceptable supportive response. Exceptions may occur in situations where a person has just experienced an extreme trauma, but this is a judicious decision that you must make with full awareness of its implications. Although most people respect personal boundaries, some people who have a serious active mental illness may not respect personal boundaries and may use too much self-disclosure as a test of the relationship or otherwise intrude into personal boundaries. It is wise, in these instances, to limit the amount of personal information that you are willing to listen to, and defer the rest to a "counselor who can help."

Preliminary conversations with people who are uncertain that they want any help generally occur in superficial ways around slow, trust-building interactions. At the point that the homeless person agrees to accept some type of service or help in obtaining services one can begin to think in terms of a client relationship. In secondary shelters this is usually a tacit reality of being in transitional housing. Nonetheless, the fact that a person is a client does not diminish the importance of building a trusting relationship nor the need to work no harder than the client, and to let the client set the pace for action and determination of goals. It does mean that a more focused interaction can take place. In many places these approaches are termed "interviewing skills" or "interviewing techniques." This wording often connotes some artificial way of communicating (wording, phrases, tone of voice) that the client will not perceive as genuine. We prefer to remain more general and designate these ways of conversation as helpful approaches to engagement.

The most fundamental approach is one of attentive listening. It requires that you, the worker, focus all of your attention on the client and what she is trying to say, and on whether there is consistency among the words, tone, volume (loudness or softness), attitude, and ambience in what the person is telling you. Avoid being distracted by others and by events around you, except as they may affect your safety, since this conveys to the client that you are giving her your true and undivided attention. Attentive listening also entails having some eye contact, but not too much, too often, or too long, because this may violate private space and be interpreted as aggressive or power seeking.

Being client focused also entails using the positive approaches espoused by noted therapists such as Carl Rogers (1966), whose client-centered approach did a great deal to focus the interaction on the needs and wishes of the client. The client-centered approach is the foundation on which you can thus build other helpful engagement skills. Many of the other skills build on attentive listening. Restating, clarifying, reflecting, identifying, and focusing are all important to conveying the message that you are listening to the client and want to understand what his concerns are. These communication techniques can be used positively, but are subject to abuse, as tables 2.2, 2.3, and 2.4 will demonstrate.

INTERVENTION SKILLS

In table 2.2 are various ways of helping to clarify the issues, noting differences between what is said and the concurrent behavior, and helping the client to identify the immediate issues of concern. In table 2.3 we note those responses that are not helpful or that are harmful to creating a trusting relationship—and why.

Dysfunctional Responses

You will notice that most of the examples in tables 2.2 and 2.3 have to do with power and control. In the world of someone who is homeless or vulnerable to housing loss, there is a prevailing sense of loss of control. Whatever the reason for the situation, inevitably this was not a choice most persons

Table 2.2. Intervention Skills and Responses (Part 1)

Skill	Helpful response. Please substitute the local ways of speaking as this makes an enormous difference in connecting with the client.
Listening	Moderate eye contact, relaxed posture. Do not cross your arms, as this is a sign of defiance, resistance, or lack of openness.
Nondirective opening	If stated by the worker; the specificity depends on the setting. In a general setting: "What brings you in today?" "What's up?" "Are you here for _____?" The last is most helpful in a specific service context. If the client says something such as, "Can you _____?," determine if you are the right person to continue the conversation, and, if so, invite the person to explain a bit further (add some details).
Clarifying	"I want to be sure that I've got it right. Can you explain this some more?" "Can you give me an example?"
Restating	"Let me see if I got this right. You are telling me _____." "So you started doing/having this _____ about six months ago?"
Focusing	"You are mentioning a lot of issues. Which would you like to deal with today?"
Identifying	Ask, e.g., "Was this a mild shower or a thunderstorm?"
Constructive silence	Sometimes the best intervention is to attentively be present with someone. However, you must be sensitive to situational cues that indicate when this is comfortable and when it creates anxiety.
Reflecting	"I get the impression that . . . ."
Observing and sharing observations	"Do you mind if I share what I see going on?"

would make, or deliberately set up as a consequence of their actions. There are some people who deliberately want and choose a life of homelessness, which is why we state that *most* persons do not choose this way of life. However, we must respect the desire of some to live this way. We continue here to reflect on those who do not want to be homeless. Along with the loss of control is a sense of powerlessness to avoid or deal with life's circumstances. This may come from many places: lack of knowledge, resources, or

Table 2.3. Intervention Skills and Responses (Part 2)

Skill	Example of improper communication	Reason for dysfunction
Listening	Maintain constant eye contact.	Misperceived as confrontational, a threat, or an intrusion.
	Allow self to be distracted, use phone, etc.	Disrespect: implicit message that the other person is not important.
Nondirective opening	"You need to deal with . . . ."	Appears to be telling a person what to do.
Clarifying	"That doesn't make sense to me."	Challenging the ability of the other person to state things well, *or* questioning the articulateness/mental health of the other person.
Restating	"You said that . . . ."	Can be misperceived as accusatory, depending on the tone of voice.
Focusing	"That's too much for now. Let's focus on your . . . ."	Directive and not considering what the other person wants to focus on.
Identifying	"I notice that you are very anxious."	May be true but can be perceived as intrusive or beyond what the person wants to acknowledge and deal with at that moment.
Constructive silence	Allowing for no silence *or* letting the silence extend to where the other person is uncomfortable.	No silence communicates control, and too much silence may be taken as not knowing what to say or do.
Reflecting	"You are feeling anxious and upset, probably because one of your buddies reminded you of your father."	The client should identify feelings, and the worker should not connect those feelings to other issues or relationships. This should be left for trained therapists.
Observing and sharing observations	"You are smiling but you say you are sad. I bet you are angry."	Interpretations are best left to trained therapists. This could be taken as very intrusive and controlling.

supportive relationships; or personal feeling of lack of self-efficacy—the ability to be personally effective in the challenges of life. One of the first tasks of the worker should be to provide feedback and support for the homeless person to be in charge of his own decisions and to provide the support to empower the person in this direction. Interactions that foster feelings of self-control, decision making, and being in charge of one's self all foster empowerment and self-efficacy.

> **Textbox 2.2. People of the Street**
>
> *Ragged Company* is written by an author who has experienced homelessness and the struggles of sleeping rough. As a result, the book offers many vignettes and depictions of characters who resonate with responses that research has also documented. The voices of the characters in this story bring this lifestyle to life. Author Richard Wagamese (2008) has added a human side to these pictures of sleeping rough and the culture of the street, and thus we refer at times to some of the characters in this book to illustrate attitudes, values, and behaviors of those who live on the street and their reactions to the Main Street people who try to help. We recommend that you read this fine and authentic depiction of life on the streets.

What are some other ways that the worker can encourage the perception of shared power? In some situations sharing is not realistic, such as when a worker represents Child Welfare or legal authorities. In these situations, the minimization of power imbalance can lead to productive outcomes. Table 2.4 provides some examples of nonverbal behavior that can minimize the power imbalance.

COMMUNICATION AND NONVERBAL BEHAVIORS

Working with a Guarded or Hostile Person

Working with guarded or cautious persons has different meanings and implications depending on the prior relationship with the potential client or the lack of any previous contact. The implications also depend on the role of the worker, so a bylaw enforcement officer or a child welfare representative will pose threats that a general outreach worker with no legal ties will not. The interactions may depend on whether this is the first contact, or one that occurs after the worker and potential client have come to know each other.

Table 2.4. Intervention Skills and Responses (Part 3)

Behavior	Description	Interpretation
Standing or sitting	Try to be at the same eye level with the person you are speaking to. Sitting is the best option when there is a considerable difference in height.	Taller people, and those who are standing when the other person is sitting, are subtly perceived as being more powerful. Don't worry about where you sit—within reason. Prepare to get dirty; you will not always be in clean places. On the other hand, avoid sofas, chairs, and bedding that may house vermin; they like to hitch rides.
Scheduled meetings	To be on time? Early? Late?	The issues around being too eager if one is early, too withholding if one is late, and too obsessive if one is on time are not as important as conveying the importance of keeping a commitment to your (potential) client. Clients may be late or miss a scheduled meeting, but will react negatively if you do the same. They are vulnerable and meetings are the first test of trust. If you must miss, have a *very* good reason.
Clothing—what to wear	Dress casually, but not provocatively, for street-level and entry-level shelter work. Avoid necklaces that someone could pull on, and any flashy jewelry, real or fake.	Dress should allow one to blend in, and not convey status, money, or power. It should be safe so that no piece can be used in a harmful way—such as a necklace. Women should avoid high heels: they are an encumbrance if you need to move quickly. Keep more formal business clothing like a suit jacket in your office or car in case you need to formalize for a meeting.
Smoking and drinking	Offers of a cigarette, coffee, tea, soda pop, or alcohol	No alcohol—*never*—on the job; you are not an undercover agent, who would handle this differently. Coffee, tea, or soda (pop) may be very welcome and a good way to share time as a "get to know you." Cigarettes are a personal choice, and may be an equalizer if you can offer someone a cigarette. Smoking, or offering a cigarette even if you as the worker are a nonsmoker, can be helpful if that person is providing important street-level information. However, many workers no longer smoke and this may be an individual issue. This is a judgment call.

They may depend on the context in which the interaction takes place: some situations produce more guardedness than others. A person's legal status as a resident, resident alien, immigrant, or refugee may also impact the response. Finally, the implications may be due to inherent personality characteristics of the potential client, whether there may be a mental health problem, or whether or not he is under the influence of alcohol or drugs. This potential situation will be further discussed in chapter 8 when we look at substance use and abuse. Indeed, the number of different factors at play in any given situation can be daunting. The ease with which a worker understands and deals with these factors improves with experience.

These are the kinds of situations where mentoring or shadowing—that is, working alongside an experienced worker—can provide valuable lessons on important intervention and relationship-building skills. Sometimes supervisors may want to come with their workers to meet their clients or homeless people and to see how they are working with this population, especially if the client is challenging. Workers may be ambivalent about supervisors meeting their clients. If the relationship with the supervisor is positive and supportive, and if the organization believes in a team approach, this may be seen as a way for supervisors to share the care and concerns of the workers. On the other hand, the intrusion of the supervisor can break continuity and trust between the worker and the homeless person. Some workers can feel devalued and judged by the supervisor's action.

So what does hostility potentially mean? If we recall that feelings of powerlessness and helplessness are prevalent in the homeless person's struggle for survival, it becomes clear that hostility may be that person's first line of defense against those feelings. The person may also be a survivor of trauma and abuse. One needs to remember, in recognizing the perspective of the homeless person, the adage that sometimes the best defense is an offense. In this instance, quiet reassurances that the other person is safe and not about to face legal or other authorities is an important first step, and must be restated as often as is necessary for the person to let her guard down. If this is a first encounter, the worker would be wise to limit the contact, stay neutral in the conversation, and mention that he will come around some other time. Be careful of using language that denotes authority or keeping track of a person such as "check back," "check in," "look you up," as the homeless person will view these negatively. People on the street will also pass along their views about the worker and, along with it, note whether you are up to date on what is going on in the street and on current language. If it appears that the person may be under the influence of alcohol or other substances, as we will look at more closely in chapter 8, keep the conversation to a minimum, back away, and leave as quickly as possible.

In the instance where you have had several or more meetings with the person and have gotten to have at least a preliminary connection, the approach that you take may be altered. For starters, this may not be usual behavior for this individual. In this case, a low-key approach with a general opening remark such as, "How are things going?," "What's up?," or "Hi there" may be a neutral beginning to the conversation. The reply to this may give you a lead-in to ask further about what is going on or if anything has happened. You also can further evaluate if the person appears to be sober or under the influence. If the person is under the influence, back away (for your safety) and then make sure that she is safe. Do not attempt a rational conversation with someone who is not sober, especially if there is a guarded or angry affect. You could endanger yourself and coworkers. If the person is not under the influence you may gently ask if the person would like to talk—or not. Don't push the conversation. But do ask if he feels safe—or needs some help. Let the answers be your guide. These are not situations that new workers should face alone, but ones where the guidance of seasoned workers can be of help.

Basic intervention strategies in unfamiliar situations are as follows:

1. Safety first.
2. Determine ability to communicate.
3. Assess for orientation, level of stress, and hypervigilance.
4. Determine ability to engage in continued conversation.

People who are homeless have an inherent caution about who they will talk with, and what they will talk about. Frontline workers should accept this as reality. The individual's caution may relax once the homeless person becomes familiar with the worker, but initially it is a significant barrier to engagement. You need to remember that for most persons who are homeless, disappointment, rejection, the failure of others to follow through on promises, fear of law enforcement, and fear of breaking bylaws are all threats to personal safety and security. At the same time, the worker may present the doorway to food and shelter for the night, so there is an inherent double-bind that a person may face. What can a worker do—and what should he not do?

ENGAGING THE CLIENT

As we previously discussed, no outreach and subsequent service will be effective if you have not arrived at an understanding with the person you seek to help about what that help consists of, and if you have not obtained the person's assent to let you help. Engaging the client also has a substantively different meaning when the engagement is on the streets, with a person who is resistant to or ambivalent about accepting help. In those situations, outreach focuses on small steps to help ease the discomforts of street life, and eventual agreement to seek permanent housing.

For the person who has already made the decision about the need for assistance in getting permanent shelter, engagement has different, more-subtle complexities. The need for respect, empowerment, and self-determination continue to play major roles in the interactions. These less-apparent expectations consist of the mutual recognition that help toward the goal of housing stability starts with acknowledgment of the client's right to self-determination, that is, the client's right to set the agenda and the priorities of any plan to work together. That right must be accompanied by an explicit understanding that some actions have to precede others (e.g., establishing a defined monthly income through entitlements such as welfare and disability), and that choice is always dependent on other circumstances (where you choose to live is limited by housing costs in specific areas). The worker should present a clear picture of current housing rental market availabilities as realities to the client, and as a situation that may present hard choices, not merely as "take it or leave it" situations. This latter style of forced choice inevitably leads to dissatisfaction and the client's desire to leave unacceptable housing.

Engaging people in finding and keeping housing must then start with where the client is—which is most often based on a *housing first* philosophy. That is, that most people would prefer to have a place of their own before tackling issues of job training, mental health, substance-abuse counseling, and so on. We will examine this further in the chapter on housing, but it is safe to state that consumer preferences strongly indicate that choice is important to stability—staying put once housed. Life on the streets is physically and psychologically demanding. Once housed, the client will have greater physical and emotional energy reserves to tackle other issues.

Motivational Interviewing: A First Step along the Road

The previous section has primarily addressed the various aspects of reaching out and engaging people who are literally homeless, including those who are sleeping in a shelter on a day-to-day basis. We now turn to situations where a person has started to move out of homelessness and has tacitly agreed to accept some services and help in locating services, and thus to accept a more formal helping relationship. At this point we refer to the individual as a client, someone who receives services that he has directly or implicitly requested.

Because a person has become a client does not imply that he is willing to accept all services. In fact, there may continue to be a considerable amount of ambivalence about the services that are acceptable, and the changes that the individual is prepared to make. For example, someone who has a drinking problem may agree to a detoxification (often called detox) program, but then become very hesitant about committing to treatment that includes total sobriety. At this point, the person is partially engaged, but not completely committed, and the process of additional treatment may not be acceptable for an additional period of time. In substance-abuse programs this would be a stage of change between partial acceptance of a problem and a commitment to fully engage in change to address the problem. We will look more at stages of change in the chapter on substance abuse (chapter 8). At this beginning phase of engagement in services the individual is most likely to leave treatment and lose sobriety again. This is the time when the frontline worker may well step into the conversation about sobriety and provide an intervention that would address the client's ambivalence to change. The best evidence-based practice to work toward change is called "motivational interviewing."

Motivational interviewing is an approach that was developed for use in substance-abuse treatment and has expanded for use in many situations where a person's motivation for change is low. Developed by Rollnick and Miller (1995), motivational interviewing uses the client-centered, empathetic relationship that was central to Carl Rogers's client-centered therapy (1966).

It deviates from the client-centered approach in that it is a more directive style, the intent of which is to explore a person's readiness to change and the ambivalence that accompanies this readiness. Motivational interviewing uses cognitive-behavioral approaches that inquire about a person's beliefs and actions and explores with the individual the discrepancies between where a person "is at" and where he would like to be. This approach does not aim to direct a person as to what course of action to take, but guides the conversation about the thoughts and attitudes toward different ways of functioning. The target behavior must be client-directed, as people do not willingly engage in talking about issues that they have no intention of exploring or changing. It begins with asking open-ended questions—that is, those that encourage further discussion, not those that can be answered with one or two words. Discussion about a person's behavior needs to explore the extent to which she wants to change (desire) and the degree to which the person believes that she can change or sees change as possible. This conversation sets the stage for exploring the pros and cons of changing behavior— that is, what is attractive about the potential changes and what is not attractive. Table 2.5 reviews some of the positive and negative ways in which interventions can proceed. A final area for exploration is the person's perceived need to change, and reasons why change is not needed. In other words, the counselor explores with the person both sides of the ambivalence to change.

What does a motivational conversation look like? Motivational interviewing uses many of the interviewing approaches common to counseling techniques. We explored some of them earlier (see table 2.2) and will briefly repeat them.

Active Listening

1. Clarify statement by rephrasing, i.e., "Do you mean . . . ?"
2. Clarify by repeating what the client has said word for word, without changing anything.
3. Ask for specific examples. "Can you describe a time when . . . ?"
4. Be careful when you restate so that you do not unintentionally misinterpret what the client has said. This is especially important when a client is likely not to agree with you.
5. Emphasize by reflecting back and deliberately overstating the comments made by the client to highlight what has been said.

Table 2.5. Intervention Skills and Responses (Part 4)

Issue	Exploring the Positive	Exploring the Negative
Smoking—identifying the need	When do you most enjoy smoking? Can you think of other ways in which you could have the same pleasant feeling?	What comes to your mind when you think about an unpleasant part of smoking? Have you thought about how to deal with these unpleasant parts? Is quitting the only way?
Excessive alcohol use	You agree that you often drink too much beer. What is the best thing about drinking too much? What would it look like for you to stop drinking? Where would you have a good time?	What is unpleasant about drinking too much? Do you ever think about quitting altogether? What would you miss about drinking?
Taking prescribed meds (medication for a mental illness)	When you take your meds regularly, how do you feel? Is that feeling good for you? Does it help you to deal differently with other people?	Is that different from how you feel now? What is the best thing about not taking your meds? Is that better than taking them?
Preparing for change in a specific behavior	What good do you hope that this change will do?	What will you have to give up if you change your behavior?
Looking forward	If you change, what will you look like five years from now?	If you don't change, what will you look like five years from now?

6. Keep the interaction on a conversational level. There is nothing worse than a worker/counselor who seems to be using a technique from a book. You need to find ways to use the above without sounding artificial.

Looking for Change

1. "Why do you want to . . . ?"
2. "What would be the benefit of . . . . ?"
3. "How much does this really matter to you?"
4. "What do you think you have to do in order to . . . . ?"

5. "Can you think of change as a series of small steps? What would they look like?"

Developing an Action Plan
1. "What is the first thing you would have to do . . . ?"
2. "Do you think your first step is realistic? Is it doable?"
3. "How would you feel if you took the first step and succeeded?"
4. "How much of this action plan is up to you—and not anyone else?"
5. "Is there anything that would prevent you from taking the first step?"

The above examples are intended to help you develop basic approaches in working with people who are not yet in treatment and are still either in denial or just beginning to contemplate change. Because the motivation to change may emerge very slowly, it is important for the worker to keep in mind that each interaction is an opportunity, that you don't know what or when there will be an "ah ha!" moment for the client. Change is possible, no matter how ingrained the behavior, and positive support is essential to establishing the lifelines that will facilitate change.

EXERCISES

1. In groups of three assign each person a role: an outreach worker, a homeless person (street living), and an observer. Have a beginning conversation on first meeting to try to engage the homeless person. Have a conversation on the assumption that this is a person the worker has spoken to on at least three occasions. How would you begin? What would be your purpose?
2. The observer reviews his observations and offers feedback on language, tone, and style of interaction. The interviewer and interviewee discuss their reactions and observations using a format that notes tone, style, language, and body posture. The group discusses the above.
3. Change roles then repeat.
4. Have the designated homeless person sit on the ground during the above exercise.
5. Ask students to get together with those they know and are comfortable with. Ask each group to pair off. Have the pairs separate, with

each person going to the opposite end of the room. Ask the pairs to walk toward each other, one step each, alternating one step at a time. Have each person stop when she begins to feel too close for comfort. Discuss the experience.

6. Repeat the exercise with people who do not know each other. Reflect on the differences between the two experiences. Experiencing personal space allows one to become aware of what this means in different situations.

7. On a sheet of paper draw overlapping circles. Place yourself in a middle circle (see figure 2.1 for an example) and mark it as "ME." Label each other circle with family, friends, coworkers,

Figure 2.1. How Close Are Our Relationships?

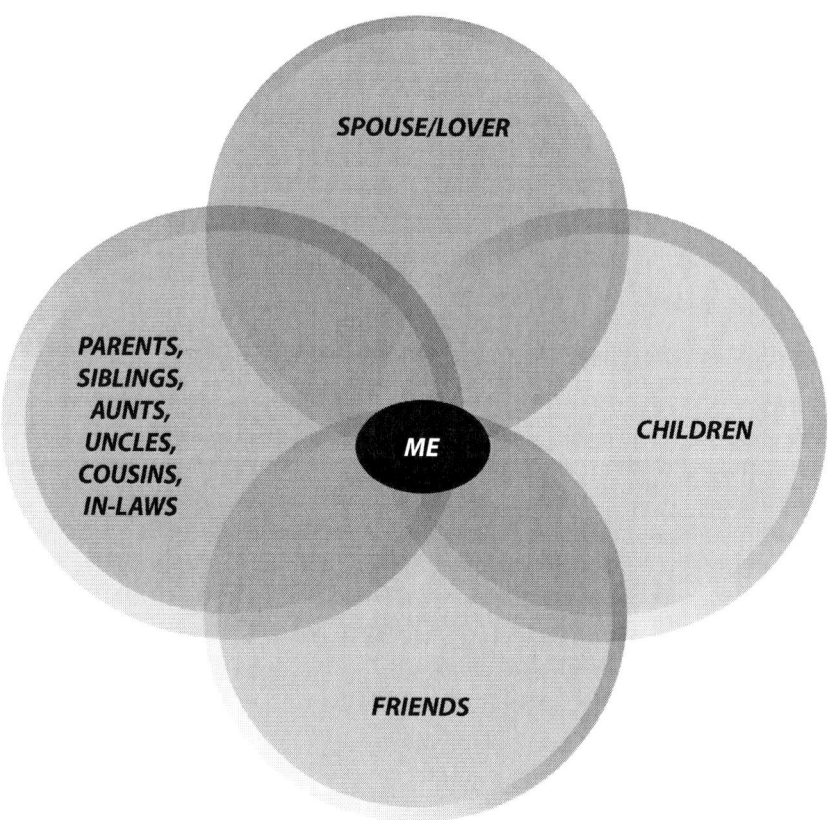

acquaintances, neighbors. Repeat this exercise noting where you would put people in describing your emotional closeness, or your legal closeness, or your physical nearness.

The aim of this exercise is to have you examine your own motives and attitudes for helping, as these are the hidden drivers that determine the ways in which you will reach out to vulnerable persons.

JOURNALING

1. How do you feel when someone tries to help you do something—and you haven't asked for help?
2. Do you like to be helped or do you prefer to be in charge? Does being helped make you feel as though you have less control? How does this preference affect your ability to help others?
3. Answer the following questions:
    a. Helping makes me feel . . . .
    b. When I want to help and I can't I . . . .
    c. When someone helps me I feel . . . .
    d. The most important help that I ever got was . . . .
    e. One time when I needed help . . . .

CHAPTER 3

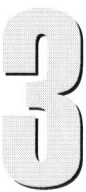

Homelessness and Health

KEY ISSUES

Overview of common infectious diseases including HIV, hepatitis, tuberculosis, skin infections, common cold, and influenza

Different routes of infection

Assessment of environmental hazards

Safe handling of body fluids and sharps

Understanding the multiple stressors that social service workers encounter

Appreciating the more work-specific stressors encountered working with homeless persons

Awareness of the various safety concerns in the work place and in the community and threats to physical safety

Hand washing and use of antiseptics

Universal precautions and means to remain safe

Infection control: pandemic responses

Psychological safety

Worker self-care, stress, and burnout

Understanding the workplace-related stressors that are linked to burnout

Exploration of coping strategies for dealing with work-related stress

Understanding of self-care strategies

Acceptance of the importance of self-care behaviors for effective work

---

OVERVIEW

In the following pages we provide awareness of common medical conditions among the homeless and substance-addicted populations. This understanding will allow workers to develop awareness and safety practices in order to minimize the risk of community health workers' exposure to and development of common infectious diseases. We then focus on understanding the stressors that workers face and ways in which to mitigate the impact of those stressors. We then turn to a brief exploration of the various aspects of worker health and self-care.

Health and homelessness are intertwined. Being homeless impacts both physical and psychological health. In this chapter we explore the various dimensions of health that affect people who are homeless and people who have precarious living conditions. We then look at the importance of self-care and healthy living and coping for frontline providers, whose health can quickly and easily be overtaken by the stressors of the intense work of helping those who live precarious lives.

Being homeless impacts every aspect of a person's life, beginning with food insecurity, lack of access to regular hygiene practices, and health-related problems. Some of the earliest research about the plight of contemporary homeless people focused on their health and access to adequate medical care (Bachrach, 1987). Research on the psychosocial determinants of health presents strong evidence that poverty, lack of education, poor living conditions including inadequate shelter, and lack of cleanliness all contribute to poor health outcomes. These outcomes are passed down through generations of people who live with deprivation of basic needs (Braveman, Egerter, & Williams, 2011).

The health status of homeless persons is rather dismal even when universal health care is available, as Hwang and his colleagues have pointed out through numerous studies of health-related problems that unhoused and fragilely housed persons experience (Hwang et al., 2010).These health concerns range from chronic conditions such as respiratory, heart, and circulatory conditions, to those directly attributable to smoking, drug use, and alcohol use. In an extensive review of the literature, O'Connell (2005) notes that together these chronic health conditions account for a seven-fold increase in premature death for those living in shelters and temporary and rooming house accommodations. In addition, communicable diseases such as influenza, tuberculosis, skin diseases, sexually transmitted diseases

(STDs), and parasitic infections create major health risks for those who are homeless and the workers who address their needs.

The health of homeless people is a quantity and quality of life issue and is frequently minimized in their quest for housing stability. Health issues can be both a cause and a result of homelessness. In this chapter we focus on issues related to physical health and will explore mental health challenges and problems in chapter 7. We have known for quite some time that people can lose their housing as a result of poor health or chronic health and mental health issues (Frankish, Hwang, & Quantz, 2005). Ill health can also be a consequence of life on the streets. Reports consistently show that those who are homeless have higher rates of many diseases and a shorter life span than those housed, even when socioeconomic factors are considered (Hwang, 2001). Lack of consistent and adequate shelter and diet aggravates underlying issues and can create some additional illnesses. Life on the streets and in many shelters is highly stressful and not always safe. In addition to the physical dangers of threats, bullying, and theft of belongings, close contact with many people leads to high rates of disease transmission. It is more difficult to avoid human contact at soup kitchens and in places to stay warm during cold weather, and thus many persons fall ill to a variety of diseases that are spread by close proximity to others. Lack of adequate hand washing and bathing facilities, both strongly recommended to stop disease transmission, can aggravate the spread of disease-bearing germs and vermin such as fleas and bedbugs, which easily hop from one victim to the next.

Several groups of homeless persons have even higher rates of health-related problems than the general homeless population. These include women, youths, the elderly, and those with persistent mental illnesses and substance abuse disorders. Women, including those who are still youths, are more likely to have been physically and sexually assaulted, to have STDs, to have unwanted pregnancies, to struggle with alcohol and drug abuse, to have conditions aggravated by shelter life, and to have conditions worsened by lack of adequate and timely treatment (Burg, 1994). Those with mental illness find their medical conditions minimized or overlooked by medical providers who concentrate on the mental illness, even though it is widely reported that those who have a mental illness are more likely to suffer from additional medical conditions.

Reports on the health of homeless youths indicate that more than one-third have been sexually abused before becoming homeless and that a further one-third are sexually abused after becoming homeless (Coates & McKenzie-Mohr, 2010). Their health is further compromised by an inability

> **Textbox 3.1. Quick Facts**
>
> - Mortality rates for homeless youths in Montreal are nine times higher for young males and thirty-one times higher for females.
> - In Toronto the death rates for homeless youths eighteen to twenty-four are 8.3 times higher than for youths in the same age cohort who are housed.
> - The death rate for homeless men in the United States is twice that of the same age cohort in Canada. Much of this difference may be attributable to gun violence and a higher homicide rate in the United States than in Canada.
>
> (Hwang, 2001)

to provide consent for treatment if they are under age (usually eighteen), unless there is an emergency (Keeshin & Campbell, 2011).

Although the elderly constitute a small percent of the total housing fragile population, their numbers appear to be growing (Sermons & Henry, 2010). This growth points out the need to recognize their special health-related problems, which include, in addition to the physical health problems of the elderly, a higher proportion of mental illness, substance abuse, and cognitive disorders (dementias). Furthermore, Hecht and Coyle (2001) suggest that because those who are homeless tend to age more rapidly, these conditions appear at an earlier age. This indicates that the concept of what constitutes being elderly occurs at a younger age for the homeless than in the general population and thus programs for the elderly need to make accommodation for those who have prematurely aged because of prolonged experiences of being homeless.

The concept of health involves physical and psychological health and safety for both the worker and the homeless and housing vulnerable. Workers often are exposed to unsafe conditions when doing outreach services. Homes may not be physically safe, may be structurally hazardous, or may be filthy and mold-ridden, or tenants may have pets that may pose a risk. Animal odors and excrement, including those from vermin such as rats and mice, pose additional hazards. Fleas and bedbugs can easily hitch a ride back to the office or home. There may be unsafe chemicals and contaminants in the environment. Neighborhoods may be prone to gang and drug violence, which add to worker risks. In this chapter we also explore some of the ways in which to ensure worker safety and protection. We will examine ways in which workers can mitigate some of these risks, and ways to work in a self-protective manner.

THE PSYCHOSOCIAL DETERMINANTS OF HOUSING AND HEALTH

The relationships among poverty, inadequate nutrition, and poor health have been widely documented. There are a number of ways in which health is influenced by housing. Although the relationships between housing and health are complicated and not well studied, especially as they apply to marginally and unhoused persons, there are some facts that stand out (McCormarck, Johnston, Boivin, & Thompson, 2010). The physical safety and cleanliness of housing, its psychological safety (internally and in the immediate environment), and its accessibility to basic amenities (food stores, services), are paramount to improved lifestyle and reduced poor health. Airborne illnesses and the effect of pollution on asthma and other respiratory conditions are well documented. The availability of safe food storage ensures that food has not deteriorated with storage. A physically safe environment reduces the possibility of falls and injuries due to neglect of necessary repairs; and a dependable, safe water supply provides basic cleanliness necessary for personal hygiene as well as for food preparation. The proximity to others in shelters means that communal eating and bathing and lack of ready access to hand washing and sanitary facilities increase the likelihood of disease transmission. For those who live in marginal housing, health and the physical environment are closely intertwined. For those who are literally homeless, they are inseparable.

Decades of research have established that psychosocial factors are also important health determinants. Of these, stress is notably the biggest factor. Numerous studies have shown that the events listed in the Stressful Life Events Scale (Holmes & Rahe, 1967) provided in table 3.1 are related to physical and mental health outcomes.

This scale was developed over forty-five years ago and reflects a middle-class lifestyle; we suggest that there are some additions and modifications that would fit with contemporary stressors that people are likely to experience. We have noted items that should be modified for contemporary society with an asterisk. Newer items, for which we suggest a range depending on personal circumstance, include those listed in table 3.2.

A quick scan of these events will show that homeless persons generally have high scores on this scale and its newer components and are thus at high risk for developing stress-related illnesses.

Table 3.1. Stressful Life Events

Stressful Life Event	Stress Score
1. My spouse died.	100
2. I got a divorce.*	73
3. I separated from my spouse.	65
4. I spent time in jail.	63
5. A close family member died (not a spouse).	63
6. I had a major illness or injury* (with or without medical insurance).	58
7. I got married.	50
8. I was fired at work.	47
9. I had a marital reconciliation.	45
10. I retired.	45
11. A family member experienced a change in health (not myself).	44
12. I became pregnant.	40
13. I experienced sexual problems.*	39
14. My family gained a new member.	39
15. I experienced an upheaval in my business affairs.	39
16. I experienced a change in my financial state.	38
17. A close friend died.	37
18. I changed to a different occupation.	36
19. My spouse and I argued significantly more (or significantly less).	35
20. I obtained a loan or mortgage over $50,000* (update to current dollars).	31
21. A loan or mortgage of mine was foreclosed.*	30
22. My responsibilities at work changed.	29
23. My son or daughter left home.	29
24. I had trouble with my in-laws.	29
25. I had an outstanding personal achievement.	28
26. My spouse began or stopped working.	26
27. I started or finished high school or college.	26
28. I had a change in my living conditions.	25
29. I had a change in my personal habits.	24
30. I had trouble with my boss.	23
31. My working hours or conditions changed.	20
32. I changed residences.	20
33. I changed schools.	20
34. I changed recreational activities.	19
35. My church activities changed.	19
36. My social activities changed.	19
37. I took out a loan for less than $50,000.*	17
38. My sleeping habits changed.	16

Table 3.1. (Continued)

Stressful Life Event	Stress Score
39. We had a change in the number of family get-togethers.	15
40. My eating habits changed.	13
41. I took a vacation.	13
42. I celebrated Christmas.*	12
43. I had minor violations of the law (traffic or parking tickets, etc.).	11

Source: Based on Holmes & Rahe (1967, 214).
* = Items that should be modified for contemporary society.

PHYSICAL HEALTH

The health status of all homeless persons is poorer in both Canada and the United States than the health status of people who are housed. In the United States the National Health Care for the Homeless Council (O'Connell, 2005) reports that homeless persons are three to six times more likely to develop serious health problems than are housed persons, primarily because of poor environmental conditions, high-stress lives, and lack of basic care They are also much more likely to die at a significantly younger age than the housed population. In the United States a person living on the streets has an average life expectancy of forty-two to fifty-two years, compared to an average of seventy-eight for a housed person. Data from Canada are comparable (Hwang, 2001). Studies of health conditions in homeless persons concentrate primarily on those living in a few larger cities; they paint a picture of

Table 3.2. Contemporary Stressful Events Supplement

New Items	Value Range
I became homeless.	80–100
My family and I became homeless.	90–100
My child developed a serious mental illness.	50–80
My pet dog (cat) died.	60–80
My spouse developed a substance-abuse problem.	50–65
My spouse developed a gambling problem.	50–80
My child developed a substance-abuse problem.	60–80
A disaster destroyed my housing (with insurance to rebuild).	60–80
A disaster destroyed my housing (without insurance to rebuild).	75–90
My spouse (or child) developed a life-threatening illness.	60–80
My child was diagnosed with a serious developmental disability.	60–80

> **Textbox 3.2. Life Expectancies for Homeless Persons**
>
> In the United States, a person living on the streets has an average life expectancy of forty-two to fifty-two years, compared to an average of seventy-eight years in the general population.
>
> In Canada homeless adults age twenty-five to forty are 3.7 times more likely to die than those of the same age who are housed.

urban homelessness that may not represent the situation of the homeless in rural areas (Waegemakers Schiff & Turner, 2014). The health problems encountered by homeless people are those commonly seen among those who live in poverty; who live in close proximity to those infected with contagious diseases; whose physical energy is spent in dealing with cold or wet or extremely hot climates and hostile environments; and who have limited access to health care, healing drugs, the diet needed for recovery, and the rest required for attaining health.

There has been some discussion about the degree to which lack of universal health-care coverage is responsible for the poor health status and outcomes of homeless persons. However, research on the health of the homeless in Canada where health care is universally available indicates that health outcomes have not been much different than in the United States where universal access to care regardless of income or ability to pay has not, to date, been available.

Four factors may account for this finding. First, in Canada many persons who become homeless lose their personal ID and health-care card and number. Without adequate documentation of residence and a mailing address, homeless people have difficulty replacing this vital ID and their health-care ID card in order to access routine services. Second, most homeless persons are too preoccupied with the challenges of finding food and accommodation nightly to be able to take the time or have the patience to go through the bureaucratic process of applying for a new card or to wait for routine and preventative health care. Thus they wait until there is an undeniable emergency before seeking care. Third, homeless people are more likely to be denied hospitalization or to face early discharge to shelters that are ill-equipped to provide adequate accommodation for those recovering from surgery or serious illnesses. This prolongs the recovery trajectory and frequently leads to rehospitalization and ongoing chronic problems. Fourth, many have difficulty in finding the money to pay for prescriptions, or fail to follow their prescribed usage, thus prolonging the illness that led to seeking treatment. Although welfare will pay for needed medicines, in both countries, following treatment recommendations of health-care providers is lower than that of the general public, and that is already unacceptably low (Hwang et al., 2010). Dental care is not usually covered under the Canadian health-care system, and is virtually nonexistent for the homeless in both countries. In cold and rainy seasons and climates, frostbite and hypothermia contribute additional risks that increase the probability of premature death eightfold in homeless persons.

> **Textbox 3.3. Case Example: Lack of Coordination of Care**
>
> John is a single man, age sixty-eight, suffered from a mixed group of mental health issues, including depression, obsessive-compulsive disorder, and Tourette syndrome. He had completed all but his dissertation for a doctorate but was unable to finish the dissertation. He had worked as a teacher and assistant high school principal for a few years but had to resign because of his multiple problems. He survived on disability income and lived in a single room of a boarding home until it was sold and demolished. Subsequently he was unable to find and retain an apartment. He eventually became homeless and sought shelter on a nightly basis. He had several medical problems including gout, heart disease, and diabetes. He received medical care at a local medical clinic and saw a psychiatrist periodically for his psychotropic medication. Eventually, after many months he also became incontinent and had no facilities to take care of his toileting and laundry needs during the day. The shelters began to refuse him a place to stay because of his incontinence. Eventually he went to the emergency room for extreme pain and was admitted to a hospital. There it was determined that excess medication had caused the incontinence and a co-occurring depressive episode had aggravated his inability to maintain self-care. As he recovered he was finally able to recognize his limitations on independence and agree to a seniors' residence placement.

COMMON MEDICAL CONDITIONS

Diseases of all types are more commonly experienced by homeless persons and are reported as more severe and persistent among the homeless than among the housed (Frankish et al., 2005). There is a consistency in the types of conditions reported. Chronic medical conditions such as high blood pressure, heart disease, diabetes, asthma, hepatitis, and emphysema, as well as diseases of the skin, foot, and circulatory system, are found at higher rates than in the general public. Many homeless people lack access to necessary medication for chronic conditions, fail to attend routine medical check-ups, have limited access to required diet, and persistently lack adequate rest to cope with their conditions. Cancer and liver and kidney disease are less frequently encountered but when present come with enormous challenges because treatment often requires additional rest and diet that is not usually available at public shelters; these conditions have significantly higher specialized care needs. Dangerous communicable diseases such as tuberculosis pose additional health risks for both shelter staff and clients as exposure to tuberculosis in crowded shelters increases the likelihood of contracting the disease. AIDS, although less frequently reported among the homeless, in part because of a system of HIV/AIDS support services, is a major concern when it presents itself.

Effective treatment also requires timely administration of medication, something that is an additional obstacle for those who do not live a scheduled life. Treatment usually requires rest, and since most shelters are not organized to provide day rest for the sick, the needed rest for recovery is often not available because sleeping in outdoor spaces invites tickets for loitering. The health risks of contracting HIV are also increased, especially for women who are forced into the sex trade and for youths who may not have enough education on safe sex, the availability of condoms, and who lack the presence of mind to use precautions when under the influence of drugs and are more vulnerable to peer pressure.

Foot Care, Skin Conditions, and Communicable Diseases

Since most homeless people rely on walking as the main means of transportation, foot conditions are not only prevalent, but also extremely disabling for them. Prolonged exposure to cold and damp conditions leads to what is called "immersion foot," a condition that causes feet to turn red or blue from poor circulation and can quickly lead to blisters and open sores. Immersion foot is different from frostbite, which results from exposure to severe cold and results in tissue damage that often leads to amputation of fingers or toes, or of limbs. Frostbite is a serious issue in northern climates; immersion foot can occur in temperatures up to 60 degrees Fahrenheit. Cellulitis, athlete's foot, and warts are also common. Skin conditions can affect both feet and other body areas. These conditions include impetigo, lice, and scabies, all of which are highly communicable in crowded and often unsanitary conditions in shelters and inadequate housing. Persons disabled by foot, skin, and circulatory problems have mobility difficulties and usually can't find ready access to services. Those with chronic conditions such as kidney failure who have no fixed address and no guarantee of the availability of the necessary specific and restricted diet may find access to dialysis unavailable. Among the most troubling conditions affecting the homeless are those easily transmittable by close approximation to disease carriers: skin conditions; parasitic diseases including lice and bedbugs; colds, influenza, and other respiratory diseases; difficult-to-control infections (discussed below); and those passed on by sharing needles and passing the bottle. For those seeking lodging at a local shelter, there may be little that can be done to avoid close proximity to others. For children, especially very young children, the health hazards can be profound as childhood communicable diseases can spread quickly.

Oral Health

The dental and oral health of homeless persons is frequently poor. Since dental care is not covered under universal health care in Canada, and only emergency care is covered under Medicare and Medicaid in the United States, the neglect of dental problems is a widespread issue among poor and homeless persons. Lack of dental care contributes to both ill health and diminished self-esteem. A recent study of adults living in shelters found that 88 percent needed fillings, 70 percent needed periodontal care, 60 percent needed prosthodontic care, and 40 percent needed emergency treatment (Figueiredo, Hwang, & Quiñonez, 2012). The result of long-time neglect, cavities, and tooth loss leaves people disfigured and reduces their self-esteem. Most medical care provides only for emergency tooth extraction and does not offer restorative services. Even those marginally housed do not have access to adequate dental care, so that the dental problems that occur are the result of years of neglect. For children it is often the beginning or a lifetime of poor oral health.

Sexual Health

Sexual health has been a long-term concern, especially among adolescents and those who work in the sex trade. While the rates of teenage pregnancy have dropped in the past several decades, young women who are homeless are far more likely to have an unplanned pregnancy than those who are housed. The causes not only include a high rate of sexual activity, but also often the dilemma of trading sex for a place to stay. Since birth control may not be readily accessible or affordable, pregnancy can be an unintended consequence. In a study of homeless youths Roy and colleagues determined that STDs, including HIV, chlamydia, syphilis, gonorrhea, and others, are prevalent among homeless youths (male and female) and those who work in the sex trade (Roy, Haley, Leclerc, Sochanski, Boudreau, & Boivin, 2004).

The problems of homeless, pregnant women are substantial and include additional health risks to both women and their unborn children. Prenatal care, essential for reducing complications in pregnancy and increasing the health of the unborn children, is the exception rather than the rule among street-dwelling youths. Adequate diet and rest are unlikely and the risk of contracting transmittable diseases on the streets is quite high. Prenatal risks may be compounded by continued sexual activity and the accompanying possibility of STDs. Homeless young women are also more likely than their housed counterparts to use street drugs and nicotine, both of which carry additional risks. For those who are addicted to alcohol, the risk of the child developing fetal alcohol spectrum disorder (FASD) is a significant and serious issue.

Communicable Diseases, Influenza, and Potential Epidemics

Being homeless inevitably entails fewer opportunities to bathe, wash clothes, and regularly wash hands. The places where one can feely go are likely to be less clean and cleaned less often than those in personal homes and residences. Inevitably the close proximity to others leads to greater exposure to bacteria and viruses that cause mild and serious illnesses. Consequently, the possibility of outbreaks of contagious disease is higher among the homeless, who are already compromised in their ability to fight off infectious diseases. Table 3.3 shows the main ways in which communicable diseases are transmitted. The possibility of an epidemic, whether it be a mild variant of a seasonal influenza, or a more virulent and deadly disease such as the SARS (Severe Acute Respiratory Syndrome) outbreak that affected Toronto and Vancouver in 2003, could be catastrophic.

A contagious illness such as tuberculosis is a good example of an infectious disease that persists among homeless people. Overcrowded shelters and low resistance to infection contribute to this alarming public health

Table 3.3. Main Ways Communicable Diseases Are Transmitted

Type of contact		Examples	Precautions
Person to person	Direct: body surface	Shaking hands: common cold, other viruses Hepatitis A Sharing body fluids, including transfusions and intercourse, e.g., HIV and hepatitis B and C Poked by needles or knives	Wear masks. Wash hands frequently. Use hand sanitizers. Use condoms. Wear gloves (winter).
	Indirect	Infectious agent (virus, bacteria, etc.) remains alive on surface touched by an infected person Hepatitis A	Avoid using common handrails, door knobs, etc., if possible. Use hand sanitizers frequently.
Airborne	Droplets: sneezing and coughing, which releases infectious agents	Influenza, common cold, upper respiratory viruses, measles, chickenpox	Wear masks. Cough into arm pit. Stand away from someone who is coughing.
Noncontact	Food-borne illnesses Water-borne illnesses Transmission via insect or animal	E-coli Giardia West Nile Lyme disease	Check source of food. Drink only treated water. Use insect repellant. Use mosquito netting.

problem. Because rates of communicable diseases are higher in homeless populations than in the housed populations, workers need to be aware of the multiple ways that they can be at risk for contracting diseases.

Use universal precautions when your area of work includes the street. These precautions refer to the guidelines that have been developed to prevent workers who are exposed to body fluids and blood from contracting diseases transmitted by these fluids. Some street people have needles or knives that are in their pockets to prevent anyone from being close to them or to deter people from pickpocketing them. This is both a physical safety issue and one that could potentially also involve transmission of disease. Keeping a safe distance is always recommended.

Textbox 3.4. The Emergency Medical Kit
Body fluids are most likely to transmit HIV, hepatitis, STDs, and other infections. Those working on the frontlines should always carry a small emergency kit that includes disposable gloves, cleaning cloths, and disinfectant for instances where contact with body fluids may be unavoidable.

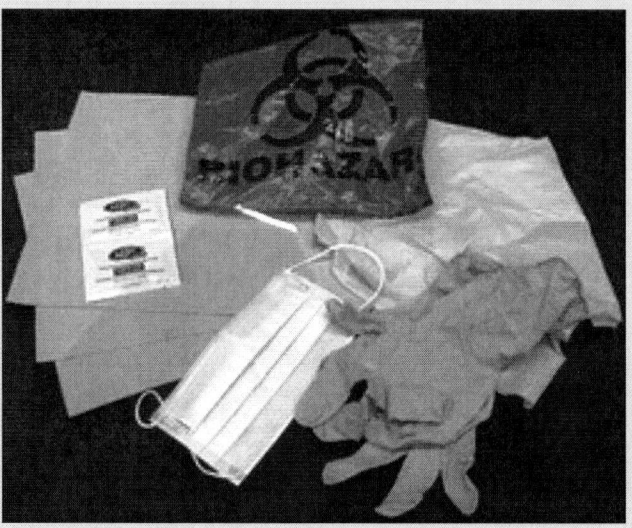

There are several important rules:

1. Any way that a bacteria or virus can enter the body and establish itself is a route of transmission. Similar to what will be further discussed in the substance-abuse section, a pathogen (something that causes disease) needs a way into the body that is favorable to its existence and growth.
2. Some pathogens such as those that cause influenza and tuberculosis prefer oral and nasal routes.
3. Skin-related pathogens often rely on contact between the host (infected person) and the recipient.
4. Some pathogens such as HIV and hepatitis are contracted through body fluids.

5. No pathway into the body is totally protected from disease-carrying agents.

Textbox 3.5. Cautions about Body Fluids

The Centers for Disease Control and Prevention (CDC; 2013) and Health Canada (2013) both recommend proactive measures to reduce the spread of illness. There are some features common to all ways of reducing the risk of infection or spreading infection. The most basic is washing hands and using antiseptic gels after all contact with people. Assume that anyone could be a possible carrier, even if that person never gets sick themselves. Follow any contact with body fluids with a complete disinfection as soon as possible. Carry and use disposable gloves for any health-related contact. Although this may be offensive to some people, it may be better to explain this as a mandatory workplace rule than to risk contracting an illness. Basic to all of these precautions is the expectation that all those who work in high-risk environments—including all those in regular contact with homeless persons—get and stay current on all vaccinations available, including all common childhood diseases, hepatitis, influenza, shingles, and so on. This is as important as requiring a construction worker to wear a safety harness.

Prevention is especially important in the light of treatment-resistant pathogens that have become prevalent and no longer respond to common antibiotics. There are three of these pathogens of special note, but as viruses have a remarkable ability to mutate, the likelihood that other resistant conditions emerge is high. These three are Methicillin Resistant Staphylococcus Aureus (MRSA), Vancomycin Resistant Enterococcus (VRE), and Clostridium Difficile (C. diff). They are often contracted in a hospital setting (CDC, 2013), but hospitals routinely discharge infected persons before they are free of infection. MRSA most often appears as a disease affecting the skin (wounds) and in the nose; VRE causes serious infection, often in the intestines; and C. diff causes diarrhea (as the most common symptoms of each, respectively). What unites these is their lack of response to usual treatments, the difficulty of locating a responsive drug, often the high cost of these drugs, and the life-threatening consequences of lack of treatment. Although usually transmitted to persons already ill with other conditions, these three are more often showing up outside the hospital setting and are thus important and dangerous sources of contagion.

Many workers receive basic training in the more common infections that are found on the streets. They do not necessarily receive training on all of these hazards that are avoidable, and they do not necessarily learn how to protect themselves. The most commonly known protective measures include avoiding all body fluids and excretions, including those that are airborne. While face masks are often worn in medical settings to protect workers from infectious contact, this is not a welcome sight in most situations where homeless people congregate. So how does one find protection in a dangerous environment?

Not everyone who is homeless—or on the edge of losing housing—lacks basic cleanliness and hygiene, but most homeless persons do as a result of their circumstance. Bathing facilities, if any, are few and far between and often use is restricted to specific times. Washrooms are not always available and, if filthy, often avoided. Thus hand washing is at a premium and not rigorously followed, even in the best of circumstances. At the same time, research has clearly demonstrated that public places and public assistances such as hand railings, door knobs, escalator rails, and the like are rife with disease-carrying bacteria. While no one lives in a totally antiseptic environment, some contaminants are likely to compromise the health of the client and the worker.

The first and most obvious approach is to avoid touching *any* surface, as it may contain contaminants and there is no way to know the extent to which the germs may be transmittable. Handshakes, while a major source of disease transmission, may be unavoidable, especially if refusing to do so may be taken as unfriendly. However, these responses come with a price, as anything that suggests that the worker is uncomfortable or fears contamination will destroy the rapport that he may have been building. Thus in this, as in other areas, there needs to be a balanced approach that accepts a certain degree of risk—and draws a line on unacceptable risk.

A second line of defense is to carry a hand disinfectant that you can use immediately after leaving a situation. Another safeguard is to carry disposable gloves for the situation where contact with possible contaminants is necessary. A backpack, oversize bag, or satchel that can be securely closed is preferable as a place to keep personal items with work-related items in a separate compartment. It should be large enough to keep important items but not so big as to be a hindrance. Finally, strip and wash when you get home, or back to the office if it has showering facilities.

- Wear clothing that can be quickly and easily washed and dried. This is explained below.
- Wear layers if the weather permits. You can always shed a layer and keep moving.
- Keep footwear comfortable, with low heels; shoes preferably should be waterproof.
- Keep a bottle of water with you for your thirst and to defer invitations to drink what may not be safe. Do not leave it unattended, do not share, and do not carry it in your hands.
- If entering a building or a person's apartment, try to go with another worker, both as a safety precaution and as a witness.
- In entering any enclosed space, whether an alley or a building, always keep yourself in line with the exit. Do not let someone get between you and your means of safe exit.
- If possible, request that household pets be placed in another room or on a leash in your presence. Some people have pets for protection and may not restrain or remove them. You will need to establish your own comfort level if a pet is present.
- Refuse offers of food and drink; you do not know if they are contaminated.
- Do not remove your shoes on entering a house. Stay near the door if you are not otherwise allowed in.
- When you come home from any questionable place, plan to completely unclothe and wash immediately. You never know what vermin may have decided to hitch a ride.

The possibility of an epidemic, whether it be a mild variant of a seasonal influenza, or a more virulent and deadly disease such as the Severe Acute Respiratory Syndrome (SARS) outbreak that affected Vancouver and Toronto in 2003 could have disastrous consequences for homeless people as well as the urban environments in which they live. Very few cities and towns have taken the needs of homeless persons into account in any planning for the possibility of a pandemic (a large-scale epidemic that is both deadly and rapidly spreading). The health, safety, and care issues in the instance of a

Textbox 3.6. Coming Home Routine

Workers who encounter questionable and dirty places usually develop a routine that includes the following:

- Have a place where you can change all clothing when you get home. This should preferably be in the laundry room of your apartment building, or lacking that, the front entry of your apartment, or the garage of your house.
- Keep a change or clothes there, as well as a garbage bag for all items that you have worn. These need to go immediately to the washing machine and then the dryer at high heat to kill any lice and bedbugs.
- Take a shower and wash your hair before doing anything else. You do not want unexpected company in your home or clothing.

Textbox 3.7. Keep Your Shoes On

In most places in Canada, but not necessarily in the United States, visitors remove their shoes upon entering another person's home. While it may be considered impolite not to do so, safety is your first concern. If your footwear is totally muddy or water drenched because of the weather, plan to stay at the door rather than imperil your safety. Do not remove your footwear in any new or unfamiliar situation. The first consideration is that you need to be able to exit quickly should the need arise. Be practical—flat comfortable footwear that will allow you to move quickly if necessary is the only practical approach on the front line. Running shoes are recommended because they are usually at least partially waterproof, have better treads for stability, are comfortable, and can be washed if necessary.

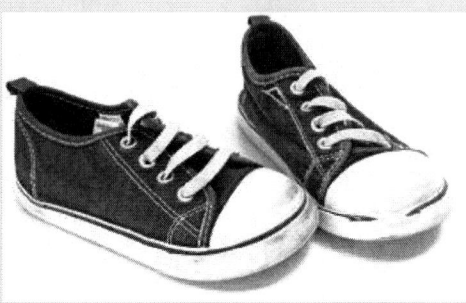

pandemic are significant. For the homeless, the daily challenges of living are multifold. Whenever a homeless person becomes ill with an easily transmittable disease, or a medical condition requires surgical intervention these challenges are greatly magnified. The obstacles to care also affect those whose health is already compromised by other chronic conditions. Table 3.4 illustrates the immediate needs of a person who becomes seriously ill while homeless. The essential responses in an outbreak of influenza or an epidemic include the isolation of the infected, the restriction of contact with potential carriers, and the limitation of the use of public spaces to prevent disease transmission. Sick people need a place to recover, one that is free of additional contamination, staffed by trained workers, and supplied with food and other essentials. Most shelters are not equipped to handle isolation protocols.

Table 3.4. Immediate Needs When Ill

Need	Access Issues
Stay in bed during an acute illness.	Limited or nonexistent sick bay facilities in shelters.
Get additional bed rest during recovery.	Shelters require everyone to be up and out of bed and out of sleeping areas during the day.
Eat a diet specific to illness and recovery.	Meals are served only in soup kitchens and shelter dining areas.
Maintain adequate intake of fluids.	Sleeping areas have no adequate storage. Access to fluids including water is limited and, other than water, often expensive (unaffordable).
Limit access to others who may carry infectious diseases.	No quarantine areas are available.
During a pandemic, obey community-wide orders to stay home and avoid outside contact. Keep five days' supply of food on hand.	No food storage facilities are available. No infectious-free facilities are available to stay in.
Reduce use of public transportation and places where people congregate.	There are no other means to get to needed services.
Appropriate place to store medication that requires refrigeration	Storage and refrigeration facilities are unavailable or difficult to access.

HEALTH RECOVERY RELATED NEEDS

Most shelters and drop-in programs, including soup kitchens, do not have the organization, space allotment, or staff skills to provide quarantine space for persons infected by highly contagious disease (Leung, Ho, Kiss, Gundlapalli, & Hwang, 2008). They lack the infrastructure to deal with dispensing medications for those who are sick, and the discharge to a convalescent location as patients pass the critical stage of the illness. Likewise, those who use shelters and food kitchens are unlikely to have other places to sleep or get food. They often need to travel by public transportation and to be in places frequented by others. They lack a place to store food and safe water for a few days in the event they get sick, and they often do not have anyone who can care for them in their illness. In many cases, except where life-threatening complications occur, hospitals and emergency rooms are not accessible. A widespread epidemic would be a disastrous event for those who are homeless.

Many of the challenges noted above also apply to those precariously housed. If a person is doubling up or couch surfing, staying in bed or getting extra rest may not be an option, or may put serious strains on the relationship that result in homelessness when the illness is over. Children who are ill are often fussy and tend to cry to express their discomfort. This often puts other adults at additional stress. Getting better often requires extra food and liquids—the chicken soup that helps recovery. Often budgets are strained to pay for this and entitlement benefits do not allow for extra dietary needs. People who are ill need a consistently comfortable temperature, which may raise the utility bill beyond affordability. Being homeless and sick is beyond misery.

Nutrition

Adequate food and nutrition are known to help disease prevention, and are often essential to dealing with chronic conditions such as diabetes, Crohn's disease, and other metabolic disorders that affect digestion, food uptake, and recovery from illness. Staff in shelters, soup kitchens, and food pantries can't always ensure that there are sufficient dietary choices and that food will be available when it is needed, and not simply according to an organization's schedule. People who have dietary restrictions, who may have kidney damage or liver impairment, and who have special needs, such as those with diabetes or gluten or lactose intolerance, can't be ensured that if eating enough means eating well enough. In all of these situations, lack of appropriate, adequate, and timely (meals at specific times) diets will compromise health and result in these conditions worsening and additional serious health problems. While there may be an adequate amount of food, it may not be of the right type, so that a person with lactose or gluten intolerance will have difficulty avoiding those substances in most meals available at soup kitchens and through food pantries or food banks. The dietary supplements that tax officials will allow to be claimed as health-related needs are of no use to a person whose taxable income may be nonexistent. Those who do not follow their diet guidelines increase the harmful effects of their condition, which will manifest itself in increased physical problems and often increased emotional problems such as anxiety and depression, both of which are associated with some uncontrolled medical conditions such as diabetes.

Impact of Trauma

Over the past decade, the impact of trauma in the lives of homeless people has come to be recognized as a significant factor that impedes their mental health, substance abuse, and behavioral stability (Sundin, 2011). These challenges are discussed in chapter 9. The reality of the transfer of trauma-related responses, known as vicarious trauma in the behavioral and mental health arena, is an important health-related condition that may impact workers. Vicarious trauma is the result of hearing about serious injury or death that occurred in a situation where the victim did not have either the opportunity to deal with the situation or the opportunity or ability to flee the situation (Mathieu, 2012). This description follows the accepted trauma definition that includes a lack of ability for fight or flight. Hearing about the extreme emotional impacts that trauma has had on some of its victims, or hearing about the impact of terror, fear, helplessness, and emotional overload, often as it is reexperienced by the victim, can result in a vicarious traumatization where the helper also experiences these feelings and their resultant physical and psychological symptoms. These situations become fundamental mental health first-aid issues for workers. Your ability as a worker to deal with and integrate these experiences forms the basis of your ability to continue to be an effective helper. While we will look more closely at self-care later in this chapter, it is important to emphasize that workers should develop a self-care plan with their supervisors as part of the work assignment.

Medical Implications of Traumatic Brain Injury

Traumatic brain injury (TBI) is caused either by a severe blow to the head resulting in an open wound or closed (thus not visible) wound such as a severe concussion, or by a variety of other factors: lack of oxygen, chemicals and other toxins, serious infection (i.e., meningitis and encephalitis), brain tumors, and stroke. Most damage occurs in the frontal and temporal lobes of the brain and result in the multiple cognitive and behavioral problems observed in those with TBI. The development of TBI by some professional sports figures has brought new attention to the pervasive effects of concussions and other head trauma. Increasingly recognized as a significant physical and behavioral health problem, TBI has been documented as significantly more prevalent among homeless persons than it is in the general public (Hwang et al., 2008; Topolovec-Vranic et al., 2012). TBI may be a cause for homelessness, as the impairments resulting from TBI may lead to an inability to maintain employment and unstable behavior that leads to financial mismanagement and resultant lack of payment of rent and utilities. The violence on the streets may also result in TBI that then renders a homeless person less able to cope with the dynamics of street life and survival.

Among homeless persons, TBI is common, frequently accompanied by a seizure disorder and associated with poor health outcomes (Hwang et al., 2008). All of these are a challenge for frontline workers who may be called on to assist with basic emergency first aid on a regular basis. Many workers will hear reports of falls and head trauma sustained during street violence, thus it is important to be aware of indications for medical intervention. Immediately following an incident when there is a possibility of TBI, any of the following observed or reported symptoms needs to be monitored: impaired consciousness or loss of consciousness for any amount of time, confusion, disorientation, or memory impairment for any time around the injury. Further signs of potential TBI include seizures, vomiting, lethargy (especially in infants and the very young), dizziness, headaches, tiredness, irritability, or poor concentration. Long-term physical complaints with a neurological origin (TBI) are reported along with problematic behaviors. The behavioral and psychosocial problems that accompany TBI will be explored further in chapter 9.

The End of Life

Homeless people have a much shorter life expectancy than those who are housed (Hwang et al., 2005). The end of life may come through violence, or much more often through the ravages of prolonged ill health. Homeless people are at higher risk of dying and of dying young than are people in the general population. While violence and infectious diseases are chief contributors, many older homeless persons suffer from terminal health issues including heart disease, liver and kidney failure, and cancer. People who have a terminal illness may be able to access the resources of palliative care, either through home care or a hospice program that is hospital-based or has a residential facility. For homeless people there are several barriers to accessing hospice care. Home hospice is unavailable to those who lack a home (i.e., a consistent and stable place to live). Those marginally housed may not have the physical and emotional resources to deal with end of life issues and thus do not access home hospice care. Residential and hospital-based hospice programs may be reluctant to admit patients with difficult behavioral or lifestyle issues. One of the major challenges for persons who are shelter dwellers is the discomfort of being confined in a place that is outside their frame of reference. Hospice belongs to Main Street and not to the streets. The unfamiliarity with the hospice surroundings makes many homeless persons uncomfortable with and unwilling to accept this type of care. As long as a person is competent, it is his decision as to what type of care he will accept. However, this freedom of choice may create ethical dilemmas for caregivers who do not want to discharge a terminally ill person to a shelter lacking appropriate support services.

While there are reports of shelters humanely and creatively creating a hospice space for long-term shelter users, as found, for example, in Ottawa (Podymow, Turnbull, & Coyle, 2006), these uniquely responsive programs continue to be the exception rather than the rule. More often a health crisis brings the person back to an emergency room, and death occurs in the hospital—because there was no other place for the person to be accommodated. Kushel reports several additional reasons for the unavailability of hospice services. Lack of medical insurance often keeps homeless persons in the United States from accessing hospice programs, either inpatient or home-based programs. Home-based programs also require a support system of family and friends that is usually not present. At the same time, the institutional environment and barriers that most people who are homeless try to avoid are ever-present in hospital-based palliative care. The development of hospital-hospice programs requires more funding than is traditionally available through Medicaid and Medicare (Kushel & Miaskowski, 2006).

Kushel goes on to point out important considerations for frontline workers who have chronically ill and terminally ill persons with whom they work (Kushel & Miaskowski, 2006). These persons often have not established health-care directives and end-of-life directives, and are unlikely to have surrogate decision makers (Song et al., 2007). Often, the involvement of a service worker or agency in end-of-life decisions presents a situation involving risks and liabilities that many organizations are reluctant to take on. In those instances the homeless person is truly left with no substantial support as her life draws to a close. The ethical implications of acting in a beneficent and moral manner are placed in stark reality in these instances, as we further explore in chapter 11 when we examine ethical issues.

Primary and Preventative Health Care

Although national health care in Canada should be able to address primary and preventative health care needs, this is not the case. Most homeless persons do not have a primary health-care physician, for several interrelated reasons. Many doctors have full practices and limit the new patients they accept. This can be an effective way of screening out high-need and low-treatment-compliant persons. Apart from the challenges of accessing a primary care physician or family doctor, the circumstances in the United States are quite similar in the use of health-care services. Primary care is infrequent and emergency care the norm.

Homeless persons have difficulty paying for prescription drugs, even when subsidized; problems following doctor's orders for special diets and adhering to specific eating times (such as for diabetes, hypoglycemia); following specific times for taking medication if this requires that the medications be taken with food; and obtaining rest for certain medical conditions. As a result many people are unable to follow medical treatment recommendations (Hwang, 2001). Most housing-challenged persons have no time or patience for doctors' waiting rooms or emergency clinics, where hours may be spent waiting to be seen. In those waiting rooms, the scornful looks of other patients is a further stigmatizing and humiliating experience. Not surprisingly, most avoid care until there is a crisis, and thus they are five times more likely to use an emergency room than are those who are housed (Frankish et al., 2005). Most homeless persons have no adequate place to go to recover if they require hospitalization and intensive care.

Access to Preventative Health Services

We know that even in countries with universal health care, access to basic health services and preventative care is not readily accessible for the homeless (Hwang et al., 2010). This access usually requires a health plan enrollment and identification of residence that many homeless people lack. Many homeless and housing-vulnerable persons lack a family doctor, the means to acquire one, or even the consistency of the same physician in a health center. Because of their unstable lifestyle and subsequent inability to always comply with doctor recommendations, because they have frequent multiple health problems, and because their unkempt appearance is discomforting to others in the waiting rooms of many doctors, most physicians are reluctant to accept homeless and fragilely housed persons as regular patients. The result is that they are often at the mercy of emergency clinics, which treat specific urgent cases and single out one ailment rather than including an assessment of all contributing conditions. Thus clinics usually do not necessarily handle all related health concerns. If there is not a single pharmacy supplying medications, people are also at risk of being prescribed multiple, and sometimes incompatible, medications. Adverse reactions, including high dosages of certain medications, may precipitate additional medical problems that may not be recognized.

Psychological Health

As we will examine in chapter 7, mental health and mental illness (mental disorders) are two different concepts. Similar to physical health, where certain markers such as blood pressure, weight, good sleeping habits, and balanced electrolytes are indicators of health, in the area of mental and psychological functioning factors such as a positive outlook on life, and interest in the well-being of self and others are indicative of (positive) mental health. The World Health Organization (WHO) has devoted considerable effort toward identifying and describing mental health as a concept distinctly different from mental illness (Herrman, Saxena, & Moodie, 2005) Like physical health, being mentally healthy does not depend on total absence of a disability (i.e., the individual with loss of a limb, or someone whose diet is restricted because of gluten intolerance). It does imply that a person is not currently experiencing or dealing with significant impairment caused by signs and symptoms of mental illness. As we shall explore, mental health is important for both workers and homeless persons. Mental health provides much of the emotional energy needed to reach out and create positive interventions and events. These are the foundations on which lives can be rebuilt.

Issues such as the feeling of hopelessness that one faces in the aftermath of losing one's housing, or the anxiety experienced in waiting to qualify for job training, are within the realm of normal and understandable reactions to life stresses. Along with the loss of housing, homeless persons experience loss of dignity that is often exacerbated by negative reactions of those on Main Street. For the many who have long-term housing loss, this loss of self-esteem becomes a major barrier to the prospect of integrating into a normalized life that permanent residence allows.

Hope is a nourishment for the soul that all persons need to survive and thrive. It is instrumental in an individual's ability and willingness to fight whatever disease has afflicted the body or the mind. While not in and of itself enough to restore health, hope has been observed to be a significant player in healing (Chiu, Emblen, Van Hofwegen, Sawatzky, & Meyerhoff, 2004). Together with values of empowerment and belief in recovery, hope is a significant factor motivating people to stable health and housing. We also know that those housed face better care and health outcomes than those living in shelters and on the street (Hwang et al., 2005). This reinforces the importance of the immediate provision of housing since many of the obstacles of medical care and convalescence can be addressed by the reality of a stable residence—a place to rest, store adequate food, and maintain a recommended pattern of nutrition and care.

Companion Pets

There are quite a number of people who have pets, lose their housing, and keep their pets with them. They may refuse housing or shelter that will not let them keep their pets, or they may refuse to leave housing that is in poor condition or a health hazard because they refuse to be separated from their pet. They may be couch surfing or sleeping rough, as shelters as a rule do not accept pets, no matter what size or how well trained. Pets are invaluable companions to many people and have been shown to reduce health and heart problems, increase feelings of belonging, and lower stress (Kidd & Kidd, 1994). Youths especially have indicated that pets reduce their loneliness and isolation, and provide both comfort and companionship (Rew, 2000). Pets also provide a powerful way to connect and communicate with youths who are wary of adults. For example, you may be able to engage a youth in speaking about experiences through her pet. Because shelters usually will not admit pets, and many landlords often do not accept pets, they are seen by many workers as a barrier to effective outreach and help. However, for those who have lost much of their lives, who have little left for themselves and who lack human companionship, a pet can be life-saving. The challenge for the frontline worker is to accept this relationship as a sign of strength and an essential part of what helps a homeless person, and then to find ways to accommodate this additional homeless being.

PROVIDER HEALTH: SELF-CARE, COMPASSION FATIGUE, AND BURNOUT

In the previous section we examined the many ways in which being homeless can affect the physical and mental health of clients and those we would like to engage in a helping relationship. In chapters 7–9 we will also look at the many ways in which mental health, addiction, and varieties of traumatic experiences are also major influences in the lives of homeless persons. Before we do that, though, we turn to examine the stressful impact direct service work has on frontline workers, the greatest contributors to stress, and how workers can address these work-related stressors before they become overwhelming. We see these factors as following an intertwined spiral that usually begins with unresolved stress and worsens, possibly evolving into compassion fatigue and emerging as burnout, or possibly proceeding directly to burnout. The process may be rapid, or slow and insidious, depending on personal factors as well as those contributed by the organizational environment in which one works, and the external environment of the homeless community that one is trying to serve. Many workers, deeply engaged in their work, do not sense its effects until they have begun to take a toll on personal and work life, including relationships in both places. We hope that this section will remind workers of the importance of self-awareness and self-care in a highly challenging environment.

High levels of stress and the almost inevitable consequences of compassion fatigue and possible burnout are major contributors to the high levels of staff turnover often experienced by organizations working with persons who have mental health and/or substance-use problems (Paris & Hoge, 2010). Turnover is a serious disruption to relationships that have been built with clients, to coordination of tasks within the organization, and to working relationships outside the organization. Staff replacement is both time-consuming and costly, from both a financial and personnel turnover perspective. Many would suggest that stress, burnout, and staff turnover are higher in those organizations that serve persons who are homeless for a number of fundamental reasons.

1. Many frontline providers, regardless of how skilled they are in interpersonal communication and establishing relationships, lack the training to effectively use these approaches with very troubled people.
2. Entry-level workers with some preprofessional or professional training (e.g., social work, nursing, psychology, rehabilitation counseling) most often have no background preparation specific to working in settings with homeless people.
3. Frontline services are generally not well funded. This results in low salary levels for frontline staff, few resources, and lack of adequate training and support.
4. Supervision is often minimal and focused on administrative aspects of the job, leaving workers with little instrumental and emotional support, especially in difficult situations.
5. Few supervisors have the training and skills to support workers who have encountered various traumas, or the death of a client. They often overlook the fact that these work-related crises affect others in the organization, in addition to the direct worker.

6. Frontline work is often hazardous and workers frequently encounter instances and reports of trauma, abuse, and violations of personal and civil rights, as well as physical and health hazards in unsafe houses and on the streets. One of the challenges for workers is to be able to self-monitor for signs of hypervigilance. While this may be a necessary street life strategy, when it flows over into one's personal life it can have repercussions in personal relationships.
7. Many frontline workers are in the field alone, without important support and back-up. This increased isolation adds to feelings of lack of value and support.
8. Without adequate support, some workers may turn to those they are trying to help for validation of their work and worth. In so doing they lose their sense of boundaries and may come to rely on the support of those they are trying to help. This form of codependency will lead to greater damage to both client and worker.
9. Management is often not aware of the negative impact of an organizational culture where staff is not valued and trusted.
10. Few organizations address issues of turnover and burnout. Even fewer have staff wellness practices and plans to support staff who are having difficulties on the job or whose personal life is impeding their ability to work effectively (Olivet, McGraw, Grandin, & Bassuk, 2010).

Stress is a universal phenomenon. At some point each of us feels the sense of being overwhelmed by too many things to do; not enough time, support, or money to do them; too many demands from different people; and too many high, possibly unrealistic, expectations put on us by ourselves or others. When stress is short term and driven by passing circumstance we cope, adapt, adjust, and look forward to relief. However, when it is unrelenting, with little escape from the pressure that it brings, stress can and does lead to counterproductive adaptations. In working with the disenfranchised, we encounter the stress faced by others on a daily basis. We also often feel helpless to change the ways in which government and organizational bureaucracies interfere or throw up obstacles that prevent rapid solutions to basic human needs of food, shelter, and clothing. In the face of additional human traumas and tragedies, we are also called on to be compassionate, to reach out and help, by giving of ourselves as real people who understand and care about the problems and feelings of others.

Causes of Burnout

Burnout comes primarily from three different sources that often overlap and create a cumulative effect: (1) the nature of the job and related work environment stressors, (2) the personality and behavioral characteristics of the worker, and (3) the lifestyle of the worker. Some jobs are inherently stressful, and working frontline with homeless people is one. The stressors are greatly increased if there is no supervisory or managerial recognition for this stress, if supervisors do not provide psychosocial support to workers, if workloads are too high, or if timelines are too short. Lack of recognition for performance, and office politics that convey lack of trust of worker activity and integrity contribute to the emotional depletion that becomes burnout. Workers who spend excessive amounts of time at work without compensatory time off, who do not take earned vacation, and who come to work even when obviously ill are clearly struggling with boundary issues between work and personal demands. Too much work without a balance of rest, recreation, and spiritual activities greatly accelerates a worker on the road to burnout. (By "spiritual activities" we mean those that rejuvenate and restore the spirit, whether through organized religion, meditation, time in nature, music, art, or any activity that refreshes your inner being.) While the need to perform, to be a perfectionist, and to work hard may all be part of a person's personality, these needs must be balanced or the worker risks becoming dysfunctional. Too much work also includes taking it home, either physically or emotionally, so that there is no rest. Too little rest also contributes to burnout. Sleep is restorative: it is essential for mental, emotional, and physical well-being. Insufficient sleep adds to cumulative fatigue and the feeling of being overburdened.

Because it usually develops slowly, rather than having a sudden onset, most people are unaware of the effects of burnout until it is highly obvious to others. There are some self-monitoring activities that can alert an individual to impending burnout:

1. Feelings of constant physical and/or emotional exhaustion that are not attributable to any recent dramatic event.

2. Contracting infectious illnesses easily and frequently is often related to stress, which lowers the immune system.
3. Spending less time with or having a lower investment in personal relationships. This may be due to disengagement because of lack of emotional energy or to spending excessive amounts of time at work.
4. A growing pessimistic attitude at work or about new expectations on proposals/activities at work.
5. Either increased absenteeism or a lack of productivity at work—just getting through the day.
6. Feeling as though work efforts don't make a difference.

Occupational stress is a major dynamic in the homeless services field. The stressors may come from having too much to do, too many difficult situations to deal with, lack of resources, and most importantly, lack of support and understanding from supervisors and management. Many jobs are stressful, but few demand empathetic engagement with others who are suffering the unfairness, indignities, and lack of caring of those with economic and social advantages, on a constant basis. We all need the opportunity to rest, emotionally and physically, from these demands, without feeling guilty that we have the privilege and ability to do so. Similarly, we need to respect personal needs for timely meals, rest, and opportunities to debrief stressful days and events.

Burnout, Vicarious Traumatization, and Compassion Fatigue

The terms "burnout," "vicarious traumatization," and "compassion fatigue" are sometimes used interchangeably, but they refer to distinct processes and require different approaches to deal with them effectively. The distinctions between burnout, vicarious traumatization, and compassion fatigue are described by Zeidner, Hadar, Matthews, and Roberts (2013). Table 3.5 provides a quick comparison of these three phenomena.

Burnout occurs when direct service workers develop a clearly defined set of responses (a psychological syndrome) as a reaction to chronic situational and interpersonal stressors on the job. There are three main components of this response: (1) an overwhelming exhaustion, (2) a sense of ineffectiveness and consequent feeling of lack of accomplishment, and (3) feelings of cynicism and detachment from the job. Vicarious traumatization

Table 3.5. Characteristics of Stress, Burnout, and Compassion Fatigue

Increased Behavioral Responses	Heightened Emotional Responses	Decreased Emotional Responses
Overreactivity to events	Blunted emotions	Preoccupation with traumatic stories/events
Failure to distinguish client/worker boundaries and overengagement as the result	Sense of detachment, disengagement	Emotional numbing or detachment
	Loss of motivation, loss of ideals	Negative change in worldview
Excessive activity in response to sense of urgency	Feelings of depression	Lack of energy
	Irritability	Loss of empathy
Resultant loss of emotional and physical energy	Frustration	Heightened sense of arousal
	Feelings of helplessness	Disrupted sleep pattern
	Lack of hope	Change in ability to trust
Increased anxiety		
Increased physical symptoms: raised blood pressure, fatigue, inability to sleep		

develops as the result of repeated exposure to the psychological impact of trauma in clients. Compassion fatigue consists of a combination of burnout and vicarious traumatization characterized by anxiety, flashbacks, nightmares, and intrusive thoughts that result from working specifically with people who have been traumatized. Two dynamics may explain these experiences: resource depletion, where workers become emotionally and physically worn out by the emotional demands of clients' experiences; and emotional contagion, where the helper experiences emotions in response to or anticipation of clients' responses. We discuss below the ways in which organizational factors play a bigger role than individual characteristics in the development of burnout.

Stress, compassion fatigue, and burnout are elements of the worker-workplace interchange that are part of the high-risk environment for front-line staff. While considerable attention has been focused on stress in the mental health workplace and burnout among professionals who work in these settings, recently some attention has become focused on the additional and unique traumatic stressors that workers face in helping highly disadvantaged and distressed homeless persons. We will discuss trauma in more detail

80 WORKING WITH HOMELESS AND VULNERABLE PEOPLE

in chapter 9. Here, we look at the potential impact on workers of hearing details about traumatic events in people's lives, the difficult emotions that some child abuse and neglect situations involve, and the exploitation and violence that occurs on the streets. In all of these situations the worker may experience the emotional upheaval that has befallen clients or feel the helplessness of those who struggle and yet are unable to achieve a better life. While worker empathy is important to the helping relationship, the constant drain on personal feelings, without opportunities to recharge emotional batteries, can easily lead to feeling physically and emotionally depleted. This feeling of depletion is commonly referred to as compassion fatigue, and is often experienced by emergency workers, trauma workers, and nurses in intensive care settings, among others. It also affects those who work frontline with homeless persons. As you can see in figure 3.1, stress, burnout, and compassion fatigue all relate to each other, with stress being a major contributor to the other two. We may experience burnout from numerous job demands, coupled by not attending to our own emotional

Figure 3.1. The Interplay of Stress, Compassion Fatigue, and Burnout

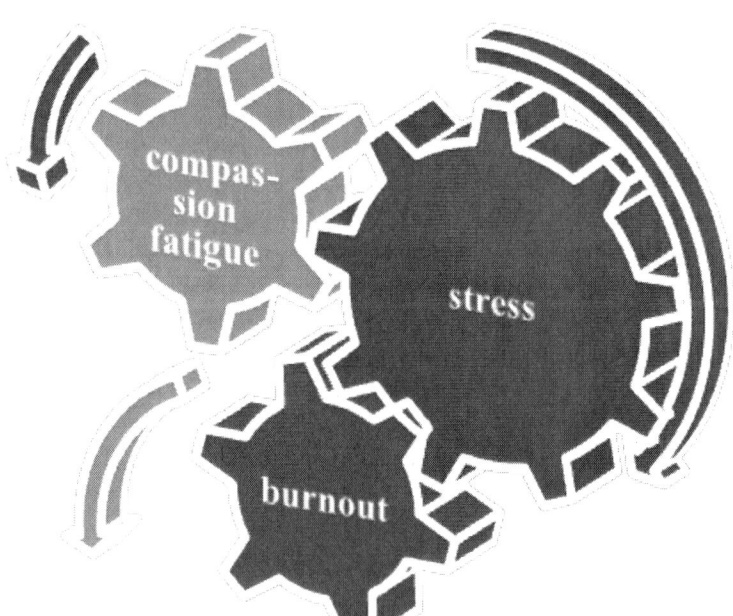

and physical needs, or we may experience compassion fatigue from working with too many people who have been badly traumatized (also referred to as vicarious traumatization). We may also feel guilty for not doing enough to safeguard homeless people from abuse, or to help house vulnerable groups such as youths and victimized persons of Aboriginal (Native American) background. This can lead to efforts to overcompensate and subsequently can lead to burnout, or we may have both burnout and compassion fatigue aggravated by excess stress caused by working with traumatized persons.

Most books written for persons working in the field of social services concentrate on the tasks and skills necessary to provide appropriate and effective services. Integral to that skill development process is the effective use of the self—that is, how best to establish empathetic relationships, reach out to vulnerable persons, and walk with them through the mazes of bureaucracy that they encounter in trying to reestablish their lives. Occasionally there is a brief mention of overload and compassion fatigue. Ways to handle issues such as burnout are most often addressed in specialty books and journal articles that few beginning workers encounter. We maintain that it is important for workers to be aware of issues around burnout and compassion fatigue early in their working careers so that they can develop self-care and coping skills and reduce the dangers of burnout (figure 3.2).

Self-care and burnout are both opposite ends of the caregiving spectrum and can act independently of each other. Fundamental to self-care is the worker's recognition of the emotional and physical toll that it takes to work with highly stressed individuals who often have multiple problems of a subsistence lifestyle, poor physical health, poor mental health, at times addictions, legal problems, and lack of access to funds to provide necessities of life. These problems may present a stress for workers whose own lives, by comparison, are relatively comfortable, with basic needs met, a measure of self-enhancing opportunities also available (e.g., entertainment, recreation, vacation), and usually income security. Beyond the differences between those who have and those who have not, there are many serious stressors that impact the worker. We will first look at those in the homeless sector and then turn to more-general issues of workplace stress that affect other social services staff as well.

Psychological health is vital for service providers. The challenges of working with very deprived persons and those who have few personal

Figure 3.2. Burnout

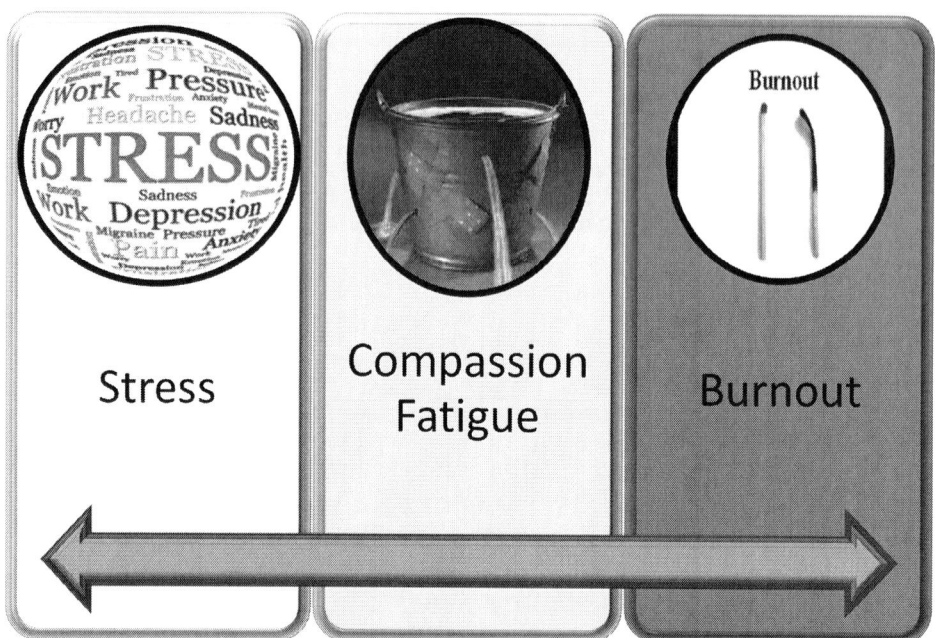

resources, the frustrations of bureaucracy that appear to inhibit fast response to urgent situations, the increased possibility of contracting a communicable disease or having to deal with a person high on drugs whose behavior threatens to go out of control, are all daily stressors for frontline workers. In addition to these stressors, workers continually face the ethical issues that present challenges and may stress the limits of their ability to walk a fine line of personal/professional, legal/illegal, moral/immoral. In appendix 2 you will find a Professional Quality of Life Scale (ProQOL) that you can use as a self-measure of the extent to which you have a balance in your life or may be in danger of burnout (Stamm, 1995). The ProQOL is a widely used and well-researched instrument that is available for your use without charge. We recommend that you refer to it and share it at work with coworkers and supervisors as a way of reminding everyone of the emotional toll that work can have. The individual items will also give you opportunities for focussed discussion about organizational- and work assignment–related responses to burnout.

Self-Care: Preventing Burnout

Given that burnout is an occupational hazard of the frontline, what are some of the ways in which you can take care of yourself? The most important issue is your recognition and acceptance that self-care is critical to your effective functioning. Lack of self-care will influence your personal life as well as your work life. You should never consider it as a weakness. The pie chart exercise at the end of this chapter is also a good way to self-assess how you are spending your time. Next, you need to develop a list of things that you *do* that make you feel good. By *do,* we mean those things that you actively participate in. For example, cooking or cleaning can be considered chores or enjoyable activities—or sometimes both; also, some physical activities may be enjoyable, others a duty. You also need a list of things that are enjoyable but require less energy such as watching a movie, reading, or listening to music (but not all at once!). Do you take time for lunch, or a brief walk over a lunch break? Do you have one day a week that you consider a day of rest and relaxation? If not, why not, and what can you do about it? Do you have comfort foods? Do you eat them regularly but in moderation?

Canadian Aboriginal and Native American people have always known about the importance of balance in one's life. We have learned from them that a respectful recognition of the importance for the four key elements in human existence is vital to a healthy life. As figure 3.3 depicts, your life needs a balance of physical, mental, spiritual, and emotional components. Do you balance sleep, work, recreation, and household responsibilities? Do you recognize your need for a spiritual life that is of your choosing and inclination? Do you have a morning ritual that gives you a short time to meditate, exercise, or read something inspirational before you leave your bedroom and begin the rest of the day's activities? Do you have a healthy diet, one that is balanced and does not rely on fast food? Have you developed activities that include recognition of when you are overworked and stressed, things that help reverse the stress, and those that promote and build your resilience?

The following are additional self-care issues. Which promote self-awareness, reversal, and resilience for you? Which allow you to set boundaries? You need to know what the realistic limits of your abilities—physical, mental, and emotional—are, and accept that overreaching these limits will set the stage for burnout. You may be able to do *it all,* but not do *all of it.*

Figure 3.3. Balance in Your Life

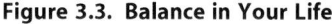

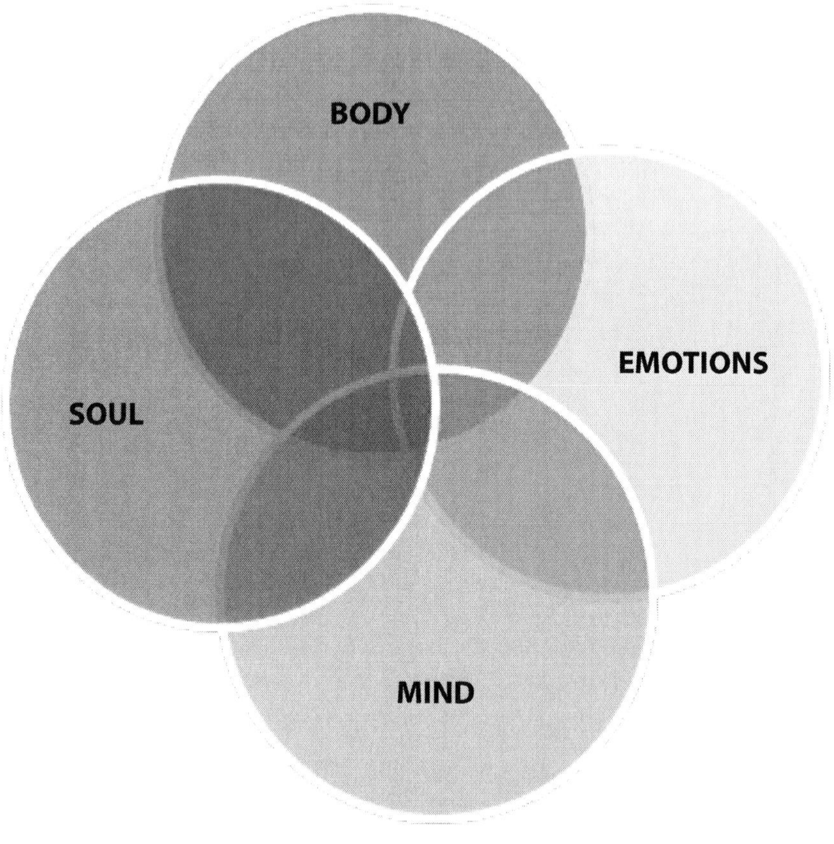

1. Delegate, learn to say *no*, recognize that others can be part of the solution. Many people in helping roles have a more difficult time asking for help than giving help. It is important for us to do both graciously.

2. Supportive supervision is essential. Supervision can often be viewed as a negative and critical assessment of one's work on the streets for several reasons. Some supervisors are far removed from their staff's work experiences or caseload and have not worked in a frontline capacity. Many have no training in mentoring supervision and see their role as administrative and task driven, rather than supportive of the process of helping. Others have not developed a strong work

relationship of trust and respect with their frontline people. If you do not have a supportive supervisor, find another person who you can speak to and who will mentor you.

3. Identify where and when you can take quick time-out breaks. Then identify what you can do on such a five-minute break: Stretching exercises. Deep breathing. A quick meditation that transports you to a favorite place. Singing a relaxing song in your head.

4. Become aware of your own limitations and boundaries around sensitive issues, such as seeing abuse of a child or dealing with a victim of sexual abuse and violence such as rape.

5. Learn what helps to relieve your stress. Sometimes it is a debriefing with a colleague or supervisor. Sometimes it is blowing off steam. Sometimes you will need to just leave work early and do something out of your ordinary routine. Watch that your stress-relieving routines do not lead into destructive habits such as alcohol, overspending, or reckless or dangerous activities.

6. Do you have a pet? If so, spend time with your pet. Animals, such as dogs and cats, have been shown to reduce stress, relax a person, evoke feelings of warmth and caring, and lower blood pressure. (Hooker, Freeman, & Stewart, 2002)

7. Tap into your creative side. How do you express your creativity? Do you have an interest or talent or hobby that needs more attention? Do you need to explore and try something new? Get a list of various hobbies, visual and performing arts, and the world of crafts. Talk to friends or surf the Internet to get some new ideas on exploring your creative side.

8. Keep a journal as part of your self-reflective life.

Managerial and Organizational Issues that Involve Burnout

The previous section focused on the ways in which a worker can become self-aware and adopt healthy activities that address issues leading to burnout. We also need to recognize the ways in which organizations either increase the chance of burnout or promote worker health. A number of organizational factors contribute to the development of burnout. These include excessive workload, time pressure, role conflict, role ambiguity, and absence of job resources (especially supervisory and coworker social support), limited job feedback, limited participation in decision making, lack of autonomy, unfairness or inequity, and insufficient rewards (Maslach, Schaufeli, & Leiter, 2001; Morse, Salyers, Rollins, Monroe-DeVita, & Pfahler, 2011; Paris & Hoge, 2010). At the organizational level, work overload, unrealistic and unnecessary timelines, detailed management of employee activities (i.e., micromanagement), and lack of flexibility with work schedules create environments in which workers feel stressed and disempowered. Organizational interventions that can reduce burnout include task restructuring and supportive supervision aimed at decreasing job demand, increasing job control, and increasing participation in decision making. One important aspect of a readily available organizational intervention is clinical supervision, which provides a way of addressing individual response to work, interwoven with educational aspects of job enhancement, and is not solely administrative oversight of job performance.

The list in table 3.6 that describes characteristics of a functional organization is not exhaustive, but presents many of the characteristics that a healthy and caring organization will have about expectations for employees and responses to support employees. In addition to contrasting expectations and behaviors, an employee-oriented organization would ensure that there is adequate time off, that holidays can be taken flexibly, and that a regular mental health day is considered an essential aspect of the work environment. Staff can also be extremely creative about the ways in which their individual and collective contributions are recognized and management should consult with staff whenever possible. In the end, the result is that these interventions build a solid team, reduce burnout, and increase reported quality of life by all members of the organization.

Table 3.6. Characteristics of a Functional Organization

	Promote Burnout	Prevent Burnout
Organizational Characteristics	Job descriptions are vague or general, or frequently change with regard to expected responsibilities.	Job descriptions are clear, specific, and relevant to the assigned position.
	Employee handbook is out of date, nonexistent, or not adhered to.	All employees have a copy of the handbook, which is updated yearly.

Table 3.6. (Continued)

	Promote Burnout	**Prevent Burnout**
	Work schedules are rigidly adhered to and nonnegotiable. Lateness is not tolerated under any circumstances. (For some shift work, punctuality may be essential.)	Work schedules depend on the assigned job and some may be negotiable. Timeliness, while valued, is balanced by weather, traffic, and personal circumstances.
Supervisor Characteristics	Information is transmitted formally and often slowly. Workers are told about changes only on a "need to know" basis.	The organization promotes transparency and communicates quickly with all staff about changes and news that affect the organization.
	Supervision is irregular and focused on administrative matters.	Supervision is regular, focused on job-related functions, and geared toward helping employee learning and growth.
	Staff training is focused on mandated topics and is management driven.	Staff training is regular and frequent, and offers a mix of management and employee-requested topics.
	Workers are assigned individual caseloads and are supervised individually.	Work assignments are made in teams to the greatest extent possible.
	Team meetings are infrequent and are department-wide rather than team or group specific.	Teams meet regularly, at least weekly, and connect informally on a daily basis.
	Crises and traumatic events are handled in a "business as usual" way, with the view that ordinary activity is the way to normalize the situation.	There are clear responses to crises, traumatic events, and extraordinary events, including serious illness and death of clients and staff. Team meetings to debrief are a part of this response and occur as soon as possible after news of the event is received.

Table 3.6. (Continued)

Promote Burnout	Prevent Burnout
The office is a functional environment.	The staff are encouraged to have a social aspect to team meetings, including bringing snacks. Teams occasionally get together for an out-of-office lunch or dinner.
Supervisors do not carry a client load.	Supervisors carry a small client load or are involved in program activities on a nominal basis and thus keep in touch with clients.
	Staff retreats are held on a regular basis and are not merely extended management meetings. Staff helps plan the content of the retreat.

EXERCISES

Health

1. In groups of three, prepare an action plan for the following scenario:

   A new flu virus has been reported in your community. It is supposed to be highly contagious and can be deadly, especially for people whose immune system is already compromised. There is no effective drug treatment or vaccine available. You need to work out a plan for handling a potential outbreak in the people in your emergency shelter. Plan for staff as well as residents.

   Types of shelters: (1) domestic violence, adult women only; (2) family shelter with elderly persons as well as infants; (3) adult-only shelter, large, with 300 persons; (4) youth shelter.

2. If you are trained in first aid and are with a homeless person who unexpectedly has a serious nosebleed, would you intervene to stop the bleeding if you did not have protective gloves available? If you are not trained in first aid what would you do?

3. Dental health is rarely available to poor and homeless people. Can you develop an advocacy project that could bring this need to the attention of dental care providers? Can you think of a way to mobilize dentists to provide free dental care?

Self-Care

List all of the activities that you do in a typical week day and the time each takes. Group them into categories: personal grooming, meal preparation, eating, sleeping, work, grocery shopping, commuting, exercise, recreation (TV, reading, sport), as examples. Calculate what percent of each day these activities occupy and put them in a pie chart (see figure 3.4). In this chart, what activities are missing that are part of your daily and weekly regular life?

Do the same calculation for a week-end day. Average the two calculations for how you spend a week.

Now examine your calculations and determine how you are spending your time. What is missing for you to have a balanced life?

Reflect on the above exercise personally and then in small groups. Can you think of ways to change your activities so that you have specific times for yourself—alone and with others—for self-care?

Figure 3.4. Time Spent in a Typical Week (in hours)

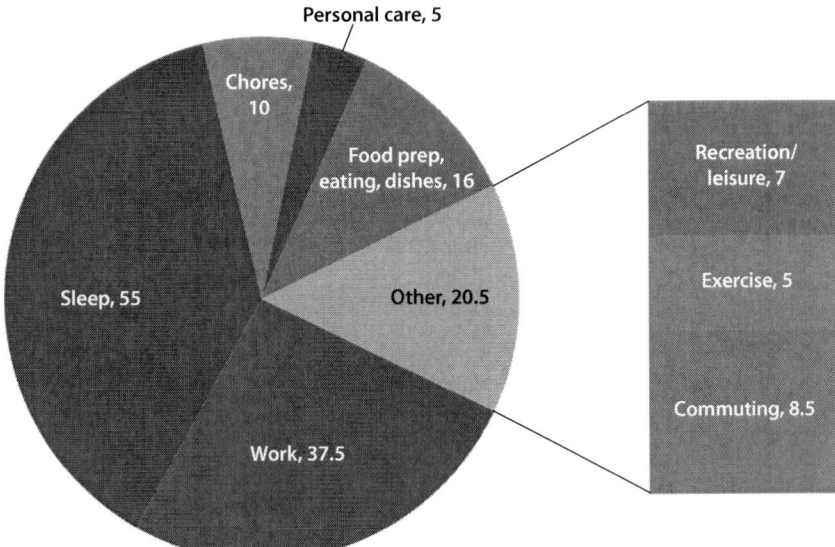

JOURNALING

Health

1. How vulnerable do you think you are personally to threats of illness contracted by associating with homeless persons?
2. Do you worry more about your physical safety or your psychological safety?
3. How vulnerable do you feel you are to the psychological stress of working with those who have serious physical problems that can be improved only with stable, permanent housing?

Self-Care

1. What are the activities that help you to unwind? Are these the best? Which would you prefer to do? What prevents you from doing them—if anything?
2. What would you like to try as a do-good, feel-good activity for yourself (not helping others—just for a change)?

CHAPTER 4

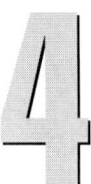

INTERPROFESSIONAL PRACTICE

KEY ISSUES
- Defining interprofessional and interdisciplinary practice
- Fundamental principle: client-centered service
- Professions and those educated in related disciplines that provide homeless and housing services
- Professional priorities, roles, and responsibilities
- How different disciplines can most effectively work together, blending client and agency concerns
- Professionalism, interagency collaboration, the etiquette of linkage conflict, and friction between different roles and professions
- Interprofessional practice: the roles of paradigm, treatment models, and theoretical foundations among diverse professionals

OVERVIEW

In chapters 2 and 3 we explored what homelessness is all about, how it is experienced, and ways of engaging people in the process of rehousing and stabilizing their lives. We now turn to a closer look at those who are the service providers. Before, during, and after securing housing a number of persons with different areas of expertise may be involved. The range of services may extend from a simple assist with a housing deposit or help securing adequately paid employment, to a complex array of services that help with health, mental health, addiction, life skills, legal problems, or a myriad of other problems. Just as we know that there is no single cause of homelessness, there is also no single solution. Once homeless, problems increase. Many people report that homelessness itself causes its own set of problems from feeling depressed, victimized, and helpless, to being exploited by those who falsely proclaim their helpfulness. In all of this complexity one thing is certain: more than a single social worker, income support worker, or frontline counselor will be needed to rehouse and keep people housed. Help will come from different professions and disciplines: social workers, addiction counselors, nurses, rehabilitation specialists, probation and parole offices, income support workers, education specialists, mental health therapists, physicians, child welfare workers, and subsidized housing providers. This list is not exhaustive but does illustrate the multiple people representing differing training, perspectives, and priorities with whom clients and workers in the homeless sector interact. Table 4.1 lists the professions and disciplines most frequently involved in providing these services.

WHAT IS INTERPROFESSIONAL PRACTICE?

When individuals from two or more different professions or disciplines work together for the benefit of a specific person, they are engaged in interprofessional practice. Not all persons working with an individual are members of a profession. Some may come from a specific disciplinary orientation related to a profession (see table 4.1). They may also come from a variety of professions, disciplines, and backgrounds not restricted to any one discipline. The result is that various perspectives, values, and priorities are brought to the helping process. Without a clear understanding of roles and responsibilities, this may lead to role conflict, confusion, and gaps in service as different workers map out areas of responsibility and assume that the vaguely defined responsibilities are covered by someone else or by another agency (see table 4.2).

Interprofessional practice occurs when two or more professionals from different disciplines jointly work to help a single individual or family unit. Its origins stem from health care where role confusion and conflict arose because of the rapid evolution of different health-care specialization and providers: from doctors and nurses to pharmacists, dieticians, physiotherapists, inhalation therapists, psychiatrists, social workers, and psychologists. This increase also came to include numerous medical specialty areas, among them cardiology, internal medicine, orthopedics, neurology, gerontology,

Table 4.1. Professions and Disciplines Providing Services

Discipline or field of practice	Profession(s) (licensed or certified)	Paraprofessional (specialized training)
Medicine	Medicine (MD) Emergency medical technician Nursing Physical therapy	Nurse's aide Home support worker
Mental health	Medicine Social work Nursing Psychology	Mental health aide Social service assistant
Legal	Law	Legal aide
Substance abuse	Social work Psychology Nursing Licensed substance abuse counselor	Substance-abuse support worker
Child care	Teacher, early education specialist	Child-care worker or aide
Child welfare	Social work Psychology	Social service worker
Criminal justice	A field of practice but not a professional designation recognized by licensing authorities	Probation officer Parole officer
Education	Teacher	Teacher's aide
Vocational training	Teacher	Vocational instructor (trades)
Peer support	Many backgrounds	Someone with lived experience

and sports medicine. Each of these specialty areas developed its own view of priorities in patient care and a specialized vocabulary and culture. Without learning ways of working together, these medical teams had difficulty coordinating care. The introduction of education to help these professionals work as teams has had a substantially positive impact on care and outcome.

> **Textbox 4.1. Interprofessional Practice in Diverse Settings**
>
> The concept of interprofessional practice originally arose in the medical field. Over the past fifty years a considerable number of medical specialties have come to play an important part in care: physiotherapists, rehabilitation specialists, pharmacists, radiologists, nursing specialists, social workers, psychologists, and chaplains, among others. This has brought about the importance of recognizing that care is not restricted to, or always dictated by, the physician in charge. Care is provided by a number of different professionals.
>
> In nonmedical settings the services may be provided by persons from different disciplines, including recognized professions and those from other backgrounds. We have chosen to use the term "interprofessional" to indicate that while there are numerous professionals involved, many workers are paraprofessional—that is, on a ladder within a professional discipline.

Similarly, social workers and others outside of health settings have begun to recognize the importance of collaborative teams where each specialty is respected and priorities are set by the group, together with the client (Littlechild, Smith, & Work, 2012). Health-care professionals recognize several themes that weave across all competencies for practice (Interprofessional Education Collaborative Expert Panel, 2011; Tashiro, Byrne, Kitchen, Vogel, & Bianco, 2011). These themes are also applicable outside of health-care settings. The themes include the ethics, values, roles, and responsibilities of each professional and represent the foundations that support the fundamental actions of team members (figure 4.1).

People who are effective in interprofessional practice have a clear idea of what their professional values and ethics are, what they share with others on the team, and how their ethical priorities may differ as a result of their

Table 4.2. Different Frontline and Direct Service Roles in Homeless Services

Outreach worker	Mental health workers
Addictions counselor	Vocational/occupational therapist
Rehabilitation counselor	Family counselor
Child welfare worker	Housing support workers
Child-care worker	Client support worker
Financial support	School counselor
Case manager in different organizations	Probation/parole officer

Figure 4.1. Professions and Disciplines Providing Services

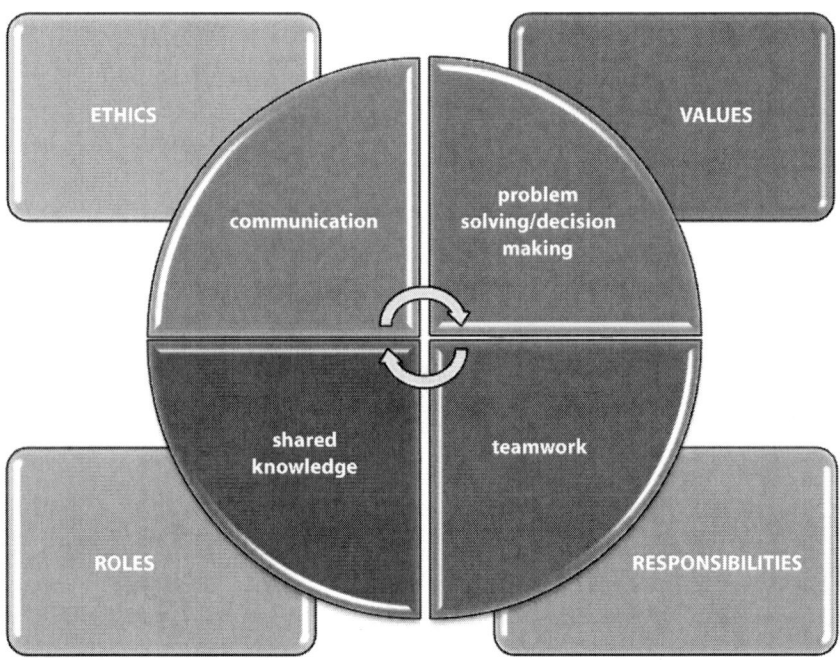

professional responsibilities. That is, a nurse and a social worker may both agree on care or intervention plans for the client, but the nurse may insist on personal safety as a primary priority while the social worker places advocacy and client empowerment as most important in client care. These values will permeate their problem solving, what and how they communicate, and what knowledge they share with others versus what is more uniquely part of their professional practice (Damron-Rodriguez, 2008). In a similar fashion, it is imperative to have a clear sense of one's own professional role and competency and the role and competency of others. Role confusion often results in turf wars about who is more knowledgeable and who is responsible. These conflicts are inevitably at the expense of good client service.

Interprofessional practice becomes an important consideration as each person involved in a care plan may bring a different perspective and different priorities to the plan. Without an understanding of the professional roles and responsibilities of team members, two possible scenarios are likely to occur: a gap in service because everyone presumed it was the responsibility of someone else, or overlaps as different people assume a specific task as their domain and turf wars result. In either event, the client loses. Understanding and being able to talk about interprofessional practice usually mitigates or helps to avoid such issues of role boundaries and responsibilities.

Interprofessional practice is a relatively recent concept in service provision. It has usually been thought of as a component of health care, where multiple professionals from different backgrounds such as medicine, nursing, social work, pharmacy, occupational and physical therapy, speech and language therapy, dietary services, and radiology, among others, work together to improve the health of specific patients. The importance of interprofessional practice became recognized as many specialties became involved with a patient's care and this care was not the exclusive domain of the doctor in charge. This forced the group of people involved with care of the patient to recognize the individual areas of expertise and competence that each brought to the table, and forced a recognition that a set of skills was necessary in order for the patient care team to function effectively (Littlechild et al., 2012). Similar concepts can be carried over into helping homeless persons where services are provided by different people with different skill sets, capabilities, and professional training. These services require a number of individual and group skills in working with diverse care providers. Some of these service providers also have the authority to provide essential assistance such as child-care supervision, food subsidies, and rent allowances. Others, such as probation officers and child-care workers, have the authority to regulate behavior. Some carry dual roles of support provision and behavioral supervision, which can entail ethical dilemmas that will be addressed in chapter 11. Recognition of both important people-oriented skills and power relations over clients that are job related is important if persons from diverse backgrounds are to work together effectively in order to help a homeless person or family.

Client-Centered Services

The foundation of all interprofessional practice is the recognition and acknowledgment that the client is the focus of the services team. This means that all actions should be with and on behalf of the client and that the client needs to be included in all discussions and decisions. Individual agendas and issues need to be kept separate from this main responsibility of the team. As we will further discuss in chapter 5, service providers have come to recognize that to be acceptable and effective any service plan must be developed together with the persons and families for whom each plan is intended and it must begin with addressing their expressed immediate needs. In order to complete a comprehensive service plan, the team, or various members of the team as needed, should meet with the client. This assessment is often time consuming, as organizing such meetings in real time can be difficult to arrange quickly. Nevertheless, experience shows that when everyone is agreeable to an action plan, it has a much greater chance of success.

In figure 4.2 the client has been placed in the middle of the circle, embraced by a host of potential helpers, each with a different specialty, expertise, and way of assistance. While there may be overlap in some areas, the point is that the client often needs someone to help navigate through multiple relationships, multiple agencies, rules, and regulations. Before this services navigation and coordination can happen, the worker needs to understand and develop the ability to interact and negotiate with people who have different values and priorities, a vocabulary specific to their own areas of specialization, and a worldview about homelessness that may differ from the worker's own.

Key Components of Interprofessional Practice

Collaboration is at the core of interprofessional practice. It is based on concepts of sharing, power, interdependency, partnership and process (D'Amour, Ferrada-Videla, San Martin Rodriguez, & Beaulieu, 2005). The competencies for interprofessional practice are usually classified into four interprofessional domains (Interprofessional Education Collaborative Expert Panel, 2011) (see table 4.3). These competencies are also referred to as practice principles. In the homeless services sector these practice principles include the following:

- Team membership: Recognition that the various persons providing services to a specific individual make up a services team. These team members may come from different service organizations.
- Access: Ensuring that all team members have access to each other.
- Member competencies: Understanding of team members' areas of competence and expertise.

Figure 4.2. Homeless Services Team

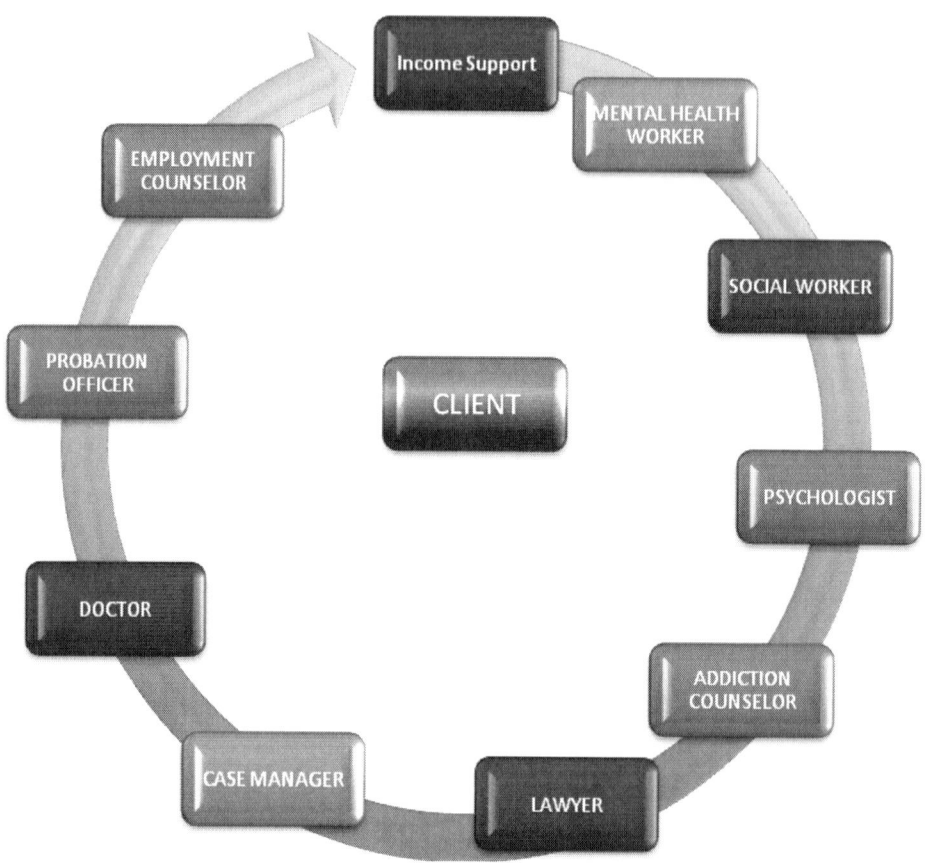

Table 4.3. Domains of Interprofessional Practice

Competency Domain 1	Values/ethics for interprofessional practice
Competency Domain 2	Roles/responsibilities
Competency Domain 3	Interprofessional communication
Competency Domain 4	Teams and teamwork

- Leadership: Identifying the team leader or the individual who acts as case manager to ensure all identified needs are addressed.
- Roles and responsibilities: Knowledge of individual team members' roles and responsibilities; the ability to clarify overlapping areas of responsibility/role; recognition of the different roles and priorities of representative organizations.
- Boundaries: Respect for professional boundaries.
- Competencies: Respect for mutual competencies and for differing competencies.
- Roles: Recognition that some basic skills and knowledge transcend specific roles and professions.
- Communication: Clear and effective communication; knowledge of common professional jargon of each member.
- Conflict resolution: Ability to identify conflict regardless of origin and negotiate resolution.

In this list, the first five items focus on team composition and various aspects of effective team work. The second set of five refer to individual skills that are necessary for working within the team. The following sections explore what is meant by each principle. Before we begin that exploration we will briefly look at the fundamental component of interprofessional practice: the nature and composition of a services team.

The Nature and Composition of a Services Team

The concept of the services team is fundamental to modern health care where a variety of specialized services are provided by multiple personnel. While it is easy to envision a hospital-based team where all members work under the same roof, outpatient teams have also become a reality because much health care is now delivered on an outpatient basis. Teams in the community are also client based. At intake or assessment, whichever is the primary fact-finding activity for a person seeking some service, the worker needs to take a complete inventory of problem areas in order to determine what additional agencies and services are involved or need to be involved in helping this particular individual. This inventory should include strengths and assets as these will be the foundation on which a plan and timeline are developed. Using the concept of client-based practice, with the client at the center of practice, figure 4.2 quickly identifies the members of this extended services team, which often extends to include several agencies. The idea that a services team consists of people who are employed by different agencies is not a traditional view of service delivery, yet it is the only configuration that fits the multiple and diverse needs of persons with complex psychosocial, health, and financial needs. Using a model of client-centered care, we need to envision who is the most appropriate and qualified person to provide each care component. Along with that comes the decision as to who takes nominal charge of coordinating team efforts.

In the community, assembling the entire team is often not practical, especially if services are time sensitive. It is also not necessarily clear who should head this team. Team leadership may be as simple as making sure everyone is informed of a team meeting, making sure that all team members have input into the action plan and that the client is involved and consents to this coordination. It may often fall on the shoulders of the identified case manager to make certain that everyone involved with this individual knows the extent and membership of the team. This individual may also need to be alert for the team-related issues that could impede the effective delivery of the service plan, especially if most members have limited time to communicate with each other.

Most workers are accustomed to thinking of teams as consisting of people in their organization who are assigned to work together. The idea of a team that includes people from different agencies makes sense when one looks at the provision of services as client centered (figure 4.2). Together, all of the people who provide services to a person with the aim of stable and permanent housing constitute a team. This team most often consists of individuals in different organizations, and members may have different mandates and priorities. Nonetheless, their actions influence each other and can either lead to success or sabotage the helping process. For example, a woman with a history of substance abuse who is being released on early parole and who is trying to regain custody of her children needs to have her parole officer, child welfare worker, and substance-abuse treatment program agree on an acceptable action plan that will result in the return of the children's custody to the mother.

The array of services that may be involved includes components of what are often separate units or departments within municipal, provincial/state, and federal governments, as well as nonprofit agencies in the social service sector (see figure 4.3). We explore the complexities of the services system in more detail in chapter 5. In a typical array of available services, some professionals, such as social workers, will be employed in many different agencies, and some, such as addiction counselors, will be employed in specialized agencies. For example, while law enforcement officers and lawyers will be found in the legal system, and nurses will be found in medical, mental health, and substance-abuse services, as well as in schools, social workers will be found in financial (income support workers), medical, mental health, substance abuse, and educational services, as well as in core services of intake, case management, housing placement, and continuing support services. Frontline workers, with or without formal training and with no specific professional identity, will also be found in outreach, frontline support,

Figure 4.3. The Interprofessional Team in a Housing First Network

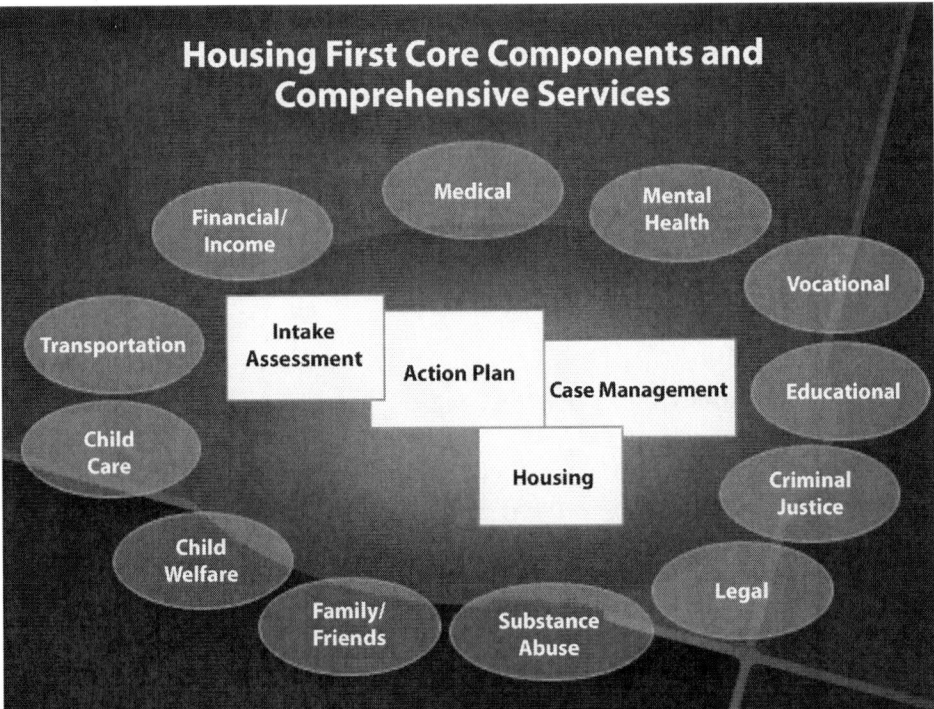

child care, substance abuse, and transportation services. Without well-connected services and communication among all service providers, a carefully constructed plan may fall apart—for lack of as basic a component as child care, transportation, or a financial management plan.

When a team member disagrees, that person can set up obstacles to service provision. When the client disagrees, there can be refusal to cooperate or engage in exploring action plans. It has long been a hallmark of social work that effective engagement must start with where the client is at. In the interprofessional team, some members may find it disconcerting to have the client present during detailed and direct discussions of problems. However, it is most often the team member and not the client whose distress is the issue. When tactfully stated, clients are generally able to deal with the issues and are usually relieved that everyone with whom they interact knows the same information, which avoids the constant repetition of issues to different team members.

The case example of Steve and Ann (text box 4.2) exemplifies some important service and support issues that should be considered in identifying the team members who work with a family.

In order for a group of diverse persons to work together as a team for a specific goal—that of housing and improving overall life of a housing-insecure person—the members must embrace a set of values, attitudes, and skills that will help all of them to work in unison. While this may sound ideal, and in many ways it is, the basic principles must exist if effective services are to be the outcome.

Working in Teams   The canoe is one of the best examples of team work that easily illustrates all essential components. In order to move effectively and efficiently across the water, all people in the boat must paddle at the same speed at the same tempo, and allow for the strengths and abilities of each team member. The crew must communicate through words and actions the timing of the strokes, the strength and power put into each stroke, and the occasional need for a crew member to take a break. The helmsperson, in the rear, needs to keep the pace and be prepared for changes in currents and for rock hazards. When one person paddles in the opposite direction, or at a different pace, it sends the boat off at different angles—and may land it on top of rocks or out in a turbulent current where it can be tossed about (see figure 4.4). The same principles apply in the services teams.

Textbox 4.2. Case Example

Steve and Ann have been a couple for the past thirteen years. Although not legally married, they have three children, ages twelve, ten, and seven, in common; the children carry Steve's last name. Both Steve and Ann have developmental delays that resulted in both of them obtaining a high school attendance certificate, but with functional skills at the fifth-grade level. They have lived independently except for two encounters with child welfare because of concern over their parenting skills, when the first two children were young. They have coped well until recently. Steve worked full time as a convenience store clerk and Ann worked part time at a fast-food restaurant. As a result of the economic downturn Steve's hours were cut in half, and he could not find other work. The result was that they could not pay their rent, and were afraid to ask for other help in fear of child welfare involvement and removal of the children. Neither abused alcohol or drugs. Since they both grew up in foster homes, they do not have extended family to turn to for support. Within three months they had exhausted all of their resources and were evicted. They now live in temporary shelters, Steve in a shelter for singles and Ann with the children in a shelter for women who are victims of domestic violence, although domestic violence has not been an issue.

What service personnel may be involved with this family? What services will they need? Is there anyone who should be designated as head of the team for purposes of case management and care coordination?

Figure 4.4. Working to Opposite Goals: Inefficient Teams

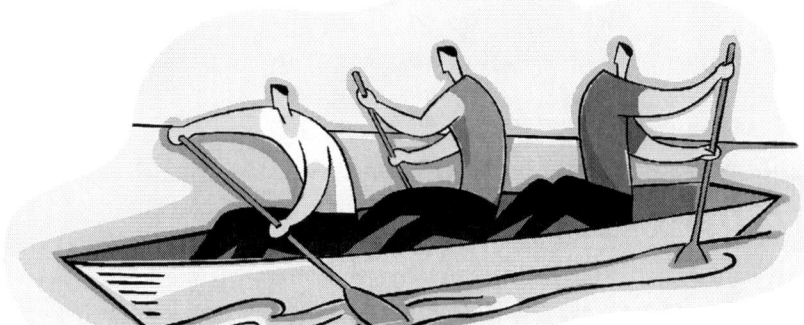

The first challenge is the identification of who constitutes the members of a team. The group or team may most often be loosely constructed of individuals representing various organizations and services, each of which is providing a specific component of an overall plan for housing and stability. Often people identify themselves as members of an organization and not as members of a group that is client-centered. Thus this concept of a team that transcends organizational boundaries is not the first and most natural way of conceptualizing service provision. A related challenge is that this virtual team is not located in one place, since providers are physically connected to different organizations with geographical distances between them. That distance entails difficulties in getting teams together for planning sessions. Another related practicality is that of delegating the role of team leader or coordinator to one of the members. This leadership might vary depending on the client priorities, it might fall to the persons with the greatest role in the client's plan, it might rotate over time as client needs change, and it might not be attached to a specific service provision. The leader, however, must accept the concept of team service, be able to allow all members to have constructive input, be willing to work with alternative means of communication when team members can't meet in person, and have a positive relationship with the client.

Team Collaboration and Interprofessional Practice While it is easy to recognize that multiple services and service providers interact in order to assemble the supports necessary for a homeless individual or family to be housed and remain housed, the idea of this support system constituting a team is new. Most of the time, we define teams in a specific workplace, organized around a set of agency-mandated activities. A good example is in a shelter for victims of domestic violence where intake counselors, child-care workers, substance-abuse counselors, and housing specialists work together to map out a plan for family support and rehousing. This internal team requires additional people to execute a service plan, among them a financial aid counselor, income support worker, housing services representative, legal aid attorney, and education support worker. Without their involvement and access to needed supports, the family will have little hope of getting and maintaining housing and independence. Similarly, each client that comes to mind will require similar needs. As this group of persons comes together, perhaps mainly in written documents and in conversations, it must be clear to all participants that the success of this family is dependent on the system of supports that are put in place.

As we discussed previously, working in teams is akin to paddling a canoe. The course of the boat is dependent on everyone paddling in the same direction and at the same time. A crew of efficient canoeists can be exemplary in navigation and speed (see figure 4.5). The same happens in teams that don't work in harmony. It is thus critical that the team respect the

- autonomy of each person who is on the team and recognize that each person can make all the difference;
- coordinate all team efforts to keep on course; and
- demonstrate mutual trust and respect of the abilities and capabilities of each members and a reliance on each individual to do his or her part properly.

Elements of Effective Teamwork

The concept of a team is the first component that must be understood and accepted by all service providers. If the definition of a team is a group of people working together for a specific purpose, then all work on behalf of homeless persons is teamwork. If work with homeless persons is to be first and foremost client centered, then this team consists of the individual staff

Figure 4.5. Efficient Team Work

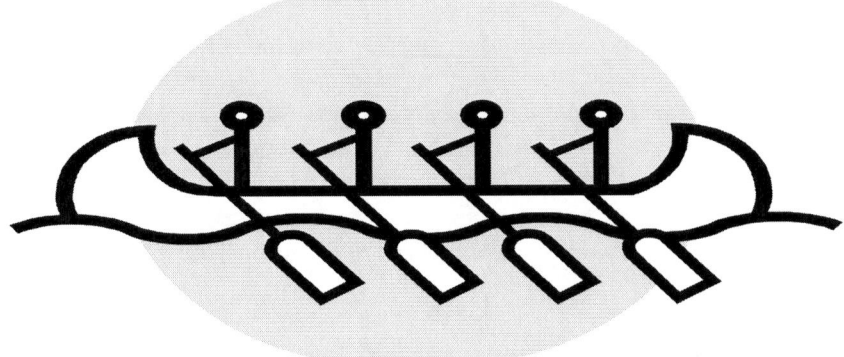

from the agencies that are providing a service for that client and is aimed at helping with some aspect of housing, support, and stability. Below are the key elements for effective teamwork (Tashiro et al., 2011). We have not listed them in any order of priority but challenge you to consider which are most important.

- Mutual trust and respect
- Assertiveness
- Autonomy
- Coordination and cooperation
- Communication
- Responsibility/accountability

Mutual Trust and Respect There are a number of components that make up effective interprofessional care, but all depend on mutual trust and respect, which are foundational to effective work. Trust is the glue that holds the fabric of human relations together. It permeates all social interactions and makes it possible for people to work effectively together. For example, an analysis of a survey that inquired about the values, attitudes, beliefs, and work practices of staff in mental health organizations revealed that trust was the dominant theme. Trust was reflected in behaviors such as being able to rely on someone for support, knowing that personal and client confidentiality would be upheld, counting on others to do their part of a project, believing what another person tells them, and so on. The helping professions all refer to the importance of establishing a positive relationship, built on trust and mutual respect. Far less is said about the equally important positive trusting relationships we need to have with other service providers, both in the same organization and with those colleagues in other agencies. In the business community the importance of trust in teams has become recognized as instrumental to team functioning and productivity. This has resulted in many training programs that use trust exercises to make staff aware of these issues. In teams where trust or lack thereof becomes a barrier to moving forward, the team will be faced with the challenge of confronting this impediment. We will return to this topic when exploring the domain of conflict resolution.

While trust guides all actions, the overarching focus should be on a client-centered approach. In order to accomplish this agreement of group

> **Textbox 4.3. Team Building**
>
> A popular way to help teams become effective is through the use of ropes or challenge exercises. These activities rely on using experiences that are outside of the realm of most people's experiences They challenge groups to learn to work together in order to solve problems and achieve stated goals. Some of these activities are easily done without technical equipment and serve as dynamic team-building experiences.
>
> (Rohnke & Buttler, 1995)

focus, those involved in providing services should see themselves as a part of a loosely constituted team that depends on everyone working together. This work requires understanding each person's role, what competencies and organizational authorities each person brings to the table, how well each person is able to work with everyone else, each person's willingness to acknowledge an informal leader for effectiveness, and his acceptance of the need to deal with conflict if that should arise. We briefly examine each competency in the context of working with disenfranchised persons with housing instability.

Assertiveness Assertiveness may at first glance seem to be an unusual characteristic to describe teamwork as it focuses on individual behavior. However, it is an aspect of effective communication that is essential to team functioning. By assertiveness, we mean those actions and words that enable us to calmly and persistently request another's attention and response. To be assertive is, then, to accept "no" as an answer only when all alternatives have been explored. It includes restating a response to make sure that you have understood correctly, and in this restatement to be clear if you perceive a violation of a person's rights or eligibilities for service. In this context assertiveness is characterized by the ability to clearly and succinctly state one's thoughts and opinions, regardless of their seeming popularity or approval from other members. It includes the ability to resist untoward and unacceptable pressure in order to assert a professional opinion. Assertiveness often means being politely persistent and refusing to be sidelined. This is especially true when issues involving ethical principles arise. Assertiveness is often the challenge for professionals whose training leads to consensus building and whose personal preferences are for avoidance of conflict. However, without the opportunity for all team members to respectfully state their views, regardless of popularity or acceptance, resentment can build if individuals feel bullied or coerced by strong-willed cohorts.

Autonomy While being a team member requires the ability and willingness to work together, all members must also be able to act autonomously, both in their area of expertise and when urgent issues require immediate action. This autonomy is a delicate balance between respecting others and having the competence and confidence to go it alone when needed.

Coordination and Cooperation Coordination and cooperation are adjuncts to autonomy as each team member needs to be aware of the priorities and concerns of other team members. The most fundamental aspect of this is the recognition that competition for power, preference, control, the team agenda, or having priority will be destructive to the spirit of cooperation that must exist if the team is to work for the mutual aim of helping a homeless individual, couple, or family.

Communication Effective communication is fundamental to working with people. We need to be able to convey in clear, unambiguous ways information that is necessary to allow all persons in the helping circle to understand the information that is presented. Communication is multifaceted, with information that comes from both what is said—the language used, how it is said, the context in which it is said—and the body language that accompanies the verbal message. Accurate communication is further complicated by language that permits multiple meanings of a single word.

> **Textbox 4.4. Nuances of How We Write and Speak**
> The title of the book *Eats, Shoots & Leaves* (Truss, 2005) is an excellent example of multiple meaning in a few words. It makes us think of three words that have different meanings depending on the context in which they are used and how punctuation also changes the written meaning. As an example, think of what happens to the meaning of three simple words when you rearrange the punctuation: "eats shoots, and leaves" or "eats, shoots, and leaves," or "eats shoots and leaves."

In interprofessional practice communication has a unique component. Working with other professions and disciplines presents challenges that arise from people having learned professional jargon as shorthand to relay information. We all use shorthand phrases in our jobs that are a way to convey to others that we come from the same professional collective. It helps us to identify with coworkers and to scope out an invisible territory of expertise around what we do. At the same time, this professional language helps us convey clear and specific information in a quick and efficient way to coworkers. Doctors and nurses provide classic examples of professional communication with such phrases as "subdural hematoma secondary to cardiac infarct," which translates to "a collection of blood on the brain following a heart attack." Doctors usually translate this information into patient-friendly language. But quite often, especially if other medical specialists are present, the temptation to speak in professional shorthand leads to confusion for the nonmedical person. By the same token, members of other professions often use terms that are unfamiliar to outsiders, or may mean different things in various settings. While this professional jargon can be of help when speaking with others in the same field, it can exclude those from other areas and can also be interpreted as a way a person may show superiority and be viewed as the only "expert." One of the first and most important things that any member of the team can do is to ask for clarification whenever a word or term is used that he does not clearly understand. This is a help to everyone because there is no guarantee that each team member will understand what is being said. It also sends a gentle reminder to everyone to keep the language simple and avoid jargon. This is especially supportive of a client who is present, may fail to follow all of the discussion, and is afraid to speak up.

Nonverbal communication is another powerful conveyor of messages. For instance, clothing is a strong communicator of status, authority, and membership in some groups. When there are representatives of several different professions present at a meeting, it is difficult to impossible to ignore the doctor's white coat, the policeman's uniform, the lawyer's dark blue suit, or the pastor's clerical collar. They convey authority, order, and competence, and can easily be mistaken as the symbols of the person in charge or the one with the "correct" and "acceptable" answers. However, in working with homeless persons the appropriate answers, if there are any, and the most acceptable responses may come from any person who is providing services to the homeless client. That person may not be the one with the visible signs of authority.

Appropriate work attire for those working with marginalized people is not likely to consist of formal dress unless there is an occasion to appear in court or similar setting. This raises the challenge of the unwarranted perception that a worker may not be as knowledgeable as someone who is in uniform or formally dressed. An important reminder to workers is that competence resides within oneself as a characteristic that develops over time and with experience. Thus nonverbal messages that convey confidence and competence (rather than arrogance) are important in assuring team members that important contributions in decisions and priorities are included.

Communication is also conveyed in where and when meetings are held, with formal settings such as a professional office being the least comfortable for the frontline worker and client. The atmosphere of authority conveyed can be intimidating; for clients who attend these more formal meetings, anxiety rises as they are expected to interact in formal ways not familiar to them. They then begin to depend on their most trusted representative to assure they can navigate this intimidation. The result is both fear and increased dependency, both feelings that workers try to reduce in those they work with.

Responsibility/Accountability Team members must also balance their responsibilities to their professional values and ethics, priorities to client service, and demands of their employers. At the same time they must also be accountable to the team for actions promised and tasks undertaken so that all members can rely on each other in the delivery of services.

Being a team members is no easy task. Some people who have played a lot of team sports can easily relate to important areas of cooperation, trust, and willingness to share the load and the glory. Others, who have entered into highly competitive professions such as business, law, and medicine, have learned the value of individual achievement and have had fewer opportunities to learn team skills. These prior experiences shape each team member; it is incumbent on the entire group to help develop these skills. For that, a bit of humor and an occasional air of lightness may help to shift the focus from winning to sharing.

Conflict Tolerance and Resolution

Different people carrying individual agendas, and all intent on the process of helping others, may readily encounter situations where views on assessment and recommendations for services and interventions differ.

Roles and Responsibilities Every profession defines certain responsibilities that are expected, those that are allowed, and those that are outside the bounds of professional practice. In many cases these responsibilities are legally defined, such as in the case of doctors, social workers, nurses, psychologists, and police. The code of ethics that each profession articulates for its members provides an excellent opportunity to understand professional priorities. These priorities provide an understanding of what importance individuals place on certain actions and decisions. Few people have the opportunity to learn about various professional roles and responsibilities before entering the workforce. Much of what we know, and a lot of what we assume, comes from word of mouth or from experience. When working together with others from differing backgrounds, we need to become aware of what people are trained to do, what they are by law permitted to do, and what additional skills they have that they share with other professionals. Since licensure and certification are state and provincial matters, each jurisdiction has similar but not identical rules and regulations about qualifications and permitted tasks. We are unable to list those for all legal jurisdictions, but strongly encourage you to look for this information in the area where you work. Most often this can be found online or through the professional association that you are inquiring about.

While licensing regulations in most jurisdictions require that people from different professional backgrounds have a specific educational preparation and be licensed to perform certain tasks such as psychosocial interventions, there are few regulations as to how these interventions are applied. In psychosocial counseling, practitioners can take various approaches and use techniques that come from different theoretical and practice orientations. For example, social workers, psychologists, nurses, and marriage and family therapists are all trained in family therapy, but have differing lenses for viewing families that are focused and perhaps biased by their professional culture. This leads to different applications of family therapy techniques.

In addition, the set of techniques used by various counselors and therapists, such as those found in family therapy and group therapy, are not always regulated by state and provincial licensing authorities if the person is working under a generic designation of "counselor." In other words, not all counselors are licensed to practice and some professionals are not properly trained in the interventions that they use. Workers and their clients need to be aware of what constitutes qualified and trained practice in psychosocial interventions. Some of the areas that employ counselors are listed in table

4.1. While this list is by no means exhaustive, it is illustrative of the various titles and worker descriptions that are found in social services agencies. The picture is complicated by the fact that some positions are held by people trained and accredited in various licensed professions who work alongside those who are not trained or licensed. While professional training always includes a practice or practicum component, many with nonprofessional backgrounds have not had this type of educational and mentorship experience. The scope and roles of some professionals are further defined by areas of specialization, such as the social worker who is employed by mental health services or works as the leader of an assertive community treatment (ACT) team, the nurse who works in a school or on an outreach team, or the mental health worker whose background may be in psychology, nursing, social work, or rehabilitation.

One of the basic mistakes made by new team members, whether they are new in the field or new to a specific job, is to assume that they know what everyone does, is allowed to do, and is supposed to do; we call this "role assumption." In addition, some professional roles overlap with those of others, such as nurses and social workers who both assume supportive roles with family members. This kind of overlap is often a source of confusion and misunderstanding in deciding the individual team member's responsibilities. Different organizations may also have internal rules about what a staff member with a specific job classification is allowed to do, irrespective of what that person's professional designation would permit him to do. One example would be of a social worker who is trained in administering a variety of questionnaires to assess client problems and needs, but whose agency will not permit this practice for social workers.

This lack of role understanding can also play out in other ways. A team can be actively involved in deciding that a particular service should be provided by a designated agency only to find out that workers there are not allowed to provide a specific service because the staff are not qualified or authorized in that capacity. Another confusion arises in agencies where counselors, who often have a bachelor's or a master's degree in a nonprofessionally designated discipline, are employed in a variety of counseling capacities, including those found in table 4.4.

In order to work effectively, all frontline staff need to recognize that they may form parts of a team working toward mutual goals of housing and living stability, despite that fact that many may represent a variety of agencies

Table 4.4. Professionals and Degree Requirements

Job Title	Degree and Qualifications Required
Attorney	LLB or JD
Dietician	BS and additional certification
Legal assistant	BA and specialized training; some jurisdictions require registration or licensing
Licensed practical nurse	Generally an associate's degree or (community) college degree
Marriage and family therapist	Usually a master's degree in marriage and family therapy or an MSW; registered in only some jurisdictions in the United States, and not registered in Canada
Nurse practitioner	BSN plus advanced training, or an MSN
Pharmacist	BS in pharmacology
Physician	MD
Physician specialist: psychiatrist	MD and additional certification
Psychologist (registered)	PhD in most jurisdictions, otherwise MS
Registered nurse	BS
Social worker (registered)	MSW or BSW (in some jurisdictions) Note: The province of Alberta allows those with a diploma to be registered.
Vocational and occupational therapists	BS

Note: BA = Bachelor of arts; BS = Bachelor of science; BSN = Bachelor of science/nursing; BSW = Bachelor of social work; LLB = Bachelor of law; MD = Doctor of medicine; MS = Master of science; MSN = Master of science/nursing; MSW = Master of social work; PhD = Doctor of philosophy.

and services. This section on interprofessional practice aims to help workers to recognize some common goals and concepts that will help their working interactions. It is not our intent for to you to become proficient in interprofessional practice by reading what follows; that will require real-time experience. Interprofessional practice begins with understanding the many ways in which different workers, representing various services and priorities, can develop mutually inclusive plans to help clients with acceptance of the various helping people involved. What we present here are some concepts central to delivering client-based services that involve multiple persons, and address the fundamental principles that this involves. The result for the reader will be a new appreciation for the complexities that a single homeless person must deal with and the ways in which a service provider becomes part of a team involved in helping the individual to solve life problems. Some fundamental principles of interprofessional practice are found in table 4.5.

In the field of health care, teams often work in the same building, although community health practitioners often find it a challenge to be connected with their hospital-based counterparts. This same challenge exists for those in the social services sector when key people on the services team may be located in different areas and different organizations. It isn't always easy to get a team together and to agree on a common action plan. Some recognized challenges include the fact that different team members have different mandates, and that some team members who have tight schedules and high workloads may have difficulty making meetings (e.g., physicians, attorneys). The team may consist of people working in different agencies with different and sometimes conflicting mandates and priorities such as medicine and law. Team members may have difficulty with accessing team members because of location, work schedules, etc. Not everyone works in the same locations or interacts frequently; also, there are infrequent times to interact and most often those times occur in the context of a specific client and an urgent situation. In addition, most people are not used to thinking of

Table 4.5. Key Components of Interprofessional Practice

Team Composition and Access to the Team	Clarity on Team Composition
Role understanding	Development of a mutually understood common language
Respect of mutual competencies and professional boundaries	Recognition of varying professional ethics and development of interprofessional ethics
Clarity on confidentiality—within the team, and outside the team	Effective communication—oral, nonverbal, and written
A culture of trust and respect, personal and professional	Conflict management and resolution

their role in client services as being a member of a team because they usually see only themselves interacting with the client, and no mutually shared record of contact is kept. Introducing team-oriented language and orientation is important. This includes the view that every member needs to make a commitment to include awareness and consideration of all members' concerns and responsibilities. This commitment will include compromises and concessions where possible for the ultimate goals of the service plan. This collaborative partnership includes recognition that differences may involve dealing with conflict. In settings where the same individuals are likely to work with mutual clients frequently, it may be very useful to have a team meeting to discuss team functioning issues.

Dealing with Conflict

Inevitably, when two or more people work together toward a mutual goal there are times when differences arise. These differences may result from a number of factors, including perceptions about the priorities of the team, the long-term goals, ways of achieving the goals, lack of commitment to the team, professional views and commitments, or basic personality differences.

When team members disagree there are some basic understandings and approaches that can clarify and resolve issues. (A person not directly involved with the main conflict should step in to moderate the dialogue.)

1. Begin by clarifying the issue(s).
2. Recognize that all views are valid.
3. Recognize that views are often guided by professional practices and priorities.
4. Recognize that views are also guided by personal values.
5. Accept that what is in the interest of the client prevails.
6. Accept that it is not always necessary to be right or to win.

Additional Practice Principles

Interprofessional work in health settings has also adopted some additional principles that resonate in the social services sector. The first is that the client is the center of the team and should be involved in all phases of problem identifications and resolution. Along with that is ensuring that each person on the team knows who is also on the team—whether in the person's own agency or in another agency. As the team develops through shared meetings and informal conversations, each member of the team should be able to describe his own role and that of the others on the team. This is vital to ensuring that there are no false assumptions about areas of expertise or legal responsibility. This also minimizes the possibility of role conflict—when two people think each alone has expertise in a specific area. Each team member should have a basic understanding of what others can (and can't) do by virtue of their training and background. It then follows that each person should recognize and observe the constraints of their role, responsibilities, and competence, yet perceive needs in a wider framework. Each team should also have a designated leader or coordinator who does not have to be the key decision maker in any specific area, but who will be responsible for team communication and meetings if necessary. When possible, this role should rotate among members so that no one person is seen as always being in charge. One final important challenge of interprofessional practice is to work with people from other professions to effect change and resolve conflict in the provision of care and treatment. That means that the team members may not always agree but will seek a consensus and will abide by the group decision.

EXERCISES

Exercise 1. Role Clarification

1. Have all students state their role/job/professional background (this will vary depending on the class composition). Write the various classifications on the blackboard or poster paper.
2. Pair students so each couple consists of two different jobs/professions, and so on. Students may elect to pair themselves, but it should be with someone they do not know.
3. Have one student in each pair explain her role/job/professional background. Then have the same person explain to the other what she thinks the other's role/job/professional background is. Ask the listener not to interrupt or contradict. Then the pairs switch and the

second person explains his job and how he sees the other's role/job/professional background. Then they compare areas of agreement and discrepancy.
4. Repeat the exercise with different pairings.
5. Group discussion. Questions:
   a. Was it difficult to describe your own job/role/professional background?
   b. Was it difficult to describe your partner's?
   c. Was it hard to remain quiet when your partner did not get it right about your role?
   d. Was it easier to do this the second time?
   e. Have you had to do this previously in your job?
6. If the opportunity allows, have the students do this as a take-home exercise. Ask them to have this conversation with a person at their agency, or at another agency if more practical, who comes from a different occupation. Have the person describe her roles and responsibilities. If the person is part of a recognized profession, explore what the profession requires, allows, and does not permit. Ask the students to write this experience as a journal entry.

Exercise 2. Communication and Jargon

Write out at least five terms that are frequently used in your job or professional world that may be unfamiliar or confusing to outsiders. In small groups of people from different backgrounds, share your lists with the group and discuss how others perceive these terms. How could students communicate these terms better?

Exercise 3. Working in Teams

This exercise is best done after exercise 1 because it requires students to be aware of the various roles and responsibilities of team members. It builds on the material presented in the case management section and thus should be presented as a follow up. This also integrates material between these two chapter parts.

Case Example Brent is a single man, age sixty-nine, who has been homeless for the past three years. Although he has suffered from serious mental illness for much of his adult life, he was able to complete graduate school and become an educator for a period of time. Eventually his symptoms could not easily be controlled and he was forced to quit his job and rely on disability income to cover his expenses. He attended a rehabilitation program part time, spent time in the library, and volunteered at a local homeless shelter once a month. In many ways he continued to function despite his disabilities and was not a typical helpless, homeless person. Nonetheless, he fell through the cracks.

He lived in a rooming house and became somewhat of a hoarder. When offered supportive housing he was unwilling to give up his self-perceived independence and saw the supportive housing as an intrusive element. Subsequently his rooming house was sold and he was assisted by staff from a rehabilitation program to find other independent housing. His symptoms gradually worsened, despite regular medical treatment, medication compliance, and lack of alcohol or substance use in his life. The result was a rapid decrease in his housekeeping and self-care skills, to the extent that he was evicted from his new residence. Housing in a seniors' independent living facility was arranged but this also fell through. He stopped regular attendance at the rehabilitation program and did not have a case manager. He was evicted from the seniors' home and had no place to go and thus wound up at the same shelter where he used to volunteer. Shelter staff were not concerned with finding housing for a single elderly man, as their efforts went primarily to families and couples. He was not referred for seniors' services and did not qualify for the limited case management services available. When he had outlasted his thirty-day welcome at the shelter he moved to another, and then another. But he was not placed elsewhere. He occasionally would come to the rehab program and he reconnected with staff there.

Shortly before this eviction, a volunteer at the last shelter took a special interest in him, and was helping him to find appropriate housing. At the same time, his physician had changed his medication and he was mentally functioning better. In this interim his health began to seriously deteriorate, as he had also developed type 2 diabetes and could not control his diet adequately. When the volunteer went on a vacation lasting several weeks, he was evicted from the shelter because his needs were greater than staff could manage. He roamed the streets, then sought medical attention, and was hospitalized for several brief stays while waiting for the volunteer to return. When the rehab staff became concerned that he had not been seen for several weeks, they started to search for him, eventually finding him hospitalized in a local facility.

In many ways this elderly man was not a typical homeless person. He had a graduate school education, and had been successfully employed as an educator for a number of years. He was never married, his parents were deceased, and he had minimal contact with distant relatives who viewed him as an embarrassment. He was well read, highly articulate, knew the local services and political structures, and had come from a stable middle-class family. He did not have a history of alcohol or drug use, but did have a serious and persistent mental illness, with acute flare-ups. He had a liveable income from his pension so that housing affordability was not the sole issue. However, adequate housing was dependent on his being in a subsidized unit. Despite his functional challenges he was fiercely independent, but ultimately was unable to manage independently. His grooming was unacceptable. He needed help—that he didn't get—for bathing, clean clothes, and the like. He looked and walked like a sad old homeless man who had lost his last friend. Yet when in conversation one could easily be touched by the gentle, intelligent, sensitive, and caring human who dwelt inside this outer shambles.

- Where did the system fail him?
- Who was responsible for his care?
- Why did shelter personnel evict him when he had no adequate place to go?
- Why did the local hospitals repeatedly discharge him to the shelter system with no social work evaluation of his needs?

Case Study Jim is a fifty-year-old man of First Nations (Native American) descent living on the streets. He was diagnosed with posttraumatic stress disorder (PTSD) related to incidents of child abuse and family violence. He frequents city shelters for food and sometimes for a place to sleep. Jim is known by shelter staff as a kind man when he is sober. However, when he drinks he becomes belligerent and is therefore often turned away from shelters.

- Who should head the team?
- Who may be involved in the team?

- Is there additional information that would be essential for the team to have?
- What community services may be available to Jim?
- Are there any support programs available to Jim?
- How would you engage Jim in working out a plan that he and the team can support?

Exercise 4. Working in Teams

This is a fun exercise and most people find it both amusing and enlightening. This exercise looks at various interactions that occur in teams that are influenced by personality and interaction styles as much as by rank and role. As preparation, the instructor should make labels (return labels for packages are a good size). The instructor should print on each label a behavioral description such as, "I am opinionated," "I am always right," "I am agreeable," "I am indecisive," "I rule!," "I don't count," "I always disagree," "Love me," and so on. Feel free to be creative with this labeling. Prepare as many packets with one of each label as there are groups of students, with preferably five or six in each group. Place the labels in an envelope.

1. Instructions: Divide the class into groups of five or six.
2. Explain that the following activity is important at work because research shows that the best teams occasionally interact socially.
3. Tell the students that their team's task is to plan an agency holiday gathering.
4. Distribute the envelopes and ask each person to take a label, not to look at their own, but to peel off the back and affix it to the forehead. Ask for help from a partner, if needed.
5. The team is to plan the picnic, but to respond to each member according to the label on that person's forehead.
6. Allow ten minutes.
7. Have the team debrief.
8. Debrief with the entire class.

Exercise 5. Role Assumptions and Misperceptions

In pairs of persons from different agencies and professions, have each pair exchange information about the following: Three common and correct assumptions about their roles and then at least two common misperceptions or incorrect expectations of their roles. Then discuss how these perceptions help and hamper services.

Exercise 6. Case Discussion and Team Planning

Case Example

Henry, a single man, age fifty-eight, with a history of mental health problems, became homeless when his boarding house was closed and he could not find affordable housing. He had no case manager and rapidly became a resident of a local emergency shelter. He did not use alcohol, drugs, or cigarettes; has a graduate-level college education; was articulate; and had a gentle, nondemanding demeanor. He was married for a short time in his twenties but after the divorce he has lived by himself. In addition to mental illness, whose symptoms were controlled by medication, he had several serious medical problems including diabetes. Medication errors led to partial kidney failure and he was hospitalized. A case worker from the shelter and one from a housing support program met to determine future plans for housing. When the program manager of a local clubhouse where the man was a long-time member found out that he had been hospitalized she called a case conference and pointed out to the workers who had previously met that their meeting was not valid in that it did not include Henry, his family, a volunteer who had stepped in to provide support, a representative from the drop-in program that he attended frequently, or a representative from senior services. The plan developed was incomplete and missed critical aspects of Henry's situation. The resulting new conference was attended by all and the new plan for Henry included his acceptance of placement in a seniors' residence where his basic needs would be met and where he would receive supervision for his medical needs.

- Who would be members of the team constructing a care plan for the client?

- What would be the immediate challenges for this team?
- Is there any natural team leader based on client need?

JOURNALING

1. For how many different professions do you understand the individual professional priorities and value systems? Which of these most closely align with your own? Which are most distant?
2. How would you go about introducing the ideas of teamwork and interprofessional practice in your work environment?
3. Reflect on a situation from work where interprofessional practice principles would have been helpful. Do you think that the outcomes would be different from what they were if interprofessional practice principles had been used?

CHAPTER 5

CASE MANAGEMENT AND SYSTEM NAVIGATION

KEY ISSUES	Understanding case management
	How to engage a person in a client-oriented individualized case plan
	How to navigate a complex system and not get lost
	Overview of government, medical, mental health, institutions, and community agencies
	Tools for effective case management
	Understanding of who gets "managed" in case management
	Entitlements and other sources of income
	How to assemble a list of resources: the toolbox of case management
	How to effectively advocate for clients

OVERVIEW

Homeless clients most often present with a variety of health, social service, legal, and other issues in addition to housing, which require attention if the individual is to be able to sustain housing and personal functioning. Meeting these needs requires a multistep process that starts with the identification of client strengths and areas by means of a thoughtful assessment. Finding and linking up with the resources to address the client's needs is a second phase, and following up to make sure the delivery of those needed services is accomplished is a third phase. A final component is the evaluation of services and how effectively they are meeting the identified needs as well as an assessment of any recently emerging issues that were not apparent in the initial assessment. This process will also, hopefully, avoid gaps in service and provide assistance for those items that are most difficult to address on initial housing placement. We explore the importance of a client-centered case-management process, the importance of empowerment for clients, and facilitation of their linkages with targeted providers. Then we examine the differences between a referral and ensuring that a linkage is made, including the situations that require direct worker intervention.

Throughout this chapter and those to follow we use the terms "agency" and "organization" interchangeably. All agencies are organizations, but all organizations are not necessarily agencies. The references in this chapter are to those organizations that deliver services intended for people to meet social, health, mental health, addiction, child development, educational, vocational, recreational, and similar life-sustaining and life-enhancing needs. In many instances these are social service agencies with specific missions, such as family preservation, child wellness, mental health or addiction services, vocational rehabilitation, a day-time meal program (soup kitchen), a night shelter for adults, or a domestic violence shelter for women and children. Homeless services may also be part of a large, multiprogram independent charitable organization such as the Salvation Army, St. Vincent DePaul Society, or the Family Service Association (in the United States) that provides (temporary or long-term) shelter, transitional programs, and meals. Others, such as community health (and mental health) centers, are usually government sponsored and funded. They may offer health as well as mental health and addiction services, some of which may also have a supportive housing program.

There are also organizations that are private or semiprivate and that operate with a mixture of government funding and private donations. These have greater flexibility than those directly served by public funds and that are part of the local, county, regional, state, provincial, or federal bureaucracy. Publicly funded and administered organizations such as income support programs, Medicaid, Veterans Affairs, and so on are subject to rules and regulations that make them dependable but highly inflexible. Some government units are called agencies; this terminology may create confusion. When we refer to agencies and organizations in this and subsequent chapters, we mean those that are free-standing, nonprofit, nongovernment organizations. The terms "agency" and "organization" do not specify the exact nature of the structure of service involved, but instead refer to nongovernment units.

Programs, on the other hand, generally refer to organizational units established to deliver a specific set of activities with the intent to target an identified client population. Agencies may have multiple programs for different groups of clients or may consist of a single program with restricted clientele (Gibelman & Furman, 2008). A soup kitchen is an example of a program that intends to provide food for the hungry. It may be a single, free-standing program, part of a shelter, or part of an agency's general mission to serve the homeless or an outreach activity of a community of faith (local church group).

PUBLICLY ADMINISTERED PROGRAMS

Agencies that help low-income (and no income) individuals and families fall into two broad categories: financial support and human services. Within government they are referred to as social welfare programs because, broadly speaking, they are intended to help human beings who live together in society; they have to do with the well-being of those people (Kahn, 1979, p. 22). These programs are provided by the government: federal, provincial (state), or local (municipal and regional). They are funded through a variety of taxation mechanisms (income tax, sales tax, business tax, real estate tax, etc.) and are meant to ensure that people have basic shelter and food for survival. Some are also intended as retraining and vocational assist programs to help individuals improve their skills and thus their employability, which leads to independence from assistance programs. These programs may be directly administered by the government or may be provided through a public/private arrangement, such as the provision of child-care supports to local agencies offering this service to low-income parents. Although there is considerable debate as to the adequacy of these supports, they are at least a first step to providing for the well-being of society.

Included in financial assistance are the programs that provide cash directly to qualified individuals (and families). Others provide vouchers for in-kind supports such as food and housing. Social services, paid through government contracts, are another source of assistance. A special group of programs consist of opportunities targeted at specific groups of people—youths, women with children, people from minority populations, persons with handicaps—to provide special training and employment opportunities. Many of these programs are based on need, such as the ability to demonstrate a financial deficit to meet basic living needs, and some are based on entitlement, such as the eligibility for support through predetermined rules. The frontline worker needs to be aware of what programs are available, which may be accessed through need, and which may be accessed through entitlement (usually by proof of or "demonstrated" need). There are many comparable programs in Canada and the United States, but not all are available in each country. Tables 5.1 and 5.2 show what these programs are, and which are available in each country. This list is not mean to be exhaustive. It also can't take into account the development of low-income housing proposals that will help meet the needs of housing-deprived people.

Most urban places, the cities and town across both nations, have an array of social services to help those who have disabilities and vulnerabilities. Not all are well developed, and many lack the ability to meet basic needs, especially for single men. In areas that are more sparsely inhabited, especially in rural and northern locations, these services may be virtually nonexistent, which becomes a major challenge for everyone—those who want to help and those who need help. Regardless of location, a first priority is to determine local resources, both those available and those that can be creatively put together.

One of the first ways to learn about the extent of services available locally is to look for an agency resource book. Many communities have handbooks of social service, health, income, educational, and child-care organizations. While telephone directories have often served this important function, as the use of paper directories diminishes local United Way organizations have taken up some of the slack. New workers will find it most valuable to use some time when they are new on the job to get to know these resources because they will speed up making referrals and finding resources.

The causes of homelessness are many, and certain risk factors are more closely linked with specific groups. Thus agencies that focus on the needs of specific groups at risk of homelessness will encounter some differing circumstances and some common problems facing their clients. Families often experience loss of housing because of lack of adequate income, sickness that reduces income, and a bit less frequently but still important, substance misuse. Youths often leave home to escape abusive family situations, which may be intertwined with substance misuse, but is predominated by parent-child discord and abuse. Youths also leave foster homes and the child welfare system ill prepared for independence, which places them at high risk

Table 5.1. Income Support Programs in the United States

Income Programs	Type of Assistance	Level of Government Responsible	Beneficiaries	Special Conditions
Disability insurance	Monthly cash payment	Federal (Social Security Administration)	Disabled workers and dependent children. Worker must have worked and contributed a specific number of quarters of the year to qualify.	Amount based on previous contributions to Social Security.
Unemployment insurance	Weekly or biweekly cash payment	Individual states	Unemployed workers actively looking for work. Must have worked a specific number of weeks to qualify.	Amount based on previous earnings.
Workers' compensation	Monthly or biweekly cash payment plus medical benefits	Individual states	Workers with employment-related injury.	Amount based on current earnings.
Old-Age and Survivors Insurance (OASI)	Monthly cash payment	Federal (Social Security Administration)	Retired workers, dependents, and survivors.	Based on past earning. Income ceilings apply.
Supplemental Security Income (SSI)	Monthly cash payment	Federal (public funds administered by Social Security Administration)	People who are blind, aged, or disabled. Must meet an income test.	Based on demonstrated need. Limits on allowed assets.
Temporary Assistance to Needy Families (TANF)	Monthly cash payment	States	Low-income families, usually women with dependent children.	Based on need. Limits on allowable assets.
General assistance	Cash, clothing, food bank eligibility, vouchers for medical care	States and local municipalities. Not available everywhere.	Available to individuals with neither source of income nor assets.	Based on need. Generally insufficient to meet basic needs without other assistance such as food and shelter vouchers.

Table 5.1. (Continued)

Housing Programs	Type of Assistance	Level of Government Responsible	Beneficiaries	Special Conditions
Section 8, Housing and Community Development Act	Housing subsidy provided as a voucher	Federal	Income dependent.	Demonstrated need.
Public housing	Housing in a government-controlled housing project	Federal, and some state or local with federal dollars	Income dependent for low-income households.	Priority to families with dependent children, those with disabilities, and the elderly.
Housing for the Elderly (Section 202)	Grants to organizations to build and operate low-cost housing for seniors	Federal	Low income. Need dependent.	Single and married elderly with an income below 50% of the region's median income.
Native American Housing Assistance and Self-Determination Act (NAHASDA)	Grants to tribal organizations for housing development	Federal	Administered by each tribal authority.	Tribal membership.
Housing Opportunities for People With AIDS (HOPWA)	Grants for short-term rental assistance	States and local jurisdictions	People with HIV/AIDS and their families.	Needs dependent. Limited availability.
Special Projects	State and local housing assists	Federal and state grants	People with low income and/or special needs.	Needs and income dependent.

Table 5.2. Income Support Programs in Canada

Income Programs	Type of Assistance	Level of Government Responsible	Beneficiaries	Benefit Level
Canada Pension Plan/ Quebec Pension Plan Disability Insurance	Monthly cash payment	Federal	Disabled workers and dependent children. Must have worked and contributed for a specific amount of time.	Amount based on previous contributions.
Employment Insurance	Weekly or biweekly cash payment	Provinces	Unemployed workers actively looking for work, or workers with a temporary illness or on maternity leave. Must have worked a specific number of weeks to qualify.	Amount based on previous earnings.
Workers' compensation	Monthly cash payment plus medical benefits	Provinces	Workers with employment-related injury.	Amount based on current earnings.
Disability income (name varies by province)	Monthly cash payment plus supplemental medical benefits	Provinces	Disabled adults over age 18. Physical, developmental, or mental health disability.	Flat amount varies by province.
Canada Pension Plan / Québec Pension Plan (CPP/QPP) for retirees	Monthly cash payment	Federal	Retired workers, spouses of deceased workers, dependents, and survivors.	Amount based on past contributions.
Old Age Security Pension (OAS)	Monthly cash payment	Federal	Retirees age 65 and over.	Flat amount.
Old Age Security Pension (OAS) Supplements A. Low-income supplement B. Survivor allowance C. Supplement	Monthly cash payment	Federal	A. Income dependent. B. Those age 60 to 64 years and spouse or common-law partner who is receiving the OAS and is eligible for the Guaranteed Income Supplement. C. Age 60–64 and widowed (income dependent).	Supplements are flat rate, and are dependent on a means test (low income). They are provided in addition to the OAS benefit.

for homelessness. Women who are victims of domestic violence often have no place to go except to a shelter (Tutty et al., 2009). As a result, being homeless is often part of multiple circumstances that require attention if rehousing is to be possible and successful. We first turn our attention to what these multiple factors may be, and then explore ways to address the solutions. In this context we will look at the importance of a service coordinator and service broker, terms we prefer to that of case manager, as we will examine further in this chapter.

SERVICES AND RESPONSIBLE ORGANIZATIONS

In order to appreciate how complex this process can be, it is important to start with an overview of the various needs that an individual or family may present. Table 5.3, which presents the areas of concern and the types of issues that may be presented, is representative but no means an exhaustive list of common issues. In putting together this list no assumptions have been made about where the responsibility for the problem may lie, but only that it is identified as a barrier to successful housing, that is, it may either prevent housing from happening or may set the stage for housing loss. Table 5.3 also indicates the local or state (occasionally federal in the United States) department that is normally responsible for this area. However, local practices may vary and thus it is important for the worker to be familiar with the specific departments responsible for each issue.

The first item in table 5.3 is worth a bit of explanation, as it is not always recognized that many homeless persons lose their ID through loss or theft of belongings or by leaving it along with other items with friends who may lack respect for other people's stuff. As further discussed in chapter 12, ID includes birth certificate, Social Security card (United States) or Social Insurance Card (Canada), alien resident (United States) card or landed immigrant card (Canada), driver's license, marriage and divorce papers, health ID card (Canada), Medicaid/Medicare card (United States), or status card (for American Indian and Canadian Aboriginal persons). Without one or more of these pieces of ID a person is unable to gain access to many income, housing, and support services to which she may be entitled. Almost all forms of ID rely on a birth certificate and/or Social Security or Social Insurance Card to obtain other forms of ID such as a driver's license. In many instances

Table 5.3. The Service System

Area of Concern	Types of Issues	Service System Involved — United States	Service System Involved — Canada
ID	Lack of ID, making it impossible to qualify for services	State: Birth certificate Federal: Social Security number American Indian: Status Card/ID Immigrant: Alien resident card Driver's license Marriage/divorce papers	Province: Birth certificate Federal: Social Insurance Card Aboriginal: Status Card/ID Immigrant: Landed immigrant card Driver's license Marriage/divorce papers
Income	Without resources but not disabled; with dependent children Dependent on entitlements because of disability Entitlements inadequate for meeting basic needs Insufficient because of lack of job skills; employment limited to minimum wage	Public welfare Social Security: Supplemental Security Income (SSI) / Social Security Disability Insurance (SSDI)	Public welfare Canada Pension Plan disability provisions
Rental assistance	Ineligible/no assistance available Long waiting list No units available Presence of extended family reduces availability and sometimes eligibility	Federal, state, and local assistance programs Section 8 housing Unavailable for immigrants, refugees, or undocumented aliens	Federal programs; some limited housing initiative through grants to provincial bodies Housing supports provincially funded and administered Available for immigrants and refugees, but not for undocumented aliens

Table 5.3. (Continued)

Area of Concern	Types of Issues	Service System Involved — United States	Service System Involved — Canada
Financial: Past housing debts and general debts	Rent owing from previous dwelling unit must be paid before eligible for rehousing Outstanding utility bills Credit card or other debtors who threaten legal action Street-level debt that threatens retaliation Poor financial management skills	Subject to state laws Bankruptcy a possible debt-relieving action, but has long-term consequences	Subject to provincial laws Bankruptcy a possible debt-relieving action, but has long-term consequences
Food	Insufficient income to provide adequate nutrition Special dietary needs because of illness and chronic conditions No available food bank or soup kitchen	USDA Supplemental Nutrition Assistance Program (SNAP) Federal funding, state administered, available but restricted for immigrants Food banks and pantries operate in most localities Breakfast and school lunch programs widely available	No federal or provincial food assistance programs Limited and restricted local support through food banks School lunch programs not widely available and offered only through local school districts and social services agencies
Health	Chronic and/or disabling health conditions that preclude employment Special living assistance required Essential medicines require too much of monthly income Unable to afford basic health-care recommendations (treatments, surgeries) Pregnancy	Department of Health and Human Services, Social Security Administration Medicaid and Medicare assistance: limits on type of assistance and types of medication coverage	Provincial health authorities and local facilities Universal coverage for medical and mental health care All legal residents (immigrants, refugees, and citizens) entitled to a health card Medication coverage: through provincial social assistance and supplementary health services available to low-income individuals

Education	Lack of training or qualified only for minimum wage jobs Unable to afford fees and living expenses to get further training School loans counted as income, thereby reducing other entitlements	Education system for children and youth Adult vocational services through state	Education system operated by provinces and funded by federal and provincial programs Some limited vocational training programs available
Mental health	Disabling mental illnesses Difficulty adhering to treatment recommendations	State and county mental health departments and their services	Provincial health departments and local services
Addiction services	Detox, inpatient, and outpatient treatment programs; continuing treatment and support programs; self-help groups	Substance Abuse and Mental Health Services Administration (SAMHSA) and contracts with individual states Publicly funded inpatient programs scarce; homeless people usually lack private health insurance to access programs	Funded through Health Canada and provincial health systems
Transportation	Unaffordable public transport to get to health, mental health, vocational, or educational services Automobile ownership unaffordable and/or renders persons ineligible for financial assistance; especially critical in rural areas where there is no public transportation	Variable state benefits	Car ownership does not disqualify for benefits

Table 5.3. (Continued)

Area of Concern	Types of Issues	Service System Involved — United States	Service System Involved — Canada
Justice system involvement (criminal and civil)	Criminal record makes it difficult to get employment Jail sentence results in housing loss; release from confinement is release to homelessness Unable to get employment if need to be bonded or have a criminal check for clearance Unable to drive because of previous record; impedes employability and access to services Legal action because of child custody, excess debt, civil cases involving lawsuits by private individuals	State and federal justice systems (depending on the nature of the crime) Challenges similar in both countries	Provincial and federal justice systems (depending on the nature of the crime) Challenges similar in both countries
Child care	Unavailable Unaffordable Need for specialized services for special needs children	Variable benefits through Department of Health and Human Services	Variable benefits through provincial programs and federal tax credits
Child welfare	Threat of removal of children because of unsanitary or unsafe living conditions Refusal to return children because of lack of adequate living arrangements, but unable to qualify for adequate arrangements if children are not in the person's custody	State child welfare authorities Bias against custodial fathers who lack the same benefits as women with children	Provincial child welfare authorities No bias based on parental sex

Household necessities	Often lost at time of eviction or move from another locality Rent usually omits furnishings, cooking and eating supplies, linens, and bedding Often no assistance for moving these items from storage, or paying for overdue storage fees	Local nonprofit organizations	Local nonprofit organizations
Access to support groups	Lack of availability near temporary shelter or housing, but essential for sobriety Shelters often located near bars and liquor stores	Same in both countries	Same in both countries
Family functioning	Family discord, problematic functioning, stress, interference, custody issues	Counseling services through nonprofit organizations with local and some national presence Cost by sliding scale	Counseling services through nonprofit organizations Cost by sliding scale; some counseling covered under health care if health issue involved

application for replacement documents requires a fee and a recognized mailing address, the first important hurdles for rehousing. Some communities have established ID programs that help homeless persons to obtain critical pieces of ID, but these programs are not universally available.

> **Textbox 5.1. Homelessness and the Ability to Vote**
>
> Becoming homeless does not take away the right to vote, but it adds encumbrances that makes it difficult to exercise this right. Voting registration requires ID in the United States. While many forms of ID are acceptable, most are not easily available to homeless persons (e.g., motor vehicle license, lease, utility bills). Residence is not an issue because shelters and even a public area can be listed, as long as there is a mailing address and some proof of residence. However, state and local elections require proof of residence, which may present an obstacle. In Canada, voting requires either ID or that a person swear an oath and have someone else attest to the individual's identity. Proof of residency also applies at provincial and local elections. A person can use a shelter as a legal address if accompanied by a letter of attestation from the shelter.

Second only to ID is the need to obtain income. While there are presently many areas where homeless persons work, full or part time, they are unable to afford the rents in market housing. Without subsidies, they are left to seek shelter in local hostels, double up, or sleep rough—in tents and cardboard boxes in parks and out-of-the-way locations. For single men there are few options: local welfare provides a minimal amount that does not cover room and board in market rental facilities unless they are supplemented by public aid. For women, social services provide a greater allowance if there are dependent children residing with the mother. Without dependents, homeless women will also not receive enough support to pay housing costs and still have enough left for food and other essentials. For women who have dependent children not currently in their care this is a dilemma: in many jurisdictions they do not qualify for housing with dependents because they do not have custody, but they can't get custody without housing adequate to accommodate a family.

Education for children, as distinct from continuing education and vocational training for adults, becomes another parental burden for homeless families. On the one hand, in all jurisdictions children are required by law to be enrolled in school or in a home schooling program. On the other hand, they usually have to be enrolled in school in the area where the custodial parent(s) reside(s). If the family is in a shelter, children may have to transfer to the school nearest the shelter, and then move to another school if the family is rehoused in a different school district. If the child is in a special or charter school that serves a wider area, then the child may be able to avoid a transfer. This is one instance where a service broker may be able to advocate for leaving the child at a designated school, especially if this is for the remainder of the school year or if there is a likelihood that the family may be again rehoused in the foreseeable future. However, transportation may then become another issue and potential barrier. Parents still have to produce ID for children, including birth certificates and proof of required vaccinations. Those not able to verify legal residency or proof of citizenship may not be able to register children for school. This creates a double jeopardy as children legally must attend school but taking them and their lack of documentation of status to officials could put parents at risk for deportation. This risk is greater in the United States than in Canada where immigrant and refugee laws are more embracing and lenient. Even when children and parents overcome these hurdles with sympathetic local administrators, they are usually prevented from opportunities for training beyond high school where document requirements are strictly enforced. In turn this places them at increased risk for housing instability because they are qualified for only low-income jobs.

This list is by no means exhaustive. The combination of people and circumstances inevitably creates situations that are unusual and complex. One of the generally neglected areas of entitlement and support programs is health and health-related issues of mobility, diet, and care requirements that require special assistance, often difficult to obtain if they are available at all. Another area of special concern is the multiple resources and special services that combat veterans need to restore stability. Adaptations to civilian life that do not accommodate the response to stressors reminiscent of battle experiences frequently misidentify and respond inappropriately to the needs of this special cohort (O'Toole, Conde-Martel, Gibbon, Hanusa, & Fine, 2003). Single men, especially those with no history of mental health problems, have historically been assumed to be able to be self-reliant, and thus few services provide the same level of support that they provide to children, women, and those with disabilities.

Social Services Usually Accessed by Homeless Persons

There are numerous organizations (nonprofit nongovernment organizations) and government agencies that are potentially involved in providing services and material assistance for homeless and indigent persons. While table 5.3 presents a comparison of publicly funded programs that are available in Canada and the United States, it is impossible to list the numerous charitable organizations in both countries that provide social services to homeless and vulnerable persons. Frontline workers and their supervisors need to develop a toolbox that includes the names, contact numbers, program description, and eligibility requirements of local programs that assist homeless people. We will refer again to the importance of a toolbox in the section on case management.

Most agencies involved with helping those without housing and those at high risk of housing loss confine themselves to a specific mission and thus a limited range of services. This does not imply that these agencies are limited in any way, but just that no single agency is equipped or sanctioned to deliver all of the services that an individual or family may require. Within each agency there is, or there should be, one or several staff members designated to keep track of client needs assessment and service delivery for each person served. The ways that this assignment is organized vary among agencies and there is ultimately no correct way for this assignment to be placed in the organizational structure. However, it must have a key role, in that the designated person, who we will call the service coordinator or case manager, is responsible for keeping track of a designated number of clients, the development of their service plans, and the implementation of these plans. This does not imply that the coordinator actually has to provide each assessment or deliver the services, because there may be several persons involved with different areas of expertise.

There are a number of potential issues that the staff may need to deal with, and some that will require referral to outside agencies. Income and education are immediately evident. There may also be issues of substance abuse, previous child welfare involvement, or legal/justice system involvement, to name some additional concerns. These will require referrals to other agencies, tracking to make certain that the client has connected with them, and working in concert with the other agencies for a mutually agreed-on plan of rehousing and supports. The critical role of the service broker (often also called a case manager) is to negotiate with all of the service providers, ensure both that there is, at minimum, the recognition of a team of

> **Textbox 5.2. Case Example**
>
> A woman, age twenty-six, with two children, ages seven and four, left her abusive boyfriend with whom she had a relationship of eight years and was admitted into a shelter for victims of domestic violence. The shelter provides up to six months of sheltered accommodation in an apartment building and has both counseling and child-care staff on site.
> - In an assessment what staff from the shelter may be involved?
> - What outside organizations may become involved?
> - Besides the presenting information, what additional information would you need to determine all of the parts of a service plan?

providers working with this individual, and that all parts of the plan are addressed.

In the event that no one is assigned the responsibility of the service broker or case manager, there is usually no one who can anticipate and attempt to monitor for service delivery, negotiate solutions to potential problems or obstacles to income entitlement, rental affordability, attempts to remain clean and sober, support through medical and mental health crises, child welfare concerns, and a myriad of living conditions from safety and cleanliness to the availability of sufficient furniture and household necessities for adequate living. Thus the service broker or case manager is the key staff person in the services plan.

CASE MANAGEMENT: SERVICE COORDINATION AND SERVICE BROKERING

Case management is a set of activities that identifies client needs, locates appropriate resources and services, and monitors their delivery. It is client centered, relies on client empowerment and involvement in implementing a service plan, and is interdisciplinary, consisting of services from multiple providers spanning various professions and disciplines. Case management came to prominence in the United States through the utilization review and managed-care focus in the health system. In Canada it also received national attention, initially through health care. Both the Commission for Case Management Certification (2013; in the United States), and the National Standards of Practice (National Case Management Network, 2009; in Canada) are health oriented. In Canada the association has forged a wide mandate covering many human services. While case management in a medical setting usually involves various medical specialties and related services, in the homeless sector, case management involves services that may be delivered in diverse agencies that have distinctly different mandates and operational procedures (Donovan, 2009).

> **Textbox 5.3. Certification in Case Management Competencies**
>
> Certification in case management competencies have been undertaken by two independent organizations. In the United States the Commission for Case Management Certification (2013) provides credentialing for qualified workers. In Canada the National Case Management Network provides standards but, as yet, no certification (Donovan, 2009). Workers are strongly encouraged to access this training and credentialing as an important component of their practice competencies.

> **Textbox 5.4. Case Managers in Various Roles**
>
> Case managers have also become associated with managed health care, where they are the gate keepers to the authorization of payments for medically necessary treatment. "Case manager" is also a term used in many hospitals to denote the nurse in charge of ensuring that all aspects of the medically prescribed treatment are delivered. In order to avoid confusing roles, we use the terms "service coordinator" and "service broker" to signify services delivered in and among agencies.

You will note that instead of the term "case manager" we refer to this role as that of a "service coordinator" and "service broker" for several important reasons. Advocates for disadvantaged persons note that people are not cases, and that this term demeans those who struggle to reclaim their individuality and their voice. The connotation of manager is that of someone who is in a position to manipulate or control another person. Homeless individuals and families need to be in charge of their destiny, to be empowered to make decisions that affect their future, to have the right to be the center of a team of service providers that assists with fundamental changes. People do not need to be managed—they need to be empowered. In that context they require the help of someone who can help to navigate the systems of services and entitlements that belong to their own service organization and the help of someone who can navigate across systems, along with the barriers that they sometimes impose. This navigation often involves searching for solutions and brokering with multiple departments internally and multiple agencies externally, and to work with their regulations. The term "service coordinator" best describes that role of someone in the organization, while the term "service broker" can describe and differentiate the role of someone who navigates across systems. "Broker" is a word used in other capacities where people need financial or housing help (such as a financial broker or real estate broker); it offers a less pejorative and more normalizing context than other terminologies. For those who work in entrenched worlds where "case manager" is the only acceptable term, please substitute "case manager" for "service broker" in order to fit your work context.

The Service Coordinator, Broker, or Case Manager

The case manager is often the coordinator or nominal leader of the services team. In some settings this role may involve counseling as well as plan implementation and monitoring. In other settings, the coordination role may predominate. The service coordinator is often charged with multiple responsibilities related to client service, but it is widely acknowledged that the case management activities include the following (Hepworth et al., 2010):

- Comprehensive assessment
- Articulation of a service plan
- Implementation of the plan
- Monitoring progress on plan delivery
- Reassessment of plan, completion of target items, and inclusion of any new items
- Termination

In work with people who do not have stable, permanent housing, the involvement of multiple service providers means that the following additional activities must also be considered:

- Client involvement at all stages
- Determination of which agencies (and professionals) need to be included in the services team

- Identification of the team leadership
- Identification of length of time that services are available
- Advocacy for those clients who are disadvantaged
- Cultural competency with the client's identified culture

Every agency will have some eligibility requirements for service, but not all agencies provide case management services. Screening for eligibility may be a simple process determined by age (i.e., children's services for those under age sixteen, or for youths from age fourteen to twenty-four), by sex (male/female), by veteran status (type of discharge), status (Aboriginal/Native American, single, or married with dependents), disability, or significant problem (mental health, substance abuse, mobility). There are also specialized programs such as those for pregnant teens, mothers with preschool children, and victims of domestic violence (usually women only), that have additional requirements. Screening may be a quick process conducted during a phone call or through a drop-in interview. It hopefully does not require an appointment: the wait to be seen, only to find out that one is not eligible, is a disappointing and frustrating experience for a person who has already experienced the slamming of many doors. An experienced worker will have a good sense of basic eligibility requirements of the local service agencies, but needs to maintain current knowledge as the eligibility rules may change quickly depending on outside regulators or internal management decisions.

Screening and assessment are often accomplished by the same person—but this is not necessarily so. They are iterative in that, while initial screening may determine eligibility and appropriateness for service, further information obtained in a detailed assessment may indicate that another organization is a more appropriate service provider. It is also important to remember that screening is the initial part of an engagement process between the client and the organization. The impressions formed at this first meeting will remain with the client and be part of how the services are both perceived and received.

Assessment is not a one-time event, but rather is an active, ongoing process that acts as a feedback loop to the client and worker. It also takes into account changing circumstances, as clients either experience additional challenges or see previously identified issues become less problematic (e.g., a relative moves to town and offers to help with day care, or the other partner obtains work at a distance and is not a daily threat). Most importantly, in addition to identifying client needs, assessment should include recognition of client assets: material, positive relationships, skills, and talents. Thus, while children may be an additional responsibility, they may provide attachment and emotional closeness that is vital to the individual. Strengths used to cope with adversity, the ability to think creatively about how to deal with problems, self-determination, and resourcefulness about how to manage on limited means and use freely available services and facilities are all assets that enhance self-esteem and promote empowerment. The ultimate aim of this assessment process is to help the client to be empowered and self-sufficient; this must build on assets already present and those that can be developed or enhanced.

Assessment should include those areas of daily living detailed in the list below. This is true not only to the extent that those needs fall within the mandate of the organizations providing services, but also because any one area, regardless of which organization is responsible for addressing the need, may represent a potential barrier to successful permanency in rehousing. Herein lies a delicate balance between getting sufficient information to determine the extent of service need in a specific area, and not obtaining more information than is necessary to ensure that services are delivered. It is not ethical—as we will examine later in chapter 11—to elicit personal information that is not required for service delivery; to do so is intrusive to personal privacy. At the same time, the worker must use some discriminate thinking to make certain that the information the individual provides is logical and consistent, and fits a coherent whole. Conflicting dates and ages of life events and large gaps in personal history that pertain to housing are examples of inconsistency of information.

Continuing Support Services after Clients Move In

After a client family moves in, provision of case management support for 6 to 12 months includes being aware of the following needs:

Tenant education
Household management
Money management
Survival skills counseling
Welfare advocacy
Legal advocacy

Family and individual counseling
Liaison with schools
Parenting education
Health/nutrition counseling
Children's special needs
Child abuse and neglect: intervention and prevention
Child-care resources
Child-care subsidies
Basic medical care
Job readiness program
Career counseling
Job training and placement
Basic remedial education
English language classes
Substance-abuse prevention

Assessment should include a brief summary of the personal presentation of the client. This should include an indication of the client's ability to articulate her problems, her understanding of the problems (insight) and their possible causes, and her ability to interact with the worker and negotiate a preliminary plan of action. The assessment should be based both on the presenting needs of the client and on the client's determination of need priority. Since clients often live with significant others and families, this assessment should also detail information about those with whom the client lives, those who may potentially live with the client in new housing, or those who influence the client's ability to remain housed. These relationships may be problematic to organizations and entitlement programs that do not recognize these extended family or informal cohabitation arrangements. Common-law relationships and care of extended family are, however, a reality of life and either circumstance needs to be considered in any services, especially those that involve housing. The other possibility occurs if these relationships have a negative influence on a person's stability as they could threaten a person's sobriety by bringing alcohol or drugs into the house, introducing criminal behavior, or moving in without permission from the resident or authorization from the landlord.

Assessment is also a continuous process that evolves as the service plan is implemented. As an initial crisis is resolved a client may have more emotional resources to acknowledge and deal with long-standing issues that have

Textbox 5.5. The Meaning of Family

This is an important place where cultural norms may differ from Western European lifestyles. Aboriginal/American Indian, Hispanic, and major African and Asian cultures live in multigenerational units and thus the nuclear family as is commonly known in North America may not apply to these lifestyles.

also impacted the ability to form a stably housed life (see figure 5.1). Such issues may take the form of a persistent physical complaint that has not been treated, the lack of reading proficiency that limits job opportunities, and lack of cooking and meal planning skills that result in the overuse of prepared meals and fast foods, which erode the monthly budget rapidly.

The service plan proceeds from an identification of need and the client's indication of which issues should be addressed first. It may be important for the worker to point out those areas where solving one issue depends on another that has not been addressed. Beyond this issue of logical primacy of addressing problems, those dealt with should be of the client's choosing for two important reasons. First, the client is the prime driver of services and needs to be able to choose what is addressed. This is in accordance with meeting client needs by placing the client first (figure 5.2) and envisioning all of the supports wrapped around. Second, clients do not like to be told what to do—no one does. So any plan that omits client preferences will fail to engage them in the service plan. This is a difficult issue for those who work in mandated services (corrections, child welfare) where clients have to meet certain objectives. However, to the extent to which even mandated goals can be negotiated with clients, workers should do so in order to maximize engagement and positive change. While the assessment may be formulated within the context of services provided by your agency, it will often include services that are the responsibility of another organization. An example of this would include income, such as welfare, entitlements, and child support payments (figure 5.3).

A second stage of the assessment is the development of a service plan that should clearly indicate what needs to be accomplished, who will be responsible (worker and client), and what timelines will be used to monitor progress and success. Ideally the action plan should state intermediate steps that can be accomplished within a few days to a week that are within the worker's and the client's abilities to handle; the steps should not be dependent on another person or chance events. They should be measurable action

Figure 5.1. The Case Management Process

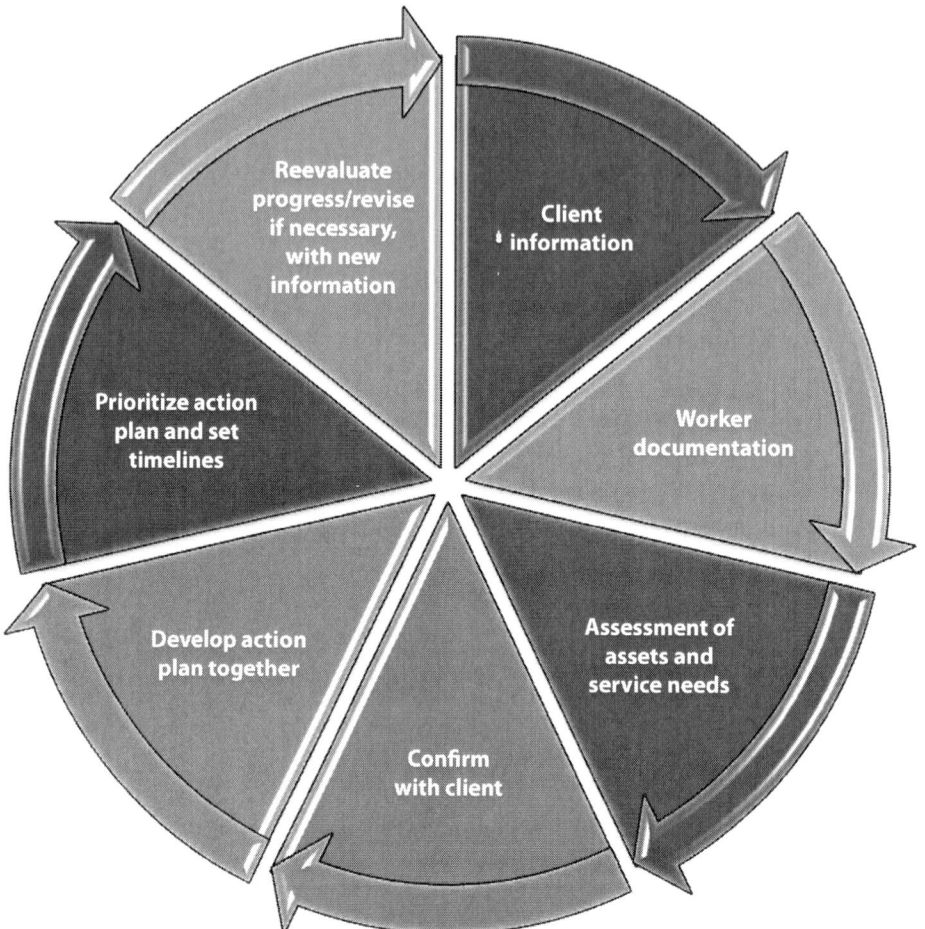

steps and not feelings. This will permit you, the worker, to monitor progress with the client and celebrate successes. For many clients who are not accustomed to long-range goals and who seek immediate response, this monitoring acts as a rapid positive feedback, which is important to continued engagement.

Many vulnerable persons are not comfortable in acting alone to take the steps to implement the service plan. They may lack self-confidence, feel

Figure 5.2. Services for Client and Family

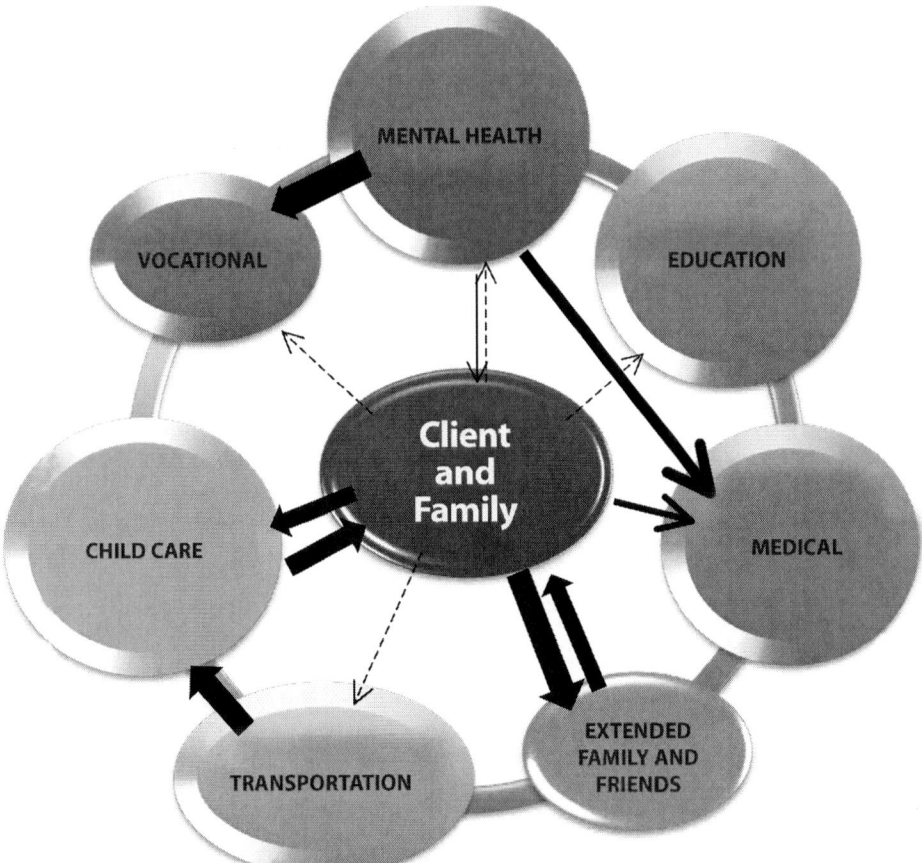

uncomfortable in formal organizations, lack reading skills to handle application forms, or have previously had unpleasant experiences where they have been ignored, neglected, disempowered, or humiliated. They will need support in order to reengage in those situations that present as personal or organizational obstacles. Failure to make these vital connections is one of the main reasons people fall through the cracks—they never get connected and no one sees them fall. Thus one critical role of the worker is to discreetly inquire about whether the client needs or will feel more comfortable with the presence of a supportive person in going to the first (or perhaps several)

Figure 5.3. Array of Individual and Family Services

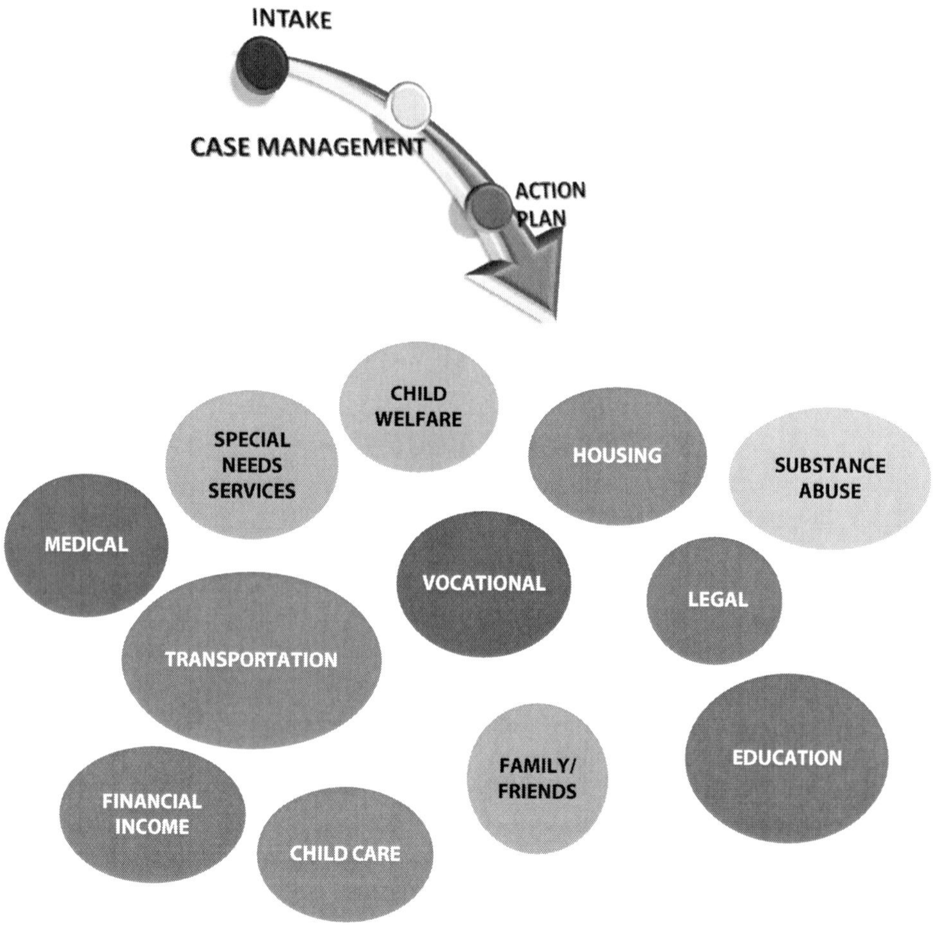

INTAKE

CASE MANAGEMENT

ACTION PLAN

- CHILD WELFARE
- SPECIAL NEEDS SERVICES
- HOUSING
- SUBSTANCE ABUSE
- MEDICAL
- VOCATIONAL
- LEGAL
- TRANSPORTATION
- FAMILY/FRIENDS
- EDUCATION
- FINANCIAL INCOME
- CHILD CARE

appointments. Discretion in determining a person's need for support is imperative as the client may be embarrassed or uncomfortable to admit that such support is important. As the worker, you must be prepared to go with the client to any appointment that may be difficult for the person to attend, and you must make this offer gently. In many cases the client may insist that he is able to handle this alone. It is only when the appointment is not kept or arranged that the admission of discomfort may come through. At other times, depending on how well you know and how comfortable you feel with the client, you can offer to go with him and deal with his minor objections. This is again another area where considerable sensitivity will help to determine the best course of action, remembering that the prime objective is to get the client connected with the services that he agrees he needs.

To understand the many different people that are part of a client's life it is helpful to establish a visual diagram, called a genogram, which depicts all of the relationships that are important in a client's life. The genogram is first mentioned by Lieberman (1973) in the context of understanding relationships in family therapy. It is now widely used by many disciplines to aid in understanding the complexities of relationships that exist in the lives of most people. In a genogram, these relationships are often with family members, including children, parents, spouses, and partners. However, the genogram can be adapted to depict close relationships in other contexts. The basic genogram is depicted in figure 5.4. There are five basic rules that are standardly used in drawing a genogram:

1. The male parent is always on the left side and the female parent is on the right side of the family. In the case of the Simple family in figure 5.5. these eldest family members are Carl and Alice, Kathy's parents, and Edward and Ruth, George's parents.
2. In case of ambiguity, assume a male-female relationship, rather than a male-male or female-female.
3. A spouse must always be closer to his or her first partner than the second partner (if any), third partner, and so on.
4. The oldest child is always at the left of the family, the youngest child at the right of the family.
5. Lines between members may be bolded to indicate strong relationships (positive), jagged to depict troubled relationships, or broken to indicate severed ties.

A variety of symbols have been developed to depict additional relationships and family events such as adoption, foster children, various living arrangements among adults, and a range of emotional relationships. However, they are not essential for basic use in the field when a worker is trying to get a graphic depiction of all relevant persons in the family and extended family. There is no firm rule as to how symbols are used so a worker can be creative in developing ways of showing different and new relationships.

Figure 5.4. Basic Genogram

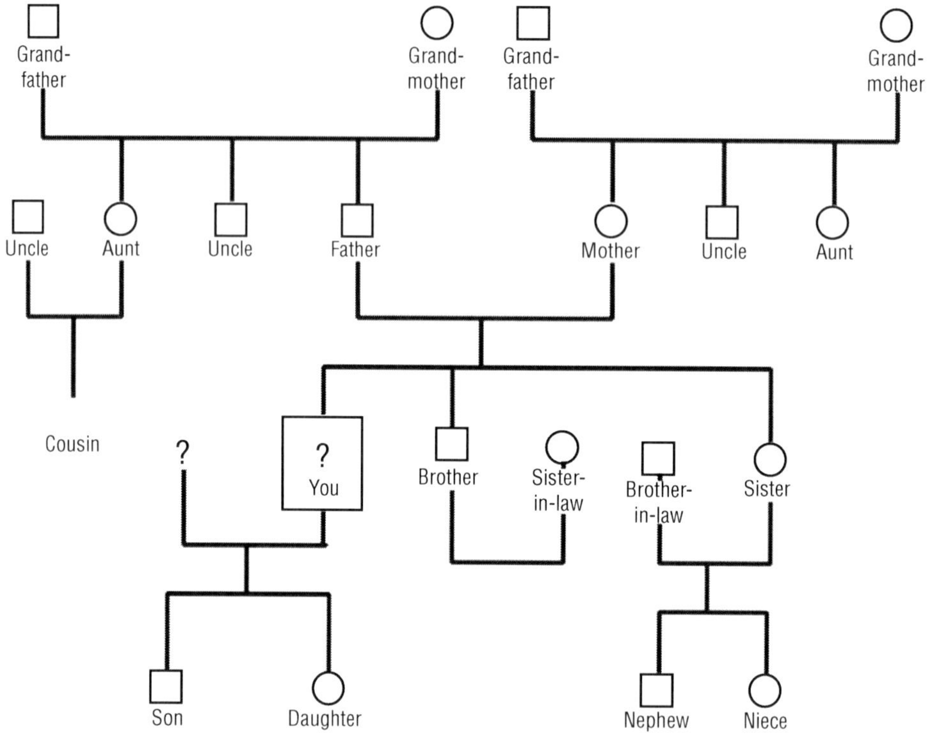

The genogram example in figure 5.5 shows basic relationships in the Simple family. Kathy and George (middle of the diagram) are divorced and George is now also deceased. They have three adult children: Melissa (reportedly pregnant but not in a relationship), Brian, and David. Kathy comes from a family of four children; she is one of the middle children. Her parents are Carl and Alice. George's parents, Edward and Ruth, have a troubled relationship and also had four children of which George is the second oldest. All family members appear to have had positive lives in business and there are no relationship disruptions such as separation or divorce in this extended family. Religion is a strong factor in both families as George's father Edward and Kathy's brother Carl and Dan are all ministers. None of Kathy and George's children are married. Genograms can be enhanced with colors to show the ethnic origins of different family members, which can be especially useful if issues of immigration, culture, and ethnicity are evident.

Figure 5.5. Genogram of the Simple Family

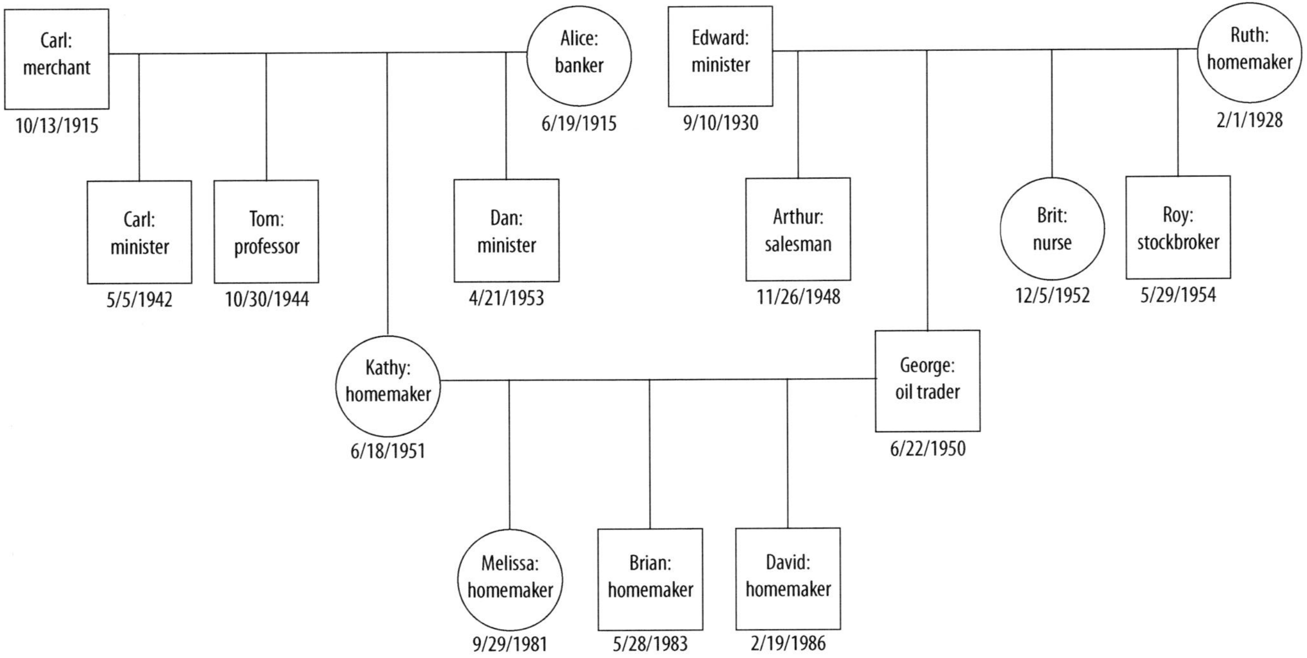

Additional symbols can be used to trace medical, mental health and substance abuse problems. The genogram is a quick and easy way to show family constellations and to provide graphic details of the complexities in and among generations.

> **Textbox 5.6. Genograms and Ecomaps**
>
> There are two ways commonly used to depict family relationships and social networks. The genogram depicts intergenerational relationships among various members of a nuclear and/or extended family. The ecomap provides a graphic depiction of the client's network, which could be social or consist of service providers (figure 5.2). Through the use of arrows and strong and broken lines the worker is able to present a graphic picture of a client's current situation, social and interpersonal supports, and conflicts.
>
> (Hartman, 1978/1995)

Equally important as visual aids are ecomaps that visually depict the service providers, and significant relationships with a client (and client family) and those in their environment. As with genograms, ecomaps use bolded (strong), dashed (weak), and jagged (conflicted) lines to illustrate the nature of these relationships so they can be quickly visualized to illustrate their strength or fragility (Hartman, 1978/1995). This allows an understanding of important relationships, extended family, and what support systems the client may have. Research strongly shows that the presence of family supports and/or strong friendships, even if there have been some previous tensions, is an important asset to rehousing and stability (Tutty et al., 2009). Thus inquiry about these extended relationships is valuable. It may also reveal the presence of persons who are likely to cohabitate with the client once housing has been secured.

The concept of an ecomap was developed by Hartman in 1978 and is now widely used in human services to aid in visually depicting the services and programs involved in helping a client (Hartman, 1978/1995).The basic idea is that the relationships and connections that a client has with service providers can be diagrammatically displayed, along with different styles of lines that can indicate the nature of the relationship (positive, supportive, mandated—positive or negative, supervisory, etc.). This ecomap (figure 5.2) provides a quick overview of potential service providers. The quality and importance of the relationships can quickly be filled in, making it easy to recognize the extent of problematic and strong connections. By putting specific names in the ecomap, it becomes easy to see who is part of the services team (and who should be included in service planning).

Systems Navigation

Navigating systems and agencies is often a challenge for service providers and frequently a daunting task for most clients. With the use of an ecomap, it is possible to explore the various means of providing effective case management and linkage within a complex system. As the list of service needs has been linked with the agencies responsible for their delivery, it now becomes possible to depict what this complexity looks like. It also makes it possible to assess the central players within this client-driven system, and to narrow down the key personnel who should be overseeing the effective linkages to ensure that needs are met.

In a client-centered approach, there are numerous agencies with which a client may be connected, or needs to be engaged, and these are depicted in figure 5.3. Some, such as income supports and child welfare services, are highly bureaucratic, and have numerous rules and regulations that are often not very flexible. Others, such as child-care services and schools may offer greater flexibility, and others, such as churches and spiritual resources, may be able to creatively organize some supports. Regardless of the degree of flexibility, the first task is to be aware of the number of organizations with which the client has to interact for services. All require specific personal information to establish eligibility and assess what services may be appropriate and available. Each organization will have gatekeepers, the frontline people responsible for intake. And each of these gatekeepers will have her own personality and way of doing business. Already one can begin to appreciate the daunting tasks of connecting with all of these resources that is facing an individual who is already depleted from the emotional stresses of dysfunctional and violent relationships. Therein lies the importance of the service broker, the person who hopefully has developed some expertise in how each agency functions at intake and, in smaller communities, may have become familiar with people who hold gatekeeper responsibilities (see the list on pp. 143-144).

Service Broker Responsibilities

The responsibilities of this service broker, or macro level of case management, start with identifying the different organizations and their points of entry—also known as the intake component of the agency. Key to the intake process is knowing whom to contact, how best to get in touch with that person or department, how to get initial appointments quickly, and how to handle an emergency. A second component is how to access the supervisor or manager of the intake service in case there are unusual circumstances or urgencies that can't wait. While it is important to recognize all housing and related services as urgent, not all have the same level of dire consequences if appointments are not immediately available. For example, a young mother with an infant who needs special formula will have to quickly be connected with a service provider or source of funding that can meet her need. On the other hand, that same mother can wait a few days longer in a women's shelter before a housing connection is made (as the shelter can often be flexible with length of stay in special circumstances).

The Toolkit of Service Brokering

Some texts on service delivery, mostly in the social work field, talk about the need to make connections and to develop a toolkit that can be used to facilitate these linkages. The toolkit is often a small notebook or computerized file of people within organizations, as well as a list of important application procedures and waiting list information that is critical for gaining entry to a specific organizational system. Some workers use smartphones to store this information. Regular back-up of this information on another computer and printing copies of these data are advised as the malfunction or loss of a phone creates a gap not easily resolved. In special cases it may include suggestions for alternative ways to gain access to services—the backdoor in—or helpful suggestions for how to receive priority services. It may also include application forms, or Internet access to these forms, as well as specific advisory notes as to what descriptions of need will gain access and which may disqualify someone.

Development of a toolkit takes time and knowledge, training in what is necessary and helpful, time to assemble the information, and the "know-how" as to what important items to include for ready and frequent access. Some items for this tool kit come from a learned set of skills such as genograms and ecomaps. Other items are acquired through hands-on experience such as effective and efficient ways to access support services systems and how to navigate across and through these complex systems. Experienced social workers who have been in the field are often some of the best sources of information for new workers seeking to build a network of reliable resources. Frontline workers who come from other backgrounds are urged to seek out social workers with this knowledge and to learn some of these basic techniques for services provision. The ability to identify and gain access to the services of an organization can be extremely time-consuming, as well as frustrating. Thus any ways to access the system will be of immense value to both worker and client.

One way to facilitate access to other systems is to use all opportunities that arise to meet workers from other organizations, whether in the context of making referrals and ensuring connections, or during consultations, meetings, and trainings. Networking becomes an essential component to getting services for other people. It also places workers in a position to be facilitators to getting clients to the intake process and into the organization they need to be involved with. A mutually respectful opening of doors is an important part of easing the flow in difficult situations and areas filled with frustrating bureaucracy. Knowing the person at the other end of a phone line or email is one of the most efficient ways of ensuring that connections are made. Their knowledge of you, your dependability, and your trustworthiness are earned, and, once established, are invaluable assets. The art of successful brokering also includes knowing senior supervisors and managers who could be called on in urgent or unique situations. However, these resources should be used with caution as they may threaten junior staff who can feel overlooked.

In addition to the services provided by official government agencies and nonprofit organizations, there are often service organizations that may step in to help in dire or unusual situations. Their availability and responsiveness will vary, with small cities and towns more likely to have a personalized response plan by churches and organizations such as the Lions/Lionettes, Kinsmen, Elks, St. Vincent DePaul Society, Mennonite Community Services, veterans clubs, and the Canadian Legion, all of which have targeted groups of persons that they assist where possible. While this list can be very long, we have provided a few examples that can be spring boards to locating local groups. Organizations such as the Red Cross and local mental health groups (Canadian Mental Health Association, National Alliance on Mental Illness in the United States) may provide some selected help on a one-time or crisis basis. The resources vary among communities and regions of both countries. It behooves a worker to make the effort to determine resources that he could call on so he can address a crisis with knowledge of some potential resources. Even better is to take the initiative to meet people who manage these resources so that a call for assistance is received by someone who already is aware of who you are, who you are trying to help, and what services you are trying to support.

The toolkit should also include some personal skills developed by a combination of individual interactive style and experience. In this realm fall assertiveness and advocacy skills. Sometimes being assertive includes requesting to speak with a person's manager or supervisor (as that person may have discretionary power to make certain decisions that frontline staff are not permitted to make). Sometimes assertiveness and advocacy require an appeal to the head of the organization, or taking your concerns to the media—where your efforts are directed at changing rules and policies that discriminate or work against helping vulnerable people. Advocacy is fundamental to helping those oppressed by aspects of society, its many and complex rules and regulations, and its failure to recognize that many people are disenfranchised because of their limited skills in navigating an increasingly technical world. Creative assertiveness and advocacy may reflect the mantra that "every door that opens is the right door," implying that if one cannot get access through intake and a reasonable waiting list (reasonable with regard to time), then a creative search for reasonable alternatives is warranted. In these instances it is the service broker who needs to be aware of alternative routes into the system or alternative but comparable services, if at all possible. While there are many times that this may not be feasible, the creative broker will try to have at least some options to explore, instead of stopping with the first refusal. Tenacity and creativity are thus additional tools for the box.

Advocating may at times require additional support from within and outside one's own organization. This may entail senior level support or may be the simple act of encouraging a client to seek help by contacting the media, which can help make others in the community aware of the service delivery problems. Appeals for help through local churches, mosques, and temples can also be successful, as these organizations have a mandate to help those in need. A final way of advocating is to support agency administrators in talking with colleagues in other organizations. When senior administrators connect across organizations, or when service-level personnel from different organizations meet with the purpose of solving interorganizational barriers (Hepworth et al., 2010) the creative and collaborative results can be surprising. One excellent example is the collaborations that have been created by homeless coalitions in the United States and community action boards in Canada to address service delivery issues for those facing homelessness.

Case management is the critical backbone of service provision. Competently executed, it scopes out the range of needs and strengths that an individual or family seeking services brings to the organization. It helps to prioritize service need and to identify the key organizations and agencies that are involved in service delivery on a client-specific basis. It reminds all workers that the center of the plan is the client and that all service provisions need to be done with the client as the focus of care.

EXERCISES

1. In groups of three—an interviewer, client, and observer—assess the services needs of (a) a homeless adult man with chronic health problems (diabetes and hypertension); (b) a female sex trade worker on parole, with addiction issues; (c) a single father with two children under the age of six; and (d) a woman fleeing domestic violence who has two teenage children.
2. Identify resources in your community for the above individuals.
3. Prepare a plan of action for how to refer and follow up on the referral for a young person who has limited English skills and needs to be enrolled in ESL classes.

JOURNALING

1. What are the most difficult obstacles that you have encountered in providing a case management approach with a homeless person?
2. How can you effectively engage a person in a case management plan?

CHAPTER

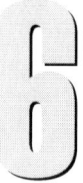

HOUSING FIRST APPROACHES AND HOUSING FIRST PROGRAMS

International human rights law recognizes everyone's right to an adequate standard of living, including adequate housing.

Office of the United Nations High Commissioner for Human Rights, 2009

KEY ISSUES
- Historical approaches to housing the poor and homeless
- Affording housing
- History of *housing first*—obstacles, successes, and change over time
- How *housing first* differs from other housing approaches
- Integrating *housing first* into agencies and staff practice
- How to help the client maintain housing
- Landlord perspectives

OVERVIEW

In the following pages we provide the historical context of housing for homeless persons, and the development and practical application of *housing first* approaches. We will describe the differences between the Housing First model of intervention that has rapidly become popular and other approaches. We also look at *housing first* as an approach that can be modified for different client groups with varying needs, and at instances where the Housing First model is a proven best practice and instances where other housing approaches may be appropriate. Then we briefly examine what services and supports are needed to help clients maintain housing. (We have chosen to denote the approach with *housing first*, and the program model with Housing First, and hope that this distinction will avoid confusion as to what is being discussed.)

BACKGROUND: HOUSING THE POOR

In North America, before the twentieth century those who could not afford housing ended up in jail or the local poorhouse, of which the Evansville County Poor House facility in Evansville, Indiana, is a typical example (figure 6.1). This picture shows that it was a large building, not too different in size and scope from contemporary shelters such as the Calgary Drop-In Centre (occupancy 1,200; figure 6.2). Most often this included women and children,

Figure 6.1. Evansville County Poor House, Evansville, Indiana

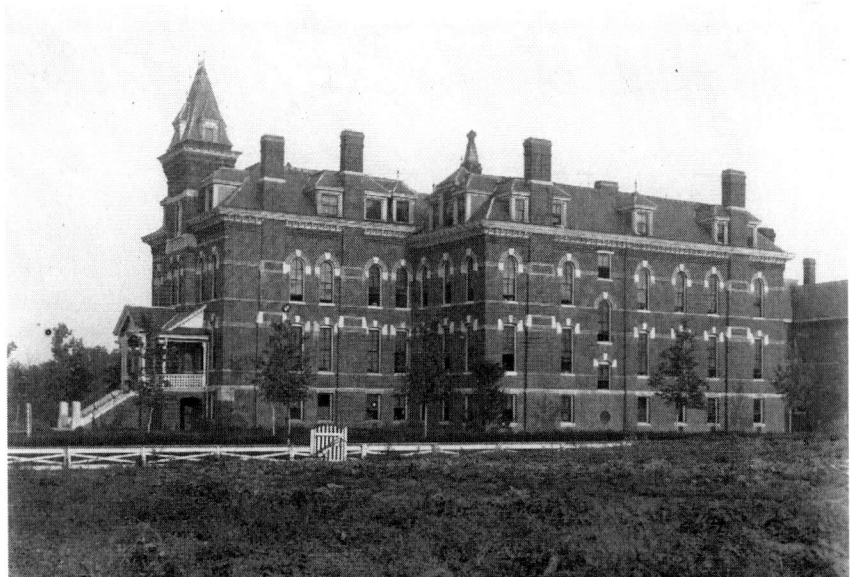

Source: Courtesy of the Willard Library Archives, Evansville, Indiana.

Figure 6.2. The Calgary Drop-In Centre: A Twenty-First-Century Special Use Building Constructed Specifically as an Urban Shelter

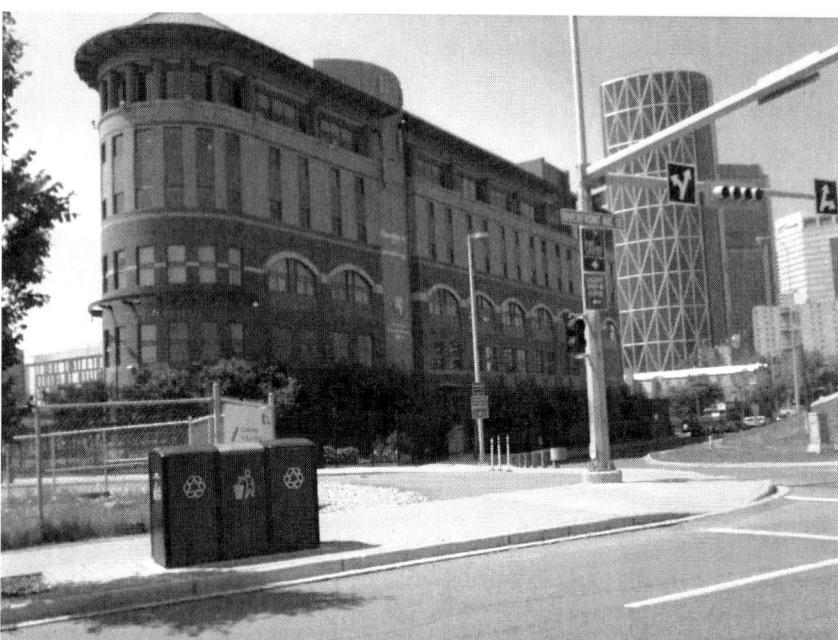

the aged, and single men with disabilities. The indigent mentally ill and "mentally deficient" who were first housed in those same poorhouses were transferred to asylums during the nineteenth century. In America asylums became the refuge for mentally and emotionally disabled persons for more than a hundred and fifty years, until the age of deinstitutionalization began in the mid-twentieth century. With the development of public assistance programs in the early twentieth century, women and children were the first to receive social housing support. Programs in the larger cities created large clusters of dense housing (town houses and apartment buildings) that eventually became urban ghettos for the poor and disadvantaged. Single people, most notably men, lived in marginal single room occupancy hotels (SROs) often near railway stations where they could "hop the rails." The poorhouse concept has not changed much in design, as the two pictures from 1882 in Indiana and 2014 in Alberta illustrate.

Until about the middle of the twentieth century, the poor, most of them immigrants, generally lived in housing that would not be acceptable by

> **Textbox 6.1. Poorhouses of the Nineteenth to Twentieth Centuries**
>
> County poorhouses and state mental health institutions of the late 1800s to mid-1900s had a similar architecture and function in similar ways. Although large and multistoried, both had a prominent entrance and few alternative exits. This design allows the housing of hundreds of people in a single location, designation of sleeping areas by sexes in different parts of the building, control of people's movement between floors, restricted areas of the building, and control over those who enter and leave through well-monitored entries. Nineteenth-century poorhouses often housed the indigent along with those deemed insane; this still occurs. Some poor were also viewed as insane. Back hallways, without direct exits, were there especially to prevent these residents from escaping. Life was strictly controlled and opportunities for release were few; this is no longer the case.

today's standards. Often referred to as cold water flats, this housing was characterized by communal toilets or outhouses and cold running water, either in the building, usually one tap per floor, or from a well. Outhouses and well water were the norm in small towns and villages. Apartment units in larger cities provided basic plumbing and sometimes also heat, but access for the poor was primarily through social housing projects for those who qualified (Hollingshead & Redlich, 1953). Demand for indoor plumbing and amenities such as running hot water led to the demolition of those basic—but affordable—units. The result was less housing at increasingly unmanageable rents. Many people, especially immigrants, coped by doubling up and living in overcrowded rental units. People dependent on public assistance, including those whose mental illness prevented them from working full time, could not pay the high rents and often could not live independently without some support. Beginning in the 1970s and stretching into current times, the serious increase in illegal drug use combined with the alcoholism of many marginal low-income persons swelled the ranks of those who can't afford housing. The result has been an ever-increasing number of people seeking refuge in homeless shelters, the twentieth-century version of the poorhouse. We now turn to a quick look at the numbers, and at how poor people can't pay the rent and meet other expenses.

Housing Affordability

Housing is first and foremost a problem of affordability. High rents and low income are two basic partners in reducing the availability of affordable housing.

There are many factors that contribute to this situation, among them

- lack of adequate employment income because of low wages,
- lack of specific skills,
- inability to afford child care,
- low government income support for those with physical and/or mental health and behavioral problems,
- escalating housing costs in areas where jobs are most plentiful, and
- little investment in low-income housing by either the government or the private sector.

A commonly accepted income standard is the one-third rule that no more than 30 percent to 33 percent of one's monthly income should be required for housing either for a mortgage or rent (see appendix 1). The average monthly rent in the United States in 2013 was $1,062 and in Canada $901. Large cities such as New York, Vancouver, Toronto, Chicago, Baltimore, Los Angeles, or Montreal have considerably higher average rents. Using the one-third rule, an individual would need an income of $3,300 a month (before taxes) to afford an average apartment in the United States. Working full time (thirty-five hours a week), a person would have to earn more than $22 an hour in order to afford to rent typical housing. These rates may change over time but the relative proportion of income spent on housing will continue to escalate unless governments take active steps to increase affordability.

Minimum wage laws in Canada and the United States differ in that American federal law governs minimum wages but states may elect to set minimum wages above the federal rates. Employers must comply with both federal and state laws. In Canada rates are set by provincial governments. While these rates are beginning to be increased in both countries, the change has been slow. The comparison of minimum wages in Canada and the United States (table 6.1) shows that a person making a minimum wage earns from one-third to less than one-half of the income needed to pay a reasonable proportion of income for her rent. In the major cities a person working for minimum wage can't afford even a single room. This situation is forecast to worsen as the income gap between the lowest wage earners and the highest continues to grow in both Canada and the United States.

People disabled by physical illness or persistent mental disorders receive disability benefits. In the United States, rates and eligibilities are set by

Table 6.1. Minimum Wages in the United States and Canada, 2014

	Federal	State/Province
United States	$7.25/hour	Most follow federal regulations. Where there is a rate difference between the federal and state laws, the higher rate prevails.
		Rates are for nonexempt employees and are lower for those who receive tips.
		Five states have no minimum wage, and the federal rate applies.
		Five have minimum wages below the federal rate.
		Twenty-two have minimum wages above the federal rate (range $7.40 to $9.32).
Canada	Does not set rates	Provinces range from $10.00 in New Brunswick to $11.00 in Ontario

federal social security benefits through SSI (supplemental security income) at $8,412 annually ($701 per month). Most states supplement this amount, and thus the benefit levels vary across the country. Alaska, for example, provides a monthly supplement of $530 per person. Government disability assistance in Canada is set provincially and ranges by province from a low of $8,665 in New Brunswick to a high of $18,402 in the Yukon. In Ontario, Canada's largest province, a person on disability would receive $12,900, or $1,075 per month. Nowhere is a single person with disabilities able to afford market rental housing. Without a rent subsidy a person with disabilities is priced out of housing and is forced into the shelter system. Without a well-identified disability that qualifies a person for disability subsidies, a single individual is qualified only for public assistance (sometimes known as social assistance or welfare), which in all cases is considerably less than income received by those with disabilities. Having children makes the situation worse because extra housing costs for more bedrooms, child-care costs, and other expenses eat away at the monthly allowance. The result is the same for all those dependent on government assistance, for whatever reason: market-level rental housing is unaffordable.

> **Textbox 6.2. Disability Supplements Vary by Region**
> The range of disability benefits in Canada takes into account the higher cost of living in northern and remote locations such as the Yukon and Nunavut. In the United States disability benefits provided by the federal government are supplemented to different degrees by each state, with some considerably more generous than others.

How do people with low-wage jobs, or who are unable to work full time, pay for their housing? Many of these people would qualify for government assistance to pay their rent. This help can come in various forms. Some arrangements are strictly through government funding and others are a combination of government, nonprofit, and private arrangements:

- Government-owned housing where the city, province, or state owns the building and charges rent equal to one-third of a tenant's income. This is often referred to as public housing.
- Housing owned by a private landlord where the government pays a subsidy directly to the landlord.
- A housing voucher provided to an individual or family by the government, which can be used to find housing in a set price range. The government then pays the landlord directly.
- Some organizations that house persons who are physically or mentally or emotionally challenged may own housing and receive government subsidies for tenants.
- Some nonprofit organizations who help to house persons with physical and mental or emotional disabilities may act as the broker or middle person with a landlord in signing a lease and ensuring that the tenant will be a responsible resident.
- Some home-ownership opportunities are provided by programs such as Habitat for Humanity where volunteers and potential homeowners buy low-income housing with sweat equity and an affordable mortgage.

Housing Vulnerability for Low-Income Persons

For the low-income wage earner, who most often works in jobs with little or no sick leave benefits, any illness that prevents the individual from working results in lost income. Low-income workers are usually only one paycheck from homelessness. Lack of savings and no umbrella of family support

> **Textbox 6.3. Habitat for Humanity**
>
> Habitat for Humanity is an international movement founded in the United States. It provides low-income people with an opportunity to work in partnership with volunteers to help build and own an affordable home of their own.
>
> http://www.habitat.org

can result in failure to pay utilities, which often results in electricity and gas being shut off, and ultimately to housing loss. Reconnection fees, in addition to hefty security deposits, may leave people with a roof but no heat, functional cooking stove, or water.

While not true for all, many people who hold low-income jobs may face additional challenges. Lack of education and basic literacy, including financial literacy skills, can trap people in poverty and low-income employment; basic household budgeting may be beyond their ability or experience. For immigrants, lack of language skills and local educational qualifications often means that they end up in low-wage jobs. They may lack familiarity with credit cards, reasonable interest rates on this type of financing, and local customs for time-based payments. While it is important not to generalize, some people, because of the presence of disabling symptoms due to a mental disorder, the impulsivity of certain personality types, or the impulsivity frequently associated with those who have FASD, find it difficult or impossible to hold on to their money and will spend it immediately regardless of the long-term consequences. When the rent money is gone before it is due, people are extremely vulnerable to losing housing, while at the same time they are unable to save for the necessary deposit to get rehoused. Rehousing for people who have accumulated unpaid rental and utility debts is one of the leading challenges in rapid housing and rehousing.

Housing Assistance: A Comparison of Two Countries

Although Canada and the United States have many similar programs and social policies, the two countries have had markedly different approaches to providing housing assistance to low-income and vulnerable people. Table 6.2 provides a brief comparison of the two.

Challenges for People Who Receive Rental Assistance

When the landlord is a public entity—such as a city, town, or nonprofit organization—there is generally no security deposit for the rent. This may

Table 6.2. Differences in Housing Assistance in the United States and Canada

United States	Canada
In the midst of the Great Depression of the 1930s the federal government became actively involved in supporting the development of affordable housing. Over the years, the provision of low-income housing became an established part of the federal housing initiative. Today, HUD is the lead agency that supplies funding and housing initiatives in a variety of forms, including specially built low-income housing as well as housing subsidies for those who seek market rental units. A focus on chronic homelessness resulted in the establishment of the Interagency Council on Homelessness. HUD now encompasses eighteen different agencies focused on housing. Two major federal legislative initiatives have focused on provision of housing and supports for homeless persons: the McKinney-Vento Homeless Assistance Act (1987) and the Homeless Emergency Assistance and Rapid Transition to Housing (HEARTH) Act 2009. Together they represent a substantial investment by the federal government in addressing the problems of homelessness. HUD programs have responded to a variety of housing and homeless issues and have recently changed titles, descriptions, and scope of some programs. While there are other specialized programs, current major HUD initiatives include the following: • Continuum of care programs aim to rapidly rehouse individuals and families. • Rural Housing Stability Assistance programs focus on counties with populations of less than 5,000. • Emergency solutions grants programs fund street outreach, emergency shelter, homeless prevention, rapid rehousing, and homeless management information systems. • A special program focuses on housing for veterans (HUD–Veterans Affairs Supportive Housing). • The Title V Program provides unused, underused, and excess federal properties as facilities that help house homeless people. • As housing programs in the United States respond to changing circumstances, you are advised to regularly check for changes and updates in these programs. (HUD, 2014)	The political responsibility for housing in Canada has historically been shared between federal and provincial governments. Through the latter half of the twentieth century, Canadian housing initiatives concentrated in policy and practice, on providing adequate housing for low-income Canadians, and on those in crisis. Following World War II the federal government's initiatives ensured affordable mortgages, investments in social housing (as government-built and -operated units are called), and subsidies for development of low-rent housing (Gaetz, 2010). In the last part of the past century federal investment in housing lagged and much responsibility was shifted to the provinces. For over twenty years, social housing in Canada was a neglected stepchild of federal initiatives and many provincial efforts. In the mid-1980s the federal government cut back on social housing programs. In 1982 development of all social housing at all levels was reported at 20,450 units annually. By 2006 this rate was 4,393 housing units (Shapcott, 2008). Provincial response to these cutbacks was uneven, with some provinces such as Ontario developing a Ministry of Housing and making a commitment to include all low-income persons, regardless of disability, as eligible for social housing. Other provinces, such as Alberta, provided no designated funds for capital development or ongoing housing support, and only minimal funds for rental supplements. This led to a homeless crisis in the 1990s when a number of dynamics converged: the reduction in the development of new social housing units (rent-supplemented) over the previous fifteen years had led to reduced availability; population increase meant that the supply of social housing could not keep up with demand; in a growing economy rental incomes soared; and many low-income and disabled persons found themselves priced out of the affordable (private and low-cost) housing market (Gaetz, 2010). Canada became the only G-8 country without a national housing policy. The results of the economic and population dynamics on the rental housing sector were the erosion of available housing for low-income people and a huge increase in poverty and homelessness.

Table 6.2. (Continued)

United States	Canada
	In response to political pressure to address the homeless issues in major cities, since 1999 the federal and provincial government response has been the funding of locally guided housing projects under the National Homeless Initiative, now called the Homeless Partnering Strategy. The approach has been to fund local community action committees to develop local responses to the need for low-income housing. The response also has led to the creation of large shelters for the homeless, with lack of attention to permanent housing needs. Some provinces and major cities have begun to develop their own approaches to helping low-income and homeless persons. The only province that did not abandon its commitment to subsidize housing costs for low-income and disabled individuals was Quebec. There, social housing continued to be developed and financial supports remained available. Throughout most of the country, local responsibility for housing has been influenced by provincial supports, or lack thereof, with most cities reluctant to supply anything other than acutely needed emergency shelters, primarily for homeless individuals. The net result is an uneven distribution of housing programs and resources across the country.
	However, Canada still lacks a formal national housing strategy and sufficient financial resources to deal with an increasing homeless population.

not be the case for utilities. For people on fixed income and receiving government assistance, even a housing subsidy does not allow for much spending flexibility, and luxuries are unaffordable. Most have to budget carefully to make ends meet. The most important priority is to pay the rent and utilities each month and then manage as best as possible with the remaining funds. Not being able to pay the rent is the major reason why people lose their housing. Not all cities and provinces protect a tenant from rapid eviction, and failure to pay the rent may result in the landlord putting furniture on the street curb. If the rent is not paid, depending on local laws, the tenant(s) may be evicted in thirty days or less.

In all Canadian provinces, a residential tenancy act regulates such matters. You can find these laws easily on the Internet for each province. In the

United States most states model their evictions laws on either the Uniform Residential Landlord and Tenant Residency Act or the Model Residential Landlord-Tenant Code. These codes are often supplemented at a local (county and municipal) level. Leases between landlords and tenants may further specify eviction practices but may not contravene local regulations (in both countries).

Another dilemma results for the person who has been evicted. The unpaid rent is considered an outstanding debt. Until it is paid, the person (or family) is not eligible to get housing from this specific landlord. The same applies to payment of gas, electricity, and water in many locations. If the landlord is a private business, negotiations of long-term repayment and some debt forgiveness are sometimes possible. If the landlord is a public entity—such as one under municipal direction—legal restriction may not allow the debt to be forgiven, even if it is ten, fifteen, or twenty years old. For a senior who suddenly has a drop in income, or an individual who develops long-term physical disabilities and now needs subsidized housing, this may be a crisis. Such legal and financial entanglements often make it difficult to impossible to rehouse a person or family unless a private social services organization or a religious group such as a local congregation steps in to help.

Textbox 6.4. Eviction Prevention Efforts

Some municipalities and provinces have rent tribunals or ombudsmen that will hear eviction appeals before a landlord can legally evict a tenant. However, these intermediaries are not nationwide; in some parts of the country people can be evicted in as little as two weeks for failure to pay rent on time. Rental tribunals are particularly lacking in small towns and rural areas.

Traditional Subsidized Housing Models

Subsidized housing is most often referred to as public or social housing. Most of these housing units are in larger cities and consist of apartments in buildings constructed for this purpose (low-income housing). Free-standing houses were occasionally available in small towns. However, the gap between those eligible and the available subsidized housing units has always been so great that in most North American cities the waiting time from application until occupancy could stretch ten years. Low-income families with two adult caregivers (in the United States most often required to be married to each other) could expect an even longer wait because they received lower priority in most instances. Single persons, regardless of sex, were generally not eligible unless they had a defined disability. Their recourse had traditionally been marginal housing in SROs. With gentrification of downtown areas around railroad stations, SROs began to be replaced by upscale apartments and the poor lost the only housing not government owned or funded that was affordable on a meager income.

> **Textbox 6.5. Public Housing**
>
> Public housing is owned by the government, federal, state, province, county, or municipality. It is rent controlled, and people eligible for residency must meet low-income guidelines. "Social housing" is a wider term, used more often in Canada and Europe, to describe rental housing that is income controlled and owned by the government or private nonprofit organizations, or a combination of the two.

Housing as part of a live-in treatment program has been a part of many residential substance-abuse programs, but these programs are usually short term and make no provision for longer tenure. Some residential treatment programs for those addicted to heroin and other hard drugs have had residential living for up to a year in facilities called therapeutic treatment communities. Beyond these intensive treatment programs, rehabilitation does not include subsidized housing. Those who are alcohol and drug dependent have few options after discharge from these programs. Supported and subsidized housing for those recovering from substance abuse are rare, despite the fact that many former substance-dependent persons lack the training and skills for competitive employment and thus the ability to afford market rental housing. In contrast, residences for those recovering from mental illnesses, as explained later in this chapter, were gradually developed as an alternative to residential institutions. Unfortunately, the availability of these units has also always been far less than needed. This reality of the lack of supply of subsidized and supported housing well below what is necessary to meet the need for those disabled by a mental disorder is quietly suppressed by governments that fail to make any reasonable assessment of housing need for this vulnerable group.

Specialized Housing Programs for Persons Recovering from a Mental Illness

The presence of a serious and persistent mental illness is extensive among homeless people, but less so than previously reported. Because those affected are most often disabled to the extent that they can't retain full-time, permanent employment, they are also unable to secure market rental housing. Their resulting poverty places them among many who cannot afford housing. Because they usually have multiple needs, the issues that they have require extra attention. The following provides an indication of the scope of this issue and some of its origins.

- Early studies on the prevalence of homelessness among those with a serious mental illness reported rates ranging from 5 percent to over 78 percent. More recent work has examined these data and recent studies consistently report lower rates than earlier reports suggested (Montgomery, Metraux, & Culhane, 2013). The first studies failed to include consideration that homeless persons with mental disorders are overrepresented among the poor and in minority groups (Folsom et al., 2005). They also examined those with mental illness among the homeless but failed to look at how many of those with a diagnosed mental disorder in a given community were among the homeless. Finally, some areas, such as Calgary, report rises in homelessness as the economy surges, primarily due to lack of affordable housing for low-income workers and not those who are mentally ill (Calgary Homeless Foundation, 2009).

- The myth that the homeless are primarily those with a mental disorder has been severely challenged by recent work.

- Before the 1960s most people with a severe or disabling mental illness were placed in public mental health institutions. Often the placement was involuntary and the process of release was long, protracted, and not favorable for the patient. These psychiatric hospitals became warehouses for some of the most disabled members of society (Torrey, 1988). Several factors resulted in a massive change in both Canada and the United States. For one, overcrowding in deteriorating facilities built one hundred years earlier led to a political rebellion against the inhumanity of long-term placement in large dehumanizing institutions (Grob, 1994).

- Development of the first psychotropic medicines that effectively reduced the most serious and disabling of psychotic symptoms provided a new ability for many previously hospitalized people to live outside of institutional care.

- The enactment of laws that narrow the circumstances under which a person could be involuntarily hospitalized greatly reduces involuntary hospitalizations.
- A large study of over 10,000 people with persistent mental illness reported a homeless rate of 15 percent (Folsom et al., 2005).
- Research suggests that the prevalence of mental disorders and substance-abuse disorders among homeless populations varies across geographic regions and major cities and may be dependent on changing social and economic environments (Montgomery et al., 2013).

> **Textbox 6.6. Asylums of the Nineteenth and Twentieth Centuries**
>
> One example of a historic asylum is that of Buffalo (New York) State Asylum for the Insane (1880–1974), which served at any one time more than 1,200 psychiatric patients in eleven buildings connected by a main administration building (figure 6.3). Men and women were housed by level of severity of their condition and on opposite sides of the complex. This was a typical arrangement for the vast majority of such institutions. Today it is known as the H.H. Richardson Complex and is a national historic landmark.

The change of automatic institutionalization of the mentally ill began as a trickle in the late 1960s and turned to a flood within a decade. People who formerly would have been admitted and retained in a psychiatric hospital for years now received treatment in local hospitals and mental health clinics or the original psychiatric institutions, and then were returned to the community. This massive shifting of care away from large, long-term care institutions to short stays in local facilities, with an emphasis on keeping people in the community, was termed "deinstitutionalization."

The major problem with this movement was not its intent to keep people close to home in a least restrictive environment. Rather, it was the failure of local and provincial (Canadian) and state (United States) governments to provide adequate community-based treatment facilities and continuing supports for those previously institutionalized. Many of those discharged from psychiatric institutions had no home or family to return to, either because of death or because the family had long ago ceased to care and be involved. There was a lack of knowledge about how much independent functioning these recently discharged people could manage, and there were no appropriate community housing facilities that could accommodate them. Moreover, there were no effective mechanisms to determine what kind and how

Figure 6.3. Buffalo (New York) State Asylum for the Insane

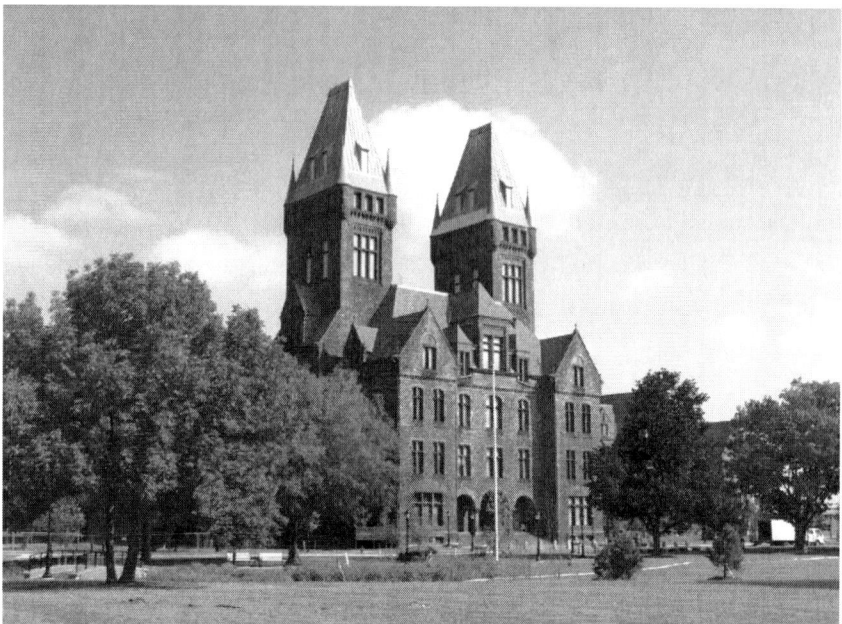

much support (housing, finances, daily living skills) these people needed. For many their entire adult lives had been spent in environments where they were told when and where to eat, sleep, bathe, exercise, and recreate. They had no skills to live on their own. Although they might not have been actively psychotic, they were unable to cope with a competitive, fast-paced society that had developed while they were institutionalized (Torrey, 1988).

Textbox 6.7. Life in the Asylum

In *Nowhere to Go*, Torrey describes the plight of the mentally ill as a result of the emptying of the psychiatric institutions throughout North America (Torrey, 1988). For another excellent and realistic view of life inside the insane asylum, watch the classic movie *One Flew Over the Cuckoo's Nest* (1975).

When these institutions were emptied, local response was to place these individuals in large boarding homes and nursing homes. For younger persons, group homes, compared to college housing, were developed in many localities. The institution–community interface was conceptualized as a continuum of care (COC). The expectation was that people recovering from a mental illness would pass through successive stages and types of accommodation (from institutional living to permanent supportive housing). The COC model grew to include, in addition to group homes and boarding homes, community residences, dedicated apartment buildings, and scatter-site supervised apartments. At each stage clients needed to demonstrate housing readiness that generally included demonstration of competence in personal care; activities of daily living skills such as cooking, cleaning, and household management; sobriety (no use of alcohol or drugs); and compliance with psychiatric treatment (Brown, 2005).

The COC model of care has received a lot of criticism. Many consumers (as those with a significant mental illness prefer to call themselves) and their significant others (family and friends) see this model of housing as one that embodies both treatment and housing and is extremely coercive (Jack & Robert, 2012). It has, these critics maintain, imposed treatment compliance as a necessity for those seeking independent living. In this way, institutional demands have been transplanted in the community, creating another form of conditional support. This restrictive housing approach also served another, hidden, purpose: there has never been sufficient social or government-assisted housing in either Canada or the United States to deal with the needs of large groups of people who are both vulnerable and poor. Thus, restrictions on those who qualified for housing reduced the visibility of those who needed it since a person did not count as needing housing until he was ready. A second function was to provide jobs for those who used to work in psychiatric hospitals. This need was created by deinstitutionalization. These huge institutions of three thousand to five thousand patients were staffed by scores of mental health aides and support staff who belonged to strong trade unions. Most of those jobs were protected even if the patient load was reduced to virtually zero. The state (or province) had to pay these salaries while trying to establish community facilities for the former patients. Clearly, the government could not afford to keep paying the enormous salary costs of institutional workers who increasingly had little to do, and at the same time establish outpatient services. The solution was to establish government-supported boarding and rooming houses and transfer these inpatient workers into the community. Subsequently their jobs could be (and were) reclassified and eliminated as necessary.

This same model of housing plus treatment (behavioral compliance) was quickly adopted by other groups seeking to help vulnerable populations. Those recovering from substance abuse or dependence were seen as needing a protracted period of living in a sober house in order not to disrupt a fragile sobriety. Women fleeing domestic violence were seen as requiring a host of household management and, where children were present, childcare education. Implicit in this view was that those who lost their housing were in some way deficient in their abilities to live independently. This view is a legacy of the Poor Laws in England on which much of the Canadian and American social assistance programs are built. The Poor Laws assumed that there was a functional, and often moral, deficiency in those who find themselves penniless, homeless, and at the mercy of the state (Trattner, 2007). The Poor Laws also mandated that assistance to the indigent should be in local poorhouses and that outdoor relief, meaning assistance in a person's home by way of food and clothing should be minimized or avoided. The "worthy poor," meaning primarily women, children, and widows, were given priority in any outdoor relief when it was made available.

While in some instances the assumptions of skill deficiencies in the poor and homeless were valid, the primary problem with these models of care for the poor was the presumption of problems with independent living. That is, no one who was vulnerable and identified as high need (also implying high risk) could be given independent housing before she proved she was ready. This continuum from institutional life to independent living is illustrated in figure 6.4. It is also important to point out that most of this housing plus treatment expectation was imposed on the poor. Middle- and upper-class individuals who had private means could choose where and how to live when a mental illness, domestic violence, or substance abuse led to broken marriages and/or lack of housing. Mentally ill persons could usually count on their financially well-off family to provide shelter and daily necessities unless their behavior had caused disruption of positive relationships.

In contrast to the COC model of housing entitlement, a harm reduction approach has been implemented in some locations for persons with both a mental illness and a substance abuse or substance dependence diagnosis. Referred to in the mental health services literature in the United States as the "dually diagnosed," these individuals were hard to house, refused the COC model of treatment compliance, and often wound up homeless. The Toronto model, developed by a program called House Link, provides housing with support services and no requirements for absolute sobriety for

Figure 6.4. The Continuum of Care Process

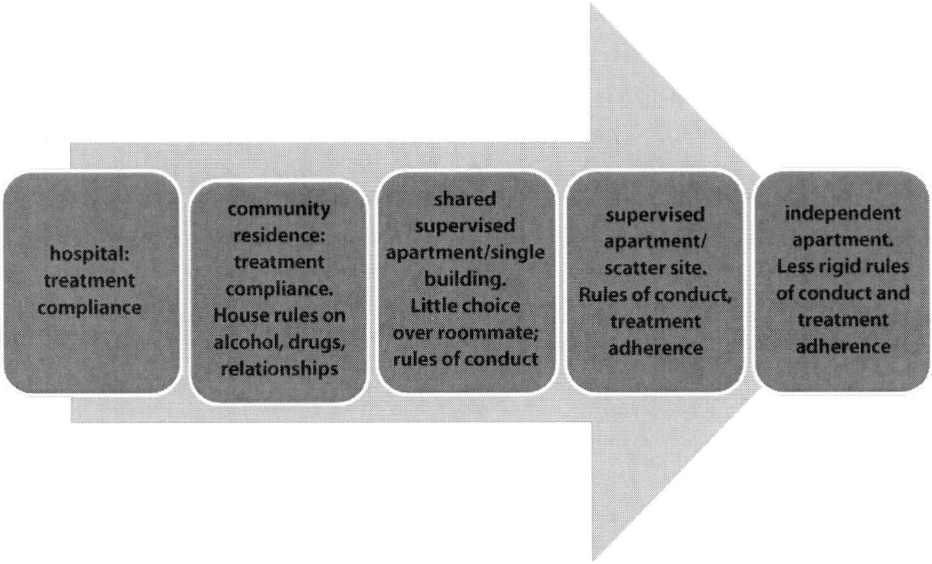

| hospital: treatment compliance | community residence: treatment compliance. House rules on alcohol, drugs, relationships | shared supervised apartment/single building. Little choice over roommate; rules of conduct | supervised apartment/ scatter site. Rules of conduct, treatment adherence | independent apartment. Less rigid rules of conduct and treatment adherence |

those with a serious mental illness and has a five-year housing retention rate of 94 percent. It has also promoted member/tenant involvement as employees in the operation of the organization (Waegemakers Schiff & Schiff, 2014). The New York City model, Pathways to Housing, has received considerable attention for promoting a *housing first* approach to helping this very vulnerable and special needs population (Tsemberis, 1999). A 2004 report of the Pathways to Housing program demonstrated that nearly 80 percent of people in the Pathways Housing First program remained housed five years later (Tsemberis, Gulcur, & Nakae, 2004). People with mental health and addiction issues do very well with a *housing first* approach and spend fewer days in the hospital; these interventions are less expensive to support. This conclusion is finding support from a national study of the Pathways Housing First model that was conducted by the Mental Health Commission of Canada (2012).

HOUSING FIRST: A HOUSING PHILOSOPHY AND A PROGRAM MODEL

There is general agreement on defining the overall concept of Housing First: it is a strategy for rapidly providing housing and at the same time building in support services that continue well after the housing has been secured (National Alliance to End Homelessness, 2011). When examining the various Housing First programs currently in operation, what becomes apparent is that, despite agreement on the overall concept or philosophy, there is a wide variation in how that concept is operationalized. In other words, different organizations and governments vary in their application of key program components and, consequently, there are numerous and different programs that all claim to employ the *housing first* approach. We have encountered extremely varied application of the *housing first* label, including substance-abuse programs that require sobriety before housing and domestic violence shelters that insist on communal living or designated apartment buildings for clients. There is a need to identify the various ways in which this term is currently used and to suggest ways in which it can be conceptually distinguished in order to determine in what context evidence-based practice exists with various populations of homeless persons.

Housing first is an approach to ending homelessness that offers homeless people a place to live with the support services needed in order for them to maintain that housing (National Alliance to End Homelessness, 2012). Table 6.3 details the basic elements of this approach. The assumption is that all people have the right to housing and it is not something a person must earn by demonstrating good behavior or proper citizenship. The difference between the *housing first* approach and traditional efforts at housing

Table 6.3. Basic Elements of a Housing First Program

Treatment Philosophy	Housing Criteria
An assertive community treatment team or an intensive case management team.	Clients have a choice in housing location: no expectations to live in a specific area or building.
Program philosophy includes a harm reduction approach.	Housing is located in scatter-site private housing.
There are no treatment contingencies attached to housing; clients do not need to be in treatment or adhere to prescribed treatment protocols.	Housing is affordable, with no more than one-third of total income devoted to housing and utilities.
Prospective tenants do not have to demonstrate housing readiness.	Housing tenure is permanent (no provisions for limited occupancy as in provisional or temporary units).
Program uses a motivational interviewing approach.	Clients have a choice about living alone or with others.

homeless people is this: The traditional shelter model is conditional on certain behavioral requirements, whereas the Housing First model is not. In the traditional homeless shelter model, a person can earn the right to move from a shelter bed to transitional housing, and then to permanency. In the COC model, a person must be compliant with agency and staff protocol before she is able to be placed in an independent apartment. Some people have recycled through this system for years, often at great expense to themselves as well as to society.

In contrast, in the *housing first* approach the goal is immediate stabilization of housing in order to prevent the development of additional problems and to avoid the reoccurrence of homelessness. Agencies using the *housing first* approach live by the mantra, "Never homeless again." Support services are individualized and often intensive. They may also be long term. Clients are offered support services, which they can reject or accept without a program condition placed on their housing. The most frequent reason for housing loss in Housing First programs is because a person fails to be a good neighbor or tenant. Drug dealing, having too many strangers couch surfing, or extra roommates moving in without invitation are frequent reasons for eviction. Research has shown that keeping someone homeless will incur system costs of $100,000 or more per year (Perlman & Parvensky, 2006). Thus it is cost effective to provide appropriate housing and supports to persons experiencing homelessness compared with traditional homeless shelter and institutional responses. Evidence is now proving that this model provides a much healthier solution for clients and is much less costly over the long term than traditional shelters (Goering et al., 2014).

As a program model, Housing First was developed by Pathways to Housing, and has a number of components that are considered essential to effective operation. These components are based on the premise that clients have both a serious psychiatric disability and a substance-use disorder. This continuum consists of homelessness to housing with ACT support (table 6.3) (Tsemberis, 2010).

The national study of the Housing First program model (figure 6.5), conducted by the Mental Health Commission of Canada in five large cities, has substantiated the Pathways findings that this approach is effective, as will be further discussed in chapter 9, for seriously mentally ill persons with co-occurring disorders (Goering et al., 2014). However, it also found that there were local variations in how the models could be successfully implemented

Figure 6.5. Housing First Continuum

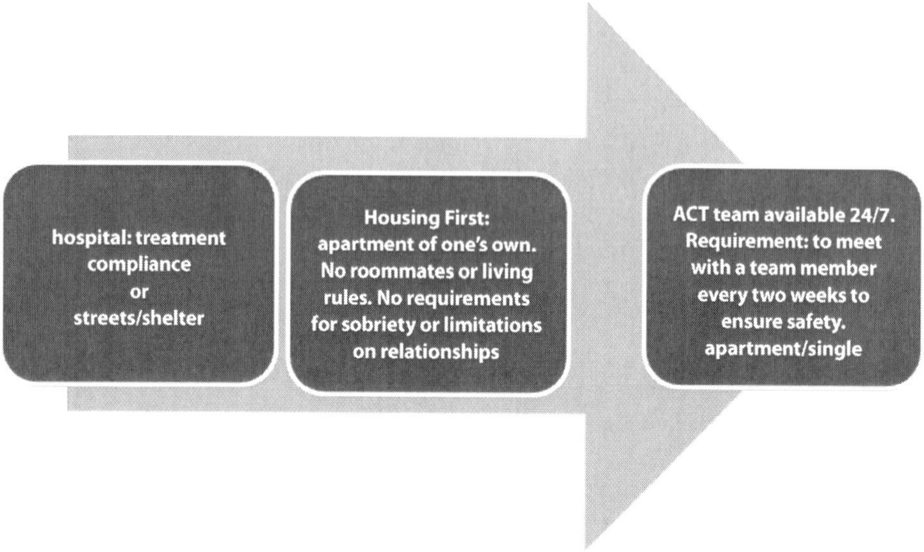

[hospital: treatment compliance or streets/shelter] → [Housing First: apartment of one's own. No roommates or living rules. No requirements for sobriety or limitations on relationships] → [ACT team available 24/7. Requirement: to meet with a team member every two weeks to ensure safety. apartment/single]

in different cities (Mental Health Commission of Canada, 2012). Finally, we note that the Housing First model has been examined for a specific group of homeless persons. At this time, there is no substantive evidence that all aspects of this program model can be applied to other groups of individuals such as those with substance-abuse problems, ex-offenders coming out of prison, emancipated adolescents fleeing domestic violence, victims of domestic violence who have dependent children, or persons from other cultures that have communal living orientations.

So what is special about Housing First? It is a radical departure from those programs that insisted on treatment compliance, sobriety, and demonstration of housing readiness because it states that "everyone has a right to housing" *before* all other issues are addressed. This type of program does not insist that a person be clean and sober (of alcohol and drugs). It does not demand that a person be in mental health or addiction treatment, or compliant with taking medication. Usually each person signs his own lease and thus is a tenant in his own housing unit. No staff person has the right of entry without prior notice and consent (thus there are no house inspections). There are two important requirements: (1) that a participant/tenant agree to meet regularly with a case manager so that important issues related to tenancy can be addressed and services can be offered, and (2) that the participant/tenant make arrangements for automatic payment of rent from any income before accessing the balance. This provision is meant to ensure that, regardless of other life circumstances, rent and utilities are paid. In the next section we take a closer look at what a Housing First model entails.

Housing First Program Components

There are several key factors that are basic to a Housing First program. They consist of elements of program structure, services, and philosophy. These are interwoven, and are based on principles of self-determination, empowerment, and choice. Important to this program philosophy is that lack of coercion is a fundamental component of all services and participant interactions. This translates to two central themes of Housing First:

1. Each person has a right to housing and the right to self-determination. The client/tenant is in control.
2. Recovery from mental illness and addiction is an individual process that begins once the client/tenant is safe and has obtained secure housing, and not before.

One of the principles of the Housing First model is that choice is an important component in housing location, furnishing, decoration, and other physical features. Program support staff work with their clients to ensure that they have the opportunity to select what will work best for them in their recovery. Choice includes realistic options based on the following:

- Affordability
- Privacy (not having to share living, dining, kitchen, and bathroom spaces)
- Location (not in areas perceived as dangerous by the participant)
- Anonymity (not in large congregate buildings designed for the handicapped)

- Permanency (not time-limited, such as found in transitional housing programs)
- Tenancy based on local land and tenant legislation, not agency rules
- The participant determines who can enter the housing unit and when, including agency staff. The only person with a key to the unit is the tenant.
- Use of unprescribed mind- and mood-altering substances is not prohibited, but a harm reduction approach is used.
- Instrumental supports such as ready access to services are offered at each visit. Supports are independent of both the right to housing and the housing location.
- While staff will help a person acquire basic household necessities, no one is forced to accept or use any item that is not personally acceptable to that person.

Textbox 6.8. Principles of Harm Reduction

Harm reduction is based on the following principles:

(1) There will always be a group of people who will engage in high-risk behavior (e.g., people who misuse alcohol or other drugs, have more than one sex partner at the same time, do not use condoms, or smoke).

(2) Harm reduction focuses on reducing or minimizing the harm associated with higher-risk behavior, such as the adverse health, social, and economic consequences.

(3) Harm reduction can complement, or be an alternative to, abstinence-based policy and programming.

As we noted in the definition of *housing first* above, an overarching feature of the *housing first* approach is the separation of treatment and services from housing. This concept has two components. In Housing First programs the participants/tenants are not required to be abstinent from alcohol or drugs to qualify for housing, and they are not expected to be in a treatment program or to be compliant with treatment recommendations. The second component is that any support services that are available are offered at a location separate from the housing itself—that is, they are not in the same building or location. Thus, housing and treatment do not fall under the same umbrella, although they may be parts of different programs in the same agency. One important exception to the "no requirements for housing" rule is that all participants/tenants must have a case manager and meet with that person regularly. This is to ensure that individuals are safe and have basic living needs of food, safety, and medical care met. There are no rules that people must be involved in specific services beyond involvement with the support of a case manager.

The Culture of Housing First

Although the use of support services is not required, support service availability has several key components:

- The array of support services offered
- The availability of support 24/7
- The composition of the support team
- The program philosophy and staff attitudes toward tenants and services provided

The last is undoubtedly the most critical component because it sets the tone for all of the other items. It may be understood as a variation of organizational culture, and thus a factor that permeates all aspects of the organization. Those who are receiving services from a Housing First program are called participants and not clients. This very deliberately sets the stage for service recipients to be regarded as central to the activities that are involved in getting and retaining housing. A basic value of Housing First programs is that the participant is the center of all decisions regarding program engagement and service planning. This leads to the fundamental principle of choice over the acceptance of any or all services available. It also means that participants have the right to refuse psychiatric or substance-abuse treatment. Choice is also based on a harm-reduction philosophy that emphasizes minimizing the risks associated with substance use and accepts the fact that some persons will not be able to totally eliminate use. This concept will be explored in greater depth in chapter 8 on addictions. Choice also implies that no one can be coerced into treatment through the threat of withholding housing or other benefits.

Textbox 6.9. Harm Reduction Strategies

Existing harm reduction strategies include the following:
- Needle and syringe exchange programs
- Public smoking restrictions
- Methadone maintenance programs
- Education and outreach programs
- Condom distribution programs
- Safer graduations and proms
- Designated driver programs
- Sex education for teens

Textbox 6.10. Organizational Culture in Housing First Programs

Organizational culture has been talked about in many business environments and has come to be seen as an important aspect of delivering human services. This concept consists of the values, attitudes, and beliefs that people in an organization jointly share and espouse, and that these in turn shape the way services are offered and the acceptability of those services to participants. The organizational culture of a Housing First program should include valuing employment of peers (persons with lived experiences) where at all possible, recovery where mental health consumers are involved, collegial teamwork, and emphasis on the importance of empowerment for staff and clients.

The essential values of a Housing First program are thus the following:

- Housing is a fundamental right.
- Participants have a right to self-determination.
- Participants are empowered to make their own decisions regarding housing type, location, and range of support services that are acceptable.
- Harm reduction, not abstinence, is the focus of substance use and treatment refusal.
- All services are based on the concept of recovery as a realistic goal.

The program also adheres to the following guidelines:

- Service recipients are participants.

- The participant is the center of services.
- Participants have a choice in what type and frequency of services they accept.
- Services are delivered by a multiprofessional team of persons that includes social workers, nurses, a physician and/or psychiatrist, and occupational and vocational counselors.
- Harm reduction accepts the importance of lowering the type and frequency of harmful behaviors as the participant indicates readiness.
- Refusal of services does not lead to housing loss.
- The array of program-delivered services includes case management; instrumental housing supports; medical services, including physical and mental health; addiction services based on a motivational counseling approach; social and vocational activities; and supported employment.

The Assertive Community Treatment Team or the Intensive Case Management Team: An Essential Aspect of Housing First Programs

A Housing First program is usually staffed by an ACT team, or an intensive case management team. Inclusion of this team is based on the original model demonstrated to help very vulnerable persons with long histories of absolute homelessness, ongoing symptoms of a mental illness, and substance abuse that interfere with recovery (Tsemberis, 2010). Programs that house a less-vulnerable and less-fragile group of people may not find it necessary to provide intensive round-the-clock services. However, there is no research to support exactly what level of need is optimal for certain groups of people such as homeless families or women fleeing domestic violence. We describe here the ACT model because it is most commonly associated with keeping people housed and out of the hospital. Intensive case management teams may be envisioned as a less intensive level of the same service components.

ACT teams have been used in community programs since 1976, when they were introduced by Test and Stein, as a means to keep de-institutionalized persons from being rehospitalized. These teams consist of groups of mental health professionals from various backgrounds (social work, nursing, medicine, psychology, addictions, community rehabilitation, occupational therapy, and vocational therapy) who provide round-the-clock community-based services (Test & Stein, 1976). These services may be provided in an ACT office or another location of the client's choosing. ACT team members provide in-home, not just office-based, support visits. In fact, service is available to the client at a location of his choosing. Services include

- medical assistance, including psychiatric consultation and follow up;
- psychosocial and substance-abuse counseling; and
- support and linkage to a variety of services.

This linkage is real and visible in that service providers will accompany clients to appointments to ensure that a referral is made effectively. Services are client centered and not time limited. They include outreach, family engagement and support, and employment support. ACT teams have been highly successful and are deemed a best practice for persons recovering from a mental illness. They support and enhance an individual's connection to and engagement in the community, and they help family members to understand and provide support through active psychoeducation programs.

Textbox 6.11. Psychoeducation

Psychoeducation is the provision of information building and skill building around the symptoms, treatment, impact, and effects of a mental disorder and how best to help persons affected by a serious mental disorder. Students of psychoeducation programs and groups can be mental health consumers or family members.

Is Housing First the Appropriate Way to Provide Housing for All Vulnerable Persons?

The evidence for the effectiveness of a *housing first* approach for housing stability has been demonstrated by a citywide randomized clinical trial that rehoused mentally ill homeless substance abusers in New York City (Tsemberis et al., 2004). In Canada, a national study on housing persons with a mental illness was conducted by the Mental Health Commission of Canada (Goering et al., 2014). Within a Canadian context, the acceptability and accessibility of housing that is culturally and ethnically suitable, as well as housing that is appropriate for families, youths, and seniors, is of utmost importance. This Canadian multicity study of Housing First programs for the mentally ill and dually diagnosed took ethnicity, age, degree of psychosocial impairment, need for supports, and other distinguishing characteristics into account in the process of recruiting study participants. The study specifically targeted immigrants at one study site and Aboriginal (First Nations) participants at another site, and distinguished between moderate and high needs participants at all sites. The effectiveness of *housing first* approaches with various groups of those with a major mental illness in differing regions has been demonstrated to provide positive and promising results (Goering et al., 2014).

Some research suggests that housing readiness—that is, the COC model—rather than Housing First models may be most appropriate for persons with a history of conflict with the law and addiction problems (Currie, 2004; Kraus, 2001; Roman, 2009; Zorzi et al., 2006). A review of housing models and approaches for other populations concluded that the efficacy of Housing First models has not been proven for those dealing with addiction or criminal justice issues (Stefancic et al., 2012). However, current efforts to link mental health and justice-involved clients to a *housing first* approach are showing considerable effectiveness in some cities.

A review of housing preferences for a group of Aboriginal women under drug court supervision found that all participants supported transitional housing (COC approach) models combined with a range of appropriate supports and services (Schiff & Waegemakers Schiff, 2010). Housing readiness programs can play a critical role in stabilizing the lives of many homeless women as it is intended to provide one or more intermediary stages between crisis and permanent independent housing. Emergency shelters provide basic needs for a short period. Transitional housing may be available as a drug-free house for women only (without dependents) offered for three months to two years (Barrow & Zimmer, 1998), and often includes services aimed at treatment and training for vocational and life skills. The premise of the congregate settings of many transitional housing models is to provide opportunities for individuals to learn or relearn those skills for daily independent living while at the same time being involved with treatment and rehabilitation services, some of which are offered on site. Research shows that those who gain permanent housing after transitional housing are likely to remain stably housed (Rog, McCombs-Thornton, Gilbert-Mongelli, Brito, & Holupka, 1995).

While proponents of a "go slow" approach argue that disadvantaged women and youths need more structure and thus often favor housing readiness interventions, some organizations are trying a *housing first* approach with youths who are homeless or aging out of the child welfare system, as well as with women fleeing domestic violence, and with some substance abusers. There is no definitive answer to what works best for these groups of people struggling to find and maintain housing. Perhaps the best answer lies in the extent to which an ACT team approach can be used as a community support and integration mechanism. One fact is undeniable: having a home of one's own is more humane, just, empowering, and cost-effective.

The Housing First model consists of finding appropriate housing facilities for an individual or family based on the United Nations Charter of Rights, which states that housing is a right. The model is employed for hard-to-house people who have been diagnosed with major mental health problems and a substance-abuse addiction. Support services are voluntary but contact with a worker is mandatory. With stable housing and ancillary support services individuals are more prepared to engage in personal healing (treatment compliance and reduction of substance misuse). The research on housing for persons with mental illness supports a Housing First model to meet the needs of most persons disabled by a mental disorder. The evidence strongly indicates that this model is associated with housing stability and tenure, but there is no strong evidence that it is equally applicable to other groups of homeless persons.

Getting and Keeping Housing

Depending on the size of your community, there may be several or many different organizations involved in keeping vulnerable people housed and preventing them from losing their housing. Some, such as local welfare offices, provide rent and utility support, although this is most often less than required for some rental units. Food banks may help with food, and voluntary agencies may have emergency funds to help with rent and utilities for someone who has suddenly become ill or disabled or who has lost her job. Others may help with child care, senior care, or assistance for those with disabilities. It is the worker's first responsibility to know what resources

> **Textbox 6.12. The Conundrum of Extended Families**
>
> An important consideration that is often overlooked in sheltering families is what to do in the case of extended families who live together. This may include a parent, adult sibling of one of the parents, aunt, or cousin who may have been living with the family for a variety of reasons. This situation is more frequently encountered in Aboriginal (American Indian) families and those from other ethnic backgrounds where extended families are integral to their lifestyles and efforts made to rapidly rehouse them need to include those beyond the nuclear family. Parents may live with children or grandchildren, especially in African American, Aboriginal (First Nations), Hispanic, and Middle Eastern and Asian ethnic communities. Families live together. An adult sibling who is disabled may be part of the family. To split up this supportive unit causes more short-term damage than to leave the family intact. Families should have consistent access to the shelter for one to four weeks while intensive efforts are made to find the most optimum living arrangement for each member and communal living preferences are considered.

there are in the community, who the contact people are, and how most quickly to contact them. These contacts are often critical to getting immediate assistance that keeps people from losing their housing. Thus knowing the key people is critical, but not enough. Keeping housing and rapid rehousing are often dependent on the extent to which a worker is able to develop positive, personal connections with these gatekeepers of resources.

WHAT ABOUT LANDLORDS?

There is a lack of extensive knowledge about the positive and negative experiences that landlords have with their formerly homeless tenants. In the past, the landlords of subsidized housing buildings were most often bureaucrats in departments of local governments, with the exception of those in the private rental market who accepted housing vouchers. As the use of housing rental subsidies has expanded, private landlords have come to be more significant partners in housing poor and homeless persons. Civil servants were constrained by government budgets in how to use rental income for property maintenance. Private landlords are caught between building maintenance and investment profit. Beyond this simple economic factor lie other important considerations.

Landlords vary in the extent to which they value provision of socially important services to society. Those who are driven by social values also see the importance of maintaining stable tenants who look after their homes and have a sense of pride in their surroundings. Economically this makes for good business as there is always a cost with tenant turnover, including additional maintenance and, frequently, unpaid rents that cannot be recovered. At the same time, landlords need to have support of local housing agencies whose staff can be instrumental in dealing with landlord-tenant disputes and addressing issues where tenants are in violation of rental agreements (Kloos, Zimmerman, Scrimenti, & Crusto, 2002).

Failure to pay rent is not always the most common problem faced by landlords. They also have to address problems that arise when tenants deal drugs from their homes, and when they fail to supervise children and adolescents who create disturbances in common areas. Noise and overcrowding become additional issues when tenants allow extended family and friends to move in. Some tenants have hoarding behaviors, which can lead to unsanitary and hazardous housing conditions. Finally, some tenants lack basic cleanliness and organization habits, leading to unsafe living situations. An example of this is the tenant who frequents places known to be infested with bedbugs, and then imports these vermin into the apartment building. It becomes a landlord's (expensive) problem to get rid of the bedbugs. How often is it realistic to expect a landlord to deal with this recurrent problem from the same tenant?

Dealing with Evictions

Evictions and abandonment of housing can occur for various reasons. While failure to pay rent and maintain utilities is a frequent occurrence, common among those recently rehoused is the nuisance created by people who know a recently rehoused person and move in, with or without invitation. Known in some areas as takeovers, these doubling-up and couch-surfing occupancies create noise and traffic, and often violate rental agreements. Those who are drug-involved often find that people crash a party and do not leave, or set up a dealing operation. Violations of this type can lead to police involvement and immediate eviction. This poses additional challenges for workers trying to help with housing stability. If the person is absolutely homeless and has no money for shelter, the first steps to rehousing should be the following (see also figure 6.6).

1. Arrange for emergency shelter (and food) with family, friends, a hotel, or homeless shelter.
2. Assess for immediate and complicating issues (see figure 6.6) that led to housing loss or that may be a barrier to rehousing.
3. Determine income available and need for housing subsidy.
4. Develop a list of priorities for obtaining housing and the persons responsible for each identified step in the process.
5. Identify any significant barriers to rapid rehousing.
6. Set timelines for addressing each issue.

If the person is at high risk for losing housing, there are a number of strategies that should be implemented. Figure 6.6 illustrates the various steps that are involved.

1. Determine the reason for the impending loss and if it can be averted with supports (i.e., rent in arrears, utility cut-off, job loss).
2. Try to negotiate with utility company, landlord, and so on, or attempt emergency housing voucher with local welfare department of a social service agency.
3. Determine if health violations can be quickly remedied or if a move is inevitable.
4. Seek a delay of eviction so that interim housing can be found.
5. As a last resource, contact the local emergency housing (shelter or hostel) to alert staff to an impending homeless situation (table 6.4).

RETAINING HOUSING

There are numerous reasons why someone loses their housing. Keeping housing once a person has been placed in a home of one's own is sometimes an old challenge and sometimes a new challenge, depending on what led to

Figure 6.6. Housing Lost

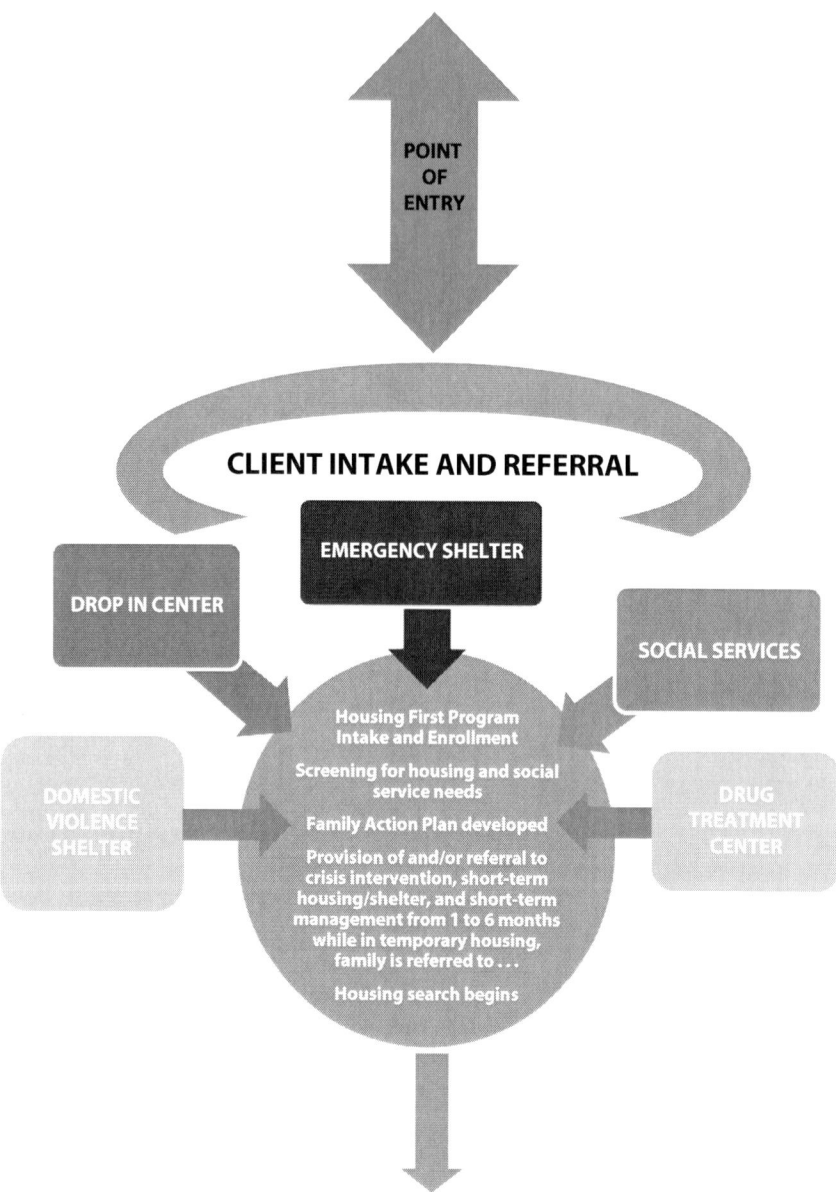

Housing First Approaches and Housing First Programs

Person or family moves to permanent housing

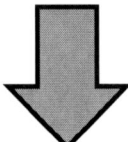

• Tenant education	• Child abuse and neglect: intervention and prevention
• Household management	• Child care resources
• Money management	• Child care subsidies
• "Survival Skills" counseling	• Basic medical care
• Welfare advocacy	• Job readiness program
• Legal advocacy	• Career counseling
• Family and individual counseling	• Job training and placement
• Liaison with schools	• Basic remedial education
• Parenting education	• English language classes
• Health/nutrition counseling	• Substance abuse prevention
• Address children's special needs	

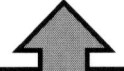

Family integrated into community, attaining improved social and economic well-being

Table 6.4. Housing Needs Assessment: Imminent Risk or Recent Housing Loss

Issue(s)	Assistance: Responsible Agency/ Person	Action(s)	Timelines	Outcome(s)
Immediate Issues				
Rent arrears				
Eviction notice				
Utilities cut-off				
Utilities threat of cut-off				
Job loss: no income				
Income earner disabled				
Death of income earner/recipient				
Housing unsuitable/ health risk				
Housing slated for demolition				
Other				
Complicating Issues				
Rent arrears of more than one month				
Chronic health or mental health issues of individual or a family member				
History of domestic violence				
Hospitalization of a family member				
Addiction issues a. Reported b. Acknowledged				

Table 6.4. (Continued)

Issue(s)	Assistance: Responsible Agency/ Person	Action(s)	Timelines	Outcome(s)
Multiple young children				
Several generations in one dwelling unit				
Previous difficulties in balancing budget				
Child welfare involvement				
Family member(s) with physical or mental handicaps				
Justice system involvement				
Family pet (dog, cat, other)				
Other				

the housing loss. In any event, the support worker needs to map out an action plan with the individual or family that includes the following:

Challenges

- Financial issues from loss of income through firing, illness, layoff, or reduction in work hours
- Financial issues from unplanned expenses: illness, death in the family, extra child care, automobile repairs, fire, theft
- Reduction in spendable income due to addictions: alcohol, drugs, or gambling
- Money management skills on a tight and limited budget: spending patterns, access to economical food if there are specific dietary requirements, and access to appropriate, weather sensitive clothing

- Psychological and emotional conflicts and crises, including those involving mental health, addictions recovery, disabilities in self, partner, or dependent children

Assets

- Stable positive relationship with another adult
- Supportive friends
- Stable income
- Spiritual connections and beliefs
- Talents, hobbies, recreational interests or pursuits
- Good physical health
- Coping skills and resiliency

Prevailing wisdom from service providers suggests that support services be in place and available for at least twelve months after move-in. In some cases, depending on multiple challenges, rehoused persons may need support for a prolonged period—several years or even a lifetime—if handicapping conditions make independence conditional on instrumental supports. Slipping through the cracks and the resulting homelessness is most likely to occur in those instances where supports were not identified or provided in a timely manner. One of the challenges in modern society will be to establish a program of extended housing supports for those who would otherwise become homeless again.

Homelessness is not a new phenomenon. It has existed in various forms for thousands of years. The primary cause of homelessness is lack of adequate income to afford housing and food. Personal difficulties such as mental health problems, lack of adequate education and job training, as well as an unstable childhood contribute to the problem of affording and keeping housing. In the twentieth century rampant drug abuse and gambling joined the age-old difficulties of alcoholism in preventing a sizable cohort of adults from holding jobs and keeping stable housing. Lack of housing is a fundamental problem but also creates and aggravates problems of physical and mental health, adequate child rearing, and self-esteem and challenges the spiritual component of hope, belief in the goodwill of others, and a positive connection to the world. Without adequate supports a formerly homeless person will continue to struggle for stability, which is the prime reason why housing begins with a roof over one's head.

EXERCISES

Since housing is the first and foremost aim in homeless programs, and since this approach is so challenging, we have provided a number of activities that you can do alone or in small groups to help build practice skills for frontline work.

A Low-Income Budget for a Family of Four: Can You Balance Their Budget?

Welfare check $1,991
Rent
Utilities (heat, electricity, phone, cable)
Food
Clothes/laundry
Transportation (private vehicle or public transport), bus fare or gas, automobile insurance and maintenance (this is a critical issue for those in rural areas)
School fees, child care, etc.
Animal food and care (see chapter 3 on the role and importance of pets)
Miscellaneous (incidental expenses)

Case Examples

Alone or in groups, read each case and identify the reasons for and against recommending a *housing first* placement for each person. Which of your reasons are based on opinion and which are based on evidence-based practices? Is there any additional information that you need before helping these people to get an apartment of their own?

Using figure 6.6 in this chapter trace the path to rehousing. Apply the service assessment in table 6.4 to determine the action plan needed to ensure housing success. Once placement is made, what would be the immediate and long-term goals? What might be the challenges?

Case Examples

1. Steve was the one in high school voted most likely to succeed. He was smart and accomplished, and had lots of friends. He started his own business but it failed during a downturn in the economy. After that he was unable to find steady work and soon lost his apartment. Now forty years old, he says, "It is pretty hard to go into a job interview carrying a sleeping bag and a knapsack." He has tried several times to get a job or retraining but something always happens to undermine his efforts. He is proud that he does not use drugs or alcohol but it is getting harder and harder to not give in to the temptation. Steve is well liked by most of the service providers but has felt bullied by the service provider at the shelter where he lives. This person is the one who is in charge of assigning beds each night and sometimes Steve does not get one. He feels as if he is being discriminated against but he does not understand why.

2. Edith and Sam are in their early fifties and have been married for twenty-eight years, with no children. They moved to the city shortly after getting married and have survived on low-income jobs all of their lives. They became homeless when their landlord sold out to developers. They have not been able to afford rent for the past five years and have managed to survive by having Edith sleep in a shelter to be safer, while Sam sleeps in a car, except when the weather is too cold, when he goes to a men's shelter. There are no shelters in town that will let both of them be together. They both work as much as they can, mostly at minimum wage jobs. All they want is to be together.

3. Nineteen-year-old Gayle was kicked out of her home when she was fourteen. She used to use drugs but is proud that she has been clean for almost two years. She has hopes for the new life that she wants to start soon. She thinks getting her high school equivalency credential might help. She lives with an older man who she describes as a "good guy." She has few supports. This relationship is physically and emotionally abusive but Gayle feels it at least protects her from excessive street violence. She also believes that, for her, there are no other options. She wants to upgrade her education but is not interested in addressing any other issues. She says, "Everything is cool." Gayle is very secretive and evasive about her past and current life situation, saying, "Really not much to tell."

JOURNALING

1. Most people have their own opinions on whether a person should be offered a place to live through a Housing First program. What did you think before reading this chapter? Did the information in this chapter change any of your thoughts or opinions?
2. Would you knowingly move into an apartment that has a *housing first* person living in the same building? On the same floor? Why and why not?
3. Are there any of the people in the case examples that you would not want as a neighbor? Why?

CHAPTER 7

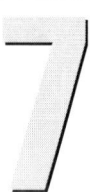

Mental Health and Mental Disorders (Illness)

KEY ISSUES
- Mental disorders and housing insecurity
- Attitudes toward the mentally ill
- Stigma
- Signs and symptoms of mental disorders
- Overview of mood, psychotic, anxiety, and behavioral disorders
- Introduction to the *Diagnostic and Statistical Manual of Mental Disorders* (DSM-5) and *International Classification of Diseases* (ICD-10)
- Impact of medical conditions on mental health, and impact of mental health on medical conditions
- Overview of explanatory causes for the development of a mental disorder
- Intervention strategies

OVERVIEW

WHO describes mental health as "not just the absence of mental disorder. It is defined as a state of well-being in which every individual realizes his or her own potential, can cope with the normal stresses of life, can work productively and fruitfully, and is able to make a contribution to her or his community" (WHO, 2007).

"Mental health" is a frequently misapplied term; most references to mental health are actually intended to address issues of mental disorder. WHO uses the term "mental disorders," and describes them as "a broad range of problems, with different symptoms. However, they are generally characterized by some combination of abnormal thoughts, emotions, behaviour and relationships with others" (WHO, n.d.). The terminology that hides mental illness under the term "mental health" arose from the stigma associated with mental illness, and the mental hygiene movement of the early 1920s in the United States. Using the term "mental *health*" made the topic more socially acceptable. As the WHO statement clarifies, mental health and mental disorders are parts of a continuum of well-being. We recognize that being homeless already impacts the mental well-being of those affected. It may also cause or increase mental disorders. Because the term "mental illness" will be most familiar with most readers, we will continue to use this term, along with the term "mental disorders," interchangeably. In the following pages we look at the end of the continuum that deals with mental disorders, and their associated difficulties in daily functioning.

What is traditionally referred to as mental health problems are those disturbances of mind, mood, and behavior that interfere with an individual's ability to handle the stressors of daily life, or to handle the responsibilities of work, education, and social relationships that are the usual part of a person's life. This chapter and the following provide an overview of the mental, emotional, and behavioral indicators of serious mental health disorders and those produced by substance use. We look briefly at outpatient mental health and addiction programs usually available for treatment and rehabilitation (for those disorders that cause some impairment) and treatment interventions used. We explore frontline approaches to working with persons with chronic disorders and those in acute distress, and introduce major mental illness and addictive diagnoses as described in the American Psychiatric Association's *Diagnostic and Statistical Manual of Mental Disorders*, fifth edition (2013; DSM-5), so that workers are familiar with the terminology and what it implies. Mental health and substance abuse (misuse) are frequent co-occurring disorders among homeless persons.

The intent of this discussion is to make you familiar with the different behaviors that are often encountered in working with homeless and near-homeless persons. In some cases the mental health or substance-use problems began before the individual lost housing or arrived at the edge of housing loss. In other situations those problems began after the loss of housing. Life on the streets is very stressful and dangerous. Even couch surfing comes with greater-than-average dangers: acquaintances may victimize the persons seeking a place to stay. It is therefore not surprising that a great majority of homeless persons have been victims of violence, abuse, and trauma that exacerbate mental health problems. We hope that this and the following chapter make you familiar with different ways that mental health and addiction issues are displayed by homeless persons.

There is a range of mental health problems and addiction issues commonly experienced by persons who are homeless and those who are extremely marginally housed and thus highly vulnerable to homelessness. It is important to recognize that while many of these problems result from risk factors for homelessness (Tutty et al. 2009), many, if not most, also result from the stressors of being homeless. Research has shown that, once housed, persons with a mental disorder and addiction problem are likely to report a decrease in mental, behavioral, and addictive problems (WHO, 2007). This chapter presents the major features of these problems and some preliminary ways of interacting with those exhibiting distressing behavior in public. It is not intended to create any diagnostic proficiency—that is, you are not expected to know all of the disorders and their criteria for purposes of diagnosis. We expect that your awareness of when problem behaviors may be linked to mental health or addiction problems will allow you to seek appropriate intervention from psychiatric professionals.

How Are Housing and Mental Health Problems Linked?

In chapter 6 on housing, we described the links between mental illness and housing instability. Here we examine in more detail the aspects of mental disorders that contribute to housing insecurity. Housing is central to successful community living. Individuals with serious mental health problems and illnesses frequently identify income and housing as the most important factors in achieving and maintaining their health. For all people, housing is a stabilizing force in everyday life that forms the foundation on which a person can establish a daily routine and begin to address other life issues. However, low incomes, stigma, and difficulties in daily functioning inherent to serious mental illness, including fluctuations in symptoms, can impact people so that they cannot compete for market rental housing or gain entry to scarce supportive housing units. Consequently, many live in substandard accommodations that are physically inadequate, crowded, noisy, and located in undesirable neighborhoods. Lack of choice in house type and location frequently leads to housing instability and loss of residence. This in turn leads to an increase in anxiety and other symptoms of mental health problems. The challenge of providing stable housing options for persons with severe and persistent mental disorders is reflected in the frequent housing loss in this population that is directly attributable to lack of affordable housing and acknowledges consumer preferences, support services, the presence of a mechanism to ensure rent is paid in a timely fashion, and an established eviction prevention initiative in the event of imminent housing loss.

Most persons at some point in their lives experience some mental health concerns. Often it is the result of personal, occupational, and family or school stress and resolves itself, but at other times it does not. Prevalence studies indicate that throughout northern North America one in five persons will, at some time in his life, experience signs and symptoms serious enough to be diagnosable as a mental disorder. In some, professional help becomes necessary. For a few, the illness results in a mental health disability (WHO, 2007). Of those afflicted, some become homeless because of the illness and/or inability to work, lack of social supports, and inability to afford housing and food. It is important to understand that mental disorders happen to people of all ages, social status, income, and education. Homelessness, especially for those who have a mental disorder, results when family and social structures are inadequate to provide supports during times of extreme stress and disability.

> **Textbox 7.1. Quick Facts on Mental Illnesses**
>
> **Some Quick Facts**
>
> One person in five in northern North American will have a mental health problem during his or her lifetime. This means that, given 20014 population rates, in Canada more than 6 million people, and in the United States more than 63.4 million people will have a lifetime experience with a serious mental disorder.
>
> - One in seven Canadians aged fifteen and older (about 3.5 million people) has an alcohol-related problem; one in twenty (about 1.5 million) has cannabis-related concerns; and some have problems with cocaine, speed, ecstasy, other hallucinogens, heroin, and other illegal drugs.
> - Mental health and substance-use problems affect people of all ages, education, income levels, religions, cultures, and types of jobs.
> - It is likely that you or a family member or friend will have a substance-use or mental health problem at some time in your life, or in his or her lifetime.

Common Misunderstandings

- *Misunderstanding:* Persons who are involuntarily admitted to a psychiatric facility do not retain all civil rights. (This is a legal and human rights/civil rights issue.)
  Comment: This is partially true. Those in psychiatric facilities do not necessarily retain the right to vote if they are deemed incompetent by the courts.

- *Misunderstanding:* By law, there are separate treatment systems for adults, children, and adolescents with mental health and addictive disorders.
  Comment: Technically there is no law in either the United States or Canada that limits services for mental health to specific age groups. In practice, child and adolescent mental health services are provided by specially designated clinics and residential treatment centers.

- *Misunderstanding:* Recovery in serious mental disorders consists primarily of symptom management. (This is a recovery issue.)
  Comment: This is a contentious issue. Many people who are recovering assert that the process of recovery is one that allows each person to achieve her potential regardless of continuing symptoms or impairments.

- *Misunderstanding:* Psychological tests are the most common way in which a person receives a psychiatric diagnosis. (This is a pathways to diagnosis issue.)
  Comment: Most diagnoses are provisionally made at intake, whether in a hospital emergency room or an outpatient clinic. Testing is not the routine route to establishing a diagnosis, although it can be invaluable in complex situations.

- *Misunderstanding:* Members of the treatment team are trained to understand each other's roles and responsibilities. (This is an interprofessional practice issue.)
  Comment: Most mental health professionals have had no training in interprofessional practice.

- *Misunderstanding:* More than 75 percent of persons with a serious mental illness abuse drugs. (This is an impact of drugs and alcohol issue.)

Comment: Fewer than half of all people with a mental illness have a co-occurring substance-use problem. Rates are somewhat higher in the homeless population.

All of these misunderstandings are part of the problems, prejudice, and bias that accompany the stigma facing persons with a mental disorder. We first need to examine what this stigma is all about because it often becomes the lens through which these disorders are viewed.

The Origins of Mental Health and Addictive Disorders

There are different explanations of what causes mental and behavioral disorders, extending from theories of nature (it is all in the genes), to nurture (how we are raised), to the environment as the cause (toxic substances and unsafe living environments such as homelessness). We briefly describe some of these causative factors, and look at examples of a vast literature in this area.

The Role of Biology and Genetics There is a considerable body of research that documents the role that biological factors and heredity contribute as significant causes in a number of disorders. Both genetic and neuroimaging studies point to the role that biology and heredity play in the development and treatment of mental disorders and addictions. The extent to which hereditary factors affect the development of mental health and substance-use disorders has been widely studied. Some disorders have a distinct genetic component, and with other disorders the evidence is less clear. A newer field of epigenetics points to the roles that environmental and biological processes have on the ways in which genes are activated or silenced. This adds a further complication by suggesting that epigenetic mechanisms act as gateways to full gene activation.

Prenatal Influences The influences of alcohol and tobacco on fetal development have been well documented. Viral illness, toxic environments, and maternal mental health all contribute to early childhood health and development.

Early Developmental Influences The literature on children's mental health has abundant examples of the influences parenting, nutrition, illnesses, childhood abuse, neglect, and trauma have on the development of mental disorders and substance-use disorders. Equally important is the concurrent risk these factors have for homelessness in adults.

Influences of Personal Characteristics and Interpersonal Relationships Concepts of resiliency and protective factors are associated with social ties. Peer influences to drink or use drugs are also powerful factors in using or abstaining. The extent to which a person is drawn to social relationships will affect the willingness to accept sober peer contacts. This in part contributes to the impact of Alcoholics Anonymous (AA) and its affiliates Narcotics Anonymous and Al-Anon (to help the families of addicts). Recently, bullying has also come under public scrutiny as a significant factor affecting child and adolescent mental health, coping, and substance-use behavior.

Environmental Influences These include both the physical and the psychosocial environment. In addition to well-documented parental influences, the social and cultural context of the country and the environment, from big city to small town and rural settings, all influence the safety and health of children and adults.

Abuse of Alcohol and Drugs Mental health problems, as previously discussed, may lead to self-medicated substance abuse. Alternatively, some substances such as amphetamines, cannabis, peyote, PCP, and so on may precipitate temporary psychosis, depression, mania, and psychosis, among others. Whether this results in a permanent mental disorder is under investigation (Weaver, Renton, Stimson, & Tyrer, 1999).

Trauma and Abuse Childhood physical and sexual abuse is widely recognized as a significant factor in the development of mental illness and addictions in adolescents and adults. In addition, the traumas caused by war, natural disasters, and violence are all now recognized as significant contributors to depressive, anxiety, and substance-abuse disorders (Mojtabai, 2011).

Socioeconomic Influences Socioeconomic influences are recognized as contributors to mental disorders. Most professionals now accept the view of multicausation in many disorders. Some influences are greater with specific disorders such as depression, where there is a strong familial pattern and bipolar disorder that has a strong hereditary link. However, usually no one factor is exclusively responsible for a specific disorder. One important consideration is the role that early childhood experiences have. There is a strong body of evidence that people from lower socioeconomic backgrounds who are more likely to experience deprived childhoods and abusive parenting are more likely to develop a mental health problem or substance-use disorder (Montgomery et al., 2013).

STIGMA

The lens through which we view others has considerable impact on the way we interpret their behavior and our acceptance of them as persons in our lives. After leprosy was largely brought under control in our society, even though it retained its fearsome associations, mental illness became the most feared and stigmatized condition that people could contact or encounter (Link, Struening, Neese-Todd, Asmussen, & Phelan, 2001). It is only recently that as a society we have begun to tackle this prejudice through education and bringing the realities of a mental disorder into the lives of everyone. One of the biggest obstacles that people with mental health problems or addictive behavior face is that of stigma. We will explore what stigma means and provide exercises to explore your attitudes toward those with a mental illness or an addiction. Many readings on mental health talk about stigma after discussing mental disorders. We reverse this order of presentation. There are several exercises at the end of this chapter that we encourage you to take the time to work through before continuing to read the following material, as this will provide a richer understanding of the pernicious and pervasive aspects of stigma. We suggest this in the belief that you will understand the following information in different ways once you have become sensitive to your own possible biases of stigma affecting those with a mental disorder.

In mental health, the term "stigma" has a specific connotation. Stigma consists of the negative attitudes and the discriminatory behaviors that people have toward those with a mental illness, and self-stigma refers to the process by which people with a mental disorder see themselves with the same negative labels (Herman, 1992). Like all prejudices, stigma begins with false information and fear of the unknown. Although mental illness, formerly called madness or insanity, has been found in all cultures since the beginning of recorded history, it was once viewed with suspicion, uncertainty, and irrational fear. The socially abnormal behavior and thoughts of those who are mentally ill have historically been associated with rash, violent, and heinous acts. The reality that most persons with a mental disorder are victims rather than instigators of violence has only recently been demonstrated. In the absence of knowledge of mental illness, most people adopted negative attitudes that discriminated against the mentally ill and have kept them from easily rejoining society. Added to that is the double dilemma of self-stigma: that is, many of those with a mental disorder also have negative self-concepts.

Because the language that historically has been used to describe the mentally ill has been, for the most part, negative and stigmatizing, we have deliberately tried to avoid negative terms that are associated with a mental disorder. Thus we do not refer to "schizophrenics" because this brings up negative images not found in most persons with a psychotic illness. Likewise, the term "people with mental illness" suggests that these problems are constant and lifelong. In fact, many disorders are one-time occurrences, or have intermittent flare-ups of symptoms interspersed with long periods of normal behavior. And yes, people do recover from mental illness. It is thus important for all of us to learn what these mental disorders look like and how to respectfully treat someone who may be having an acute episode.

Stigma is a damaging and pervasive issue that keeps many people in the closet about their emotional struggles. It prevents those with a serious mental illness from being accepted in the workplace (Rosenthal, Hellerstein, & Miner, 1992) and having workplace accommodations when their symptoms become disabling, which they might do at times. It creates the fear of being found out, and being socially ostracized. Thus stigma hinders the road to recovery and casts a shadow over all those family members and acquaintances who know of the existence of mental illness in their midst.

Indications of Stigma

Stigma occurs because of lack of knowledge and prejudicial views of people different from ourselves, fear of contamination that somehow we will develop a mental disorder by association, lack of understanding of how people regain their health, and fear that a mental illness is a permanent problem. The erroneous ideas and judgments include these:

- People with mental health and addictive problems are not like the rest of us, and are not normal.

- They cause their own problems.
- They can get over their problems if they want to.
- They are more dangerous than the rest of us.
- They would rather receive welfare than work.
- They are not as smart as other people.
- They will pass on their illness to their children.

These attitudes result in discrimination and exclusionary behaviors such as

- excluding those with problems from social and recreational activities;
- refusing to hire or work with someone who has a history of mental illness;
- avoiding those with obvious problems from fear of danger or contamination;
- not wanting someone with a mental disorder as a relative through marriage; and
- not wanting a person with mental illness as a neighbor.

An examination of various behaviors and attitudes that contribute to stigma indicates that there are at least four, and potentially six, major components to stigma as it applies to those with a mental illness (Foucault, 1988). Most of these will resonate with many of you as they apply to common prejudices that have been widely reported. The most prominent is the perception of those with a mental illness as dangerous, and the resulting personal fear of harm associated with that perception. The popular press has reinforced this perception by reporting on a person's mental health problems even when they may not be relevant to the issue. Public perception of danger is thus falsely reinforced since most persons who have a mental illness are more likely to be a victim than a perpetrator of dangerous and criminal behavior (Link, Yang, Phelan, & Collins, 2004). A second area of stigma concerns itself with a person's willingness to interact with and help a person with a mental disorder. Many people also believe—erroneously—that an individual is responsible for his illness and that forcing a person into treatment is the solution to his errant behavior. Finally, feelings of empathy toward the struggles of the mentally ill compete with feelings of aggravation, irritability, and anger. All of these reactions suggest that the causes and effects of mental illness are not widely known, and that the extent to which it impacts every family and individual in society is seriously misunderstood. Furthermore, research suggests that the best education to address this ignorance is through personal contact with those who struggle with a mental disorder.

In order to become aware of your own attitudes and behaviors toward someone with a mental disorder, we suggest that you complete the Attribution Questionnaire (AQ-27) (Corrigan, Markowitz, Watson, Rowan, &, Kubiak, 2003) at the end of the chapter, which provides a brief vignette about Jean, a man with schizophrenia; it also explores a number of commonly held attitudes toward similar people. The AQ-27 was developed to address the stereotypes about people with mental illness. These attitudes that reflect the stereotypes mentioned above are:

1. Blame: thinking that people have control over and are responsible for their mental illness and related symptom.s
2. Anger: becoming irritated or annoyed because the people are to blame for their mental illness.
3. Pity: having sympathy because people are overcome by their illness.
4. Help: providing assistance to people with mental illness on the assumption that they cannot help themselves.
5. Danger: assuming that people with mental illness are not safe.
6. Fear: being frightened because people with mental illness are dangerous.
7. Avoidance: staying away from people with mental illness.
8. Segregation: sending people with mental illness to institutions or to jails away from their community.
9. Coercion: forcing people to participate in medication management or other treatments.

IDENTIFYING MENTAL HEALTH DISORDERS

Mental, emotional, and behavioral disorders are usually identified by noting abnormalities in how a person talks, thinks, reacts, expresses feelings, and takes care of her physical self, such as how she dresses herself and takes care of her own hygiene. We must keep in mind that cultural traditions influence all of these aspects of how a person presents herself, and thus it is important to remember the circumstances of each person before concluding that a specific aspect falls outside of commonly acceptable norms in our society. Some scholars criticize the whole process of labeling a set of behaviors and feelings as abnormal since this way of identifying mental illness is not universally accepted. Nonetheless, we commonly accept the fact that certain actions, feelings, and thoughts do constitute a mental illness. We first look at what is included in this emotional and behavioral array of experiences.

> **Textbox 7.2. Universality of Feelings**
>
> Behavior is socially determined and what is acceptable varies somewhat in different societies and cultures. However, there is general agreement about what people feel, including extremes of anxiety, depression, and distortions in cognition and perception.

Common Signs and Symptoms

Table 7.1 includes many of the common signs of mental and/or emotional disturbance (that can be observed) and symptoms (that are internal experiences reported by the individual). Some of these are overlapping, in that they may be both reported and/or observed by others, while a few symptoms rely primarily on the individual to self-report their presence. All mental health disorders have one or more of the features of mood, cognition, and behaviors that fall markedly outside of the norm of social behavior, cause distress or impairment, and can be classified according to the following main clinical features. These indications are broadly categorized as the following:

- Anxiety
- Depression; mood disorders, including bipolar disorder
- Thought and emotional processing disorders; psychosis such as schizophrenia
- Cognitive and organic disorders, e.g., dementia and Alzheimer's disease, TBI, FASD

Table 7.1. Common Signs and Symptoms

Signs (observable)	Symptoms (reported)
Sad or flat affect	Mood irritability
Isolation from family and/or peers	Preoccupation with death
Little or no eye contact	Lack of interest in activities**
Low energy*	Reduced appetite**
Increased sleep, decreased sleep, disrupted sleep pattern*	Lack of interest in participating in significant activities**
Inability to fall asleep or stay asleep*	Poor concentration and indecision**
Reduced need for sleep*	Sense of detachment from others
Feelings of hopelessness, worthlessness, or inappropriate guilt	Suicidal ideation
Frequent verbalizations of low self-esteem	Hypersensitivity to criticism, disapproval, or perceived signs of rejection by others
	Heightened anxiety
Psychomotor retardation, slowed responsiveness	Flighty thoughts**
High energy and restlessness	Hypervigilance**
Pressured speech	Hallucinations or delusions
Poor attention span and susceptibility to distraction	Consistently angry or resentful**
Negativistic, hostile, and defiant behavior toward most adults (in children and adolescents)	Avoidance of certain places or people for no logical reason
	Disturbances of perception (auditory, visual, or olfactory hallucinations)
Illogical forms of thought or speech	Inadequate control over sexual, aggressive, or frightening thoughts, feelings, or impulses (blatant fantasies or acting out)
Bizarre thought content	
Affect blunted, flat, or inappropriate	

Note: * = can also be a symptom; ** = can also be a sign.

- Addictive disorders
- Developmental disorders
- Disorders consisting of mixed mood, anxiety, and psychotic features, e.g., PTSD

Mental health disorders are not mutually exclusive, and there is considerable overlap among their signs and symptoms, as figure 7.1 illustrates. This means that there are times when even the best psychiatric experts cannot agree on what disorder a specific group of symptoms may represent, and it is why the business of diagnosis remains problematic. However, because medical illnesses need a diagnosis, usually for payment and data-gathering purposes, specific combinations of symptoms, and the extent to which they are present, are commonly used to assign diagnostic labels such as major depression, bipolar disorder, and schizophrenia. We will discuss these diagnostic labels in greater detail later in this chapter.

For most social services personnel who work with homeless people, it is more important to be aware of the common signs and symptoms of a mental disorder or impairment due to substance abuse. Most of the following signs and symptoms can be caused by a mental health condition or a substance-use problem (listed in table 7.1), or by the interplay of the two conditions. Sometimes the indicator is a cause and sometimes it is a result of the

Figure 7.1. Interplay of Signs and Symptoms

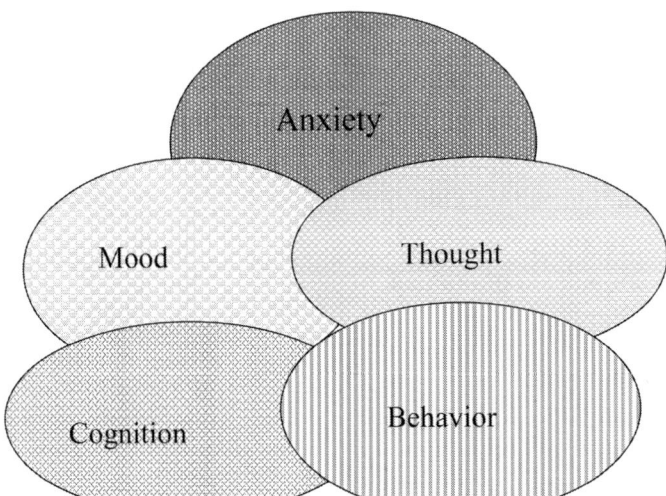

disorder. In chapter 8 we explore substance use and abuse, but caution that on the frontline it is frequently difficult to impossible to distinguish between a mental disorder and the effects of substances. For most frontline workers diagnosis is not a pressing concern but appropriate intervention is; the immediate concern is the recognition that something is wrong and that there is the need to respond quickly and appropriately.

It is important to recognize that some behaviors that may be abnormal in ordinary social settings are considered adaptive behaviors for a person who is homeless. For example, a person is initially judged by his appearance. Someone who lives on Main Street who looks unkempt may be having difficulty with self-care. The same unkempt person who is homeless may lack access to places to clean up and wash clothing. In the context of working with homeless persons, we have emphasized those signs and symptoms of a mental illness, when they may be the result of being homeless and not necessarily due to a mental disorder, by using italics to bring this to your attention. It is important that we do not make a specific issue such as personal appearance, a behavior, a mood, a feeling, or a way of looking at the world a sign of mental illness when it may be a response to being without a safe and secure place to live. In this light, some expressions of hopelessness, depression, and anxiety may be appropriate responses to a person's life circumstances, and may alleviate as those circumstances change. Nonetheless, the impact of these feelings on a person's ability to function may be pronounced.

> **Textbox 7.3. Signs and Symptoms**
>
> Mental health practitioners distinguish between *signs*, or behaviors that an outsider can readily observe, and *symptoms*, or internal feelings that a person reports but an outsider cannot as easily observe. Some mental health problems, such as anxiety, consist of both signs and symptoms. A person may report symptoms of feeling anxious, restless, and jittery, and be observed to be restless, jittery, and hypervigilant. Other symptoms, such as the cognitive distortions in psychosis, are not readily observable.

Appearance and Self-Care

The following are frequent indications of mental or emotional problems that can be observed and may be misunderstood or misinterpreted by those outside of the homeless sector. The italicized words caution you that a specific behavior may be explained as a result of being homeless.

- Does not take care of physical and oral hygiene *when the means to do so are available.*
- Does not take care of appearance or clothing *when the means to do so are available.*
- Does not eat enough, or overeats, *when adequate food is readily available.*
- Does not take care of household or personal possessions *when there is an appropriate and safe place to store them.*
- Does not attend to finances, insurance bills, vehicle, and so on. (Use with great caution. *This indication of a problem should be reserved for those who have adequate income and then fail to take care of these issues.*)
- Pays little or no attention to physical health and fails to seek health care even *when a local health clinic for homeless or low-income individuals is available.*

Thinking and Cognition

This is one important area where it is difficult to determine if the signs and symptoms are due to the influence of drugs or if the behaviors and thoughts are a combination of mental disorder and drug use. Since many persons who are absolutely homeless use substances, and since substance use is pervasive, even among those marginally housed, this is a critical consideration that we explore in chapter 8.

Difficulties in Thought and Thought Processing These are various ways in which an individual shows signs of cognitive difficulties. Information may be difficult to understand, may be misperceived, or experiences may be reported although there is no evidence of an external stimulus. Please remember that there is a distinction between those whose cognitive abilities are diminished because of developmental difficulties or brain damage, as contrasted with a mental disorder. The distinctions are not always readily observable. The following list presents many of the most common indications of cognitive difficulties. You should suspect cognitive difficulties when a person exhibits the following:

- Has difficulty in processing and remembering information.
- Processes information slowly and/or has to work hard to solve even simple problems. (Be careful that this is not due to developmental disabilities, English language problems, or lack of sleep.)
- Cannot think abstractly and is very concrete in language and how it is interpreted; for example, a person might think that a fire hall is a hall that is on fire.
- Has trouble concentrating.
- Is easily distracted.
- Is confused.
- Is unaware of day, week, month, or year. (This is also observed in those with a psychotic illness, but use with caution in those chronically homeless.)

Cognitive difficulties that may be due to psychosis will often include observations or reports of the following:

- False or odd perceptions or perceptual distortions such as claiming to be hearing loud sounds or seeing unusually bright colors when there are none. Another variation is when a person reports hearing colors and seeing sounds.
- Hears voices that are not attributable to external sounds.
- Experiences déjà vu, where new situations feel as if they were experienced before.
- Believes that TV, the radio, or public communications are sending hidden messages specifically to her.

Anxiety and depression can be disorders by themselves or they can be components of other disorders.

Symptoms of Anxiety and/or Depression A person self-reports or is observed as

- Tense and anxious (*beyond what would be expected under the circumstances, especially if someone has been sleeping rough*).

Mental Health and Mental Disorders (Illness) 215

- Hypervigilant, meaning very alert and on guard for no discernible reasons. (*This may be attributable to street culture.*)
- Excessively worried about daily events.
- Experiencing upsetting, intrusive memories or nightmares of past events. (*Check for history of trauma as this may be trauma related.*)
- Having intrusive thoughts of death or suicide.
- Unable to make decisions, concentrate, or follow through.
- Having guilty feelings over minor things.
- Having loss of interest and pleasure in most things. (*This may be adaptive to the dangers of the streets or illegal activities for subsistence. This may also be due to substance intoxication.*)
- Feeling worthless, hopeless, and helpless. (*This could be situational.*)

Signs: Observable Behaviors of Anxiety and/or Depression

- Is uncomfortable around people. (*This may depend on whether people are from the homeless or the Main Street culture, or whether they represent authority figures.*)
- Feels compelled to do ritualistic or repeated behaviors.
- Has decreased appetite and weight loss (*not due to lack of adequate, acceptable food*).
- Avoids normal activities such as taking the bus or grocery shopping. (*This may be the norm for some homeless persons.*)
- Has difficulty sleeping or interrupted sleep, or is sleeping too much. (*This may be due to street life and/or the problems with shelter accommodations.*)

Mania (Bipolar) Symptoms

Mania is frequently overlooked as a serious problem unless the behavior escalates out of control. Nonetheless, it can be disruptive and disabling, interfering with relationships and job performance. High levels of energy, rapid speech, and intense emotionality may warn the worker of a potential problem with mania. Symptoms of mania may be misidentified in homeless persons because they may mimic a drug high. Another possibility is that those who are experiencing an episode of mania may also be under the influence of drugs that could be aggravating the behavior. A person who is experiencing manic behavior can also easily be aroused because of an irritable component inherent in the disorder, and as a result he can quickly become angry. This emotionality is often referred to as mood lability (a labile mood indicates marked fluctuations of mood). This irritability can escalate to out of control behavior rather rapidly. Interacting with someone who is possibly experiencing a manic episode should include a gentle, nonconfrontational approach, acknowledging the individual's concerns, and using body language that is not threatening. Because a person in a manic state is potentially volatile, a worker should use extreme caution when interacting with someone who exhibits the following behaviors.

Behavioral Indicators of a Manic Episode

- Is excited, euphoric, or disruptive to others.
- Is overly confident and grandiose about abilities, talents, wealth, or appearance.
- Has excessive energy and needs little sleep.
- Speaks very fast. It is difficult for the worker to interrupt the person.
- Has extreme mood swings with no provocation (lability).
- Is irritable much of the time.
- Is easily angered.
- Has impaired social interactions (*not due to trauma or other street experiences*).
- Has difficulty perceiving and understanding social clues; cannot read other people (usually because of the lability of mood and not due to another condition such as an autistic, developmental, or personality disorder).
- Is anxious and afraid around others. (*This behavior may be an adaptation to the streets.*)
- Is verbally or physically aggressive. (*This behavior may be an adaptation to the streets.*)
- Has extreme variability in relationships, from overly critical to worshipful.

- Is hard to get along with.
- Reports variations in mood (from happy to sad) and energy levels that may fluctuate over days or months. Has a reported history of problems at work, school, or home.

Behavior that may have its origins in a bipolar (manic phase) disorder can be observed in the following ways, or may be reported by previous school and employment history:

- Is fired or quits frequently (work).
- Is unable to remain in a regular classroom environment (school).
- Has difficulty waiting in line such as at a soup kitchen, signing up for shelter, waiting for appointments.
- Is easily angered or irritated by normal stresses and expectations at school or on the job.
- Has difficulty with rules and requests from those in authority.
- Has difficulty in relationships with peers and superiors at work, school, or home.
- Can't concentrate or work effectively.
- Can't attend to the needs of others.
- Is overwhelmed by chores or household expectations.
- Instigates arguments and fights with family and those in close relationships, passively or actively.

Identifying Disorders: Using Labels

Unlike most physical conditions where lab tests can help pinpoint the precise condition and point to optimal treatments, most mental disorders and addictions have no definitive laboratory tests. While a specific disorder consists of a group of signs and symptoms drawn from the previous list, the precise criteria that are required for any specific mental disorder come from the consensus of a group of mental health professionals, primarily psychiatrists (Brown, 2008). Most of the information used is derived from clinical interviews, rating scales, and psychological tests. We emphasize this because misidentification or misdiagnosis of mental illnesses continues to be an obstacle in precise treatment and rehabilitation of those who are labeled with a specific disorder. The resulting stigma and inability to receive appropriate treatment remains a significant problem in the mental health community.

Even so, certain diagnoses are used frequently. We now turn briefly to discuss the methods used to classify mental health disorders and the features of the most common disorders. Worldwide, there are two major classification systems that list all medically accepted mental health and addictive disorders: The first is the *Diagnostic and Statistical Manual of Mental Disorders* of the American Psychiatric Association, and the second is the *International Classification of Diseases* (ICD) published by the WHO. In North America the DSM predominates, and in Europe the ICD is the preferred diagnostic classification system. Both the fifth edition of the DSM (DSM-5) and the tenth edition of the ICD (ICD-10) make some attempt to recognize the impact of culture on diagnosis, but stop short of a comprehensive approach that fully integrates culture and ethnicity into diagnostic considerations. Specific training is required to use the DSM and ICD accurately. It can be used by physicians, psychologists, nurses, and social workers, but in most jurisdictions in Canada and the United States only a physician (in some states and provinces also a psychologist) is legally allowed to make a diagnosis.

Structure of the Diagnostic and Statistical Manual of Mental Disorders

So far we have avoided labels that are inherent in diagnoses because of the stigma that is involved, because there continues to be considerable debate about how to classify mental illnesses, and because mislabeling continues to be a vexing problem. We briefly describe the structure of the DSM so that you are aware of what this diagnostic classification system entails. This description is intended to help you understand that a proper diagnosis should include all of these steps and that additional life circumstances are included in understanding the individual and what treatment plan is most appropriate. Diagnoses involve labeling, and it is important that no one misapply these labels.

The DSM definition of a mental disorder must include *all* of the following:

- A clinically significant behavioral or psychological syndrome or pattern that occurs in an individual *and* that is associated with present

Mental Health and Mental Disorders (Illness)

distress (e.g., painful symptom) or disability (e.g., impairment in one or more important areas of functioning) *or* with significant pain, increased risk of suffering disability, or an important loss of freedom.

- *Also,* whatever its original cause, it must currently be considered a manifestation of a behavioral, psychological, or biological dysfunction in the individual or create significant impairment and distress (dysfunction or distress criteria must be present).

For each disorder, criteria include the following:

1. The specific symptoms that must be present, and for how long (called inclusion criteria).
2. Those symptoms that must not be present (called exclusion criteria).
3. A rule-out of medical conditions that may cause the symptoms. Note: This is extremely important as many medical conditions and their treatment can include mental, emotional, and behavioral disturbances.
4. A rule-out of the influence of alcohol and/or drugs.
5. Screening to determine that symptoms are not due to an expectable and culturally sanctioned response to a particular event, (e.g., the death of a loved one).

Cultural considerations of the context of any behavior need to be included in any evaluation of a possible mental disorder. A discussion on the influence of culture in the DSM states, "the boundaries between normality and pathology vary across cultures for specific types of behaviors. Thresholds of tolerance for specific symptoms or behaviors differ across cultures, social settings, and families. Hence, the level at which the experience becomes problematic or pathological will vary" (DSM-5, p. 14).

Each disorder is characterized by a specific combination of signs and symptoms. But in order to be diagnosed with a mental disorder the following conditions *must* also exist:

1. The signs and symptoms cannot be due to a medical condition. Note: This is extremely important because many medical conditions and drugs used to treat these conditions can cause mental, emotional,

and behavioral symptoms. People can easily be treated for the wrong condition or improperly if medical problems are not first ruled out.

2. The signs and symptoms cannot be due to the effects of alcohol or drugs (legal or illegal). As we examine later in chapter 8, the effects of drugs can have similar or identical appearances to some mental disorders, but with drugs the feelings or behaviors of concern disappear when the drug effects wear off.

3. The signs and symptoms must cause either distress (to the individual) or impairment in daily functioning. (Impairment in daily functioning is more difficult to assess with a homeless person because there is usually lack of employment, involvement in educational activities, or opportunities for other common daily activities.) However, it is possible to assess if a persons is unable to independently seek the essentials of food and shelter or to follow through on agreed-on action plans for rehousing because of mental and emotional problems.

The most common disorders fall into the following groups:

- Addictions: Alcohol and substance abuse and dependence, and addictive behaviors such as gambling

    Anxiety disorders: Generalized anxiety, social anxiety, panic, phobias, traumatic stress, and PTSD

    Depressive disorders : Major depression, bipolar disorder (hypomanic, manic, and mixed episode), seasonal affective disorder

    Cognitive/developmental disorders: attention deficit/hyperactivity disorder (ADHD), Alzheimer and other dementias, TBI, developmental disorders, including FASD

    Cognitive disorders: Thought, schizophrenia, and other psychoses

    Disorders with mixed features (anxious, depressive, and cognitive features): anorexia, bulimia, obsessive-compulsive disorder

There are now some movies that give a fairly accurate portrayal of persons with certain disorders. We recommend that you take the opportunity to view some of them as this will make the behaviors and problems real in ways that the printed page cannot. One concerned with a homeless man who has schizophrenia, *The Soloist* (Foster, Krasnoff, & Wright, 2009) is an accurate and sensitive examination of struggles that many with this disorder endure. Others include *As Good As It Gets* (Ziskin & Brooks, 1997), *Waltz with Bashir* (Folman et al., 2008), *The King's Speech* (Canning, Sherman, Unwin, & Hooper, 2010), and *The Fisher King* (Hill, Obst, & Gilliam, 1991).

Personality Disorders

Personality disorders consist of a group of mental disorders that are classified separately because they include long-standing, pervasive, and inflexible patterns of behavior that are usually not changed by therapy (medication or counseling), and that cause distress or impairment for the individual. Personality disorders may be viewed as discrete categories of behaviors but may also be seen as extreme variations of deviant personality traits that flow from normalcy into severely disordered functioning (American Psychiatric Association, 2013, p. 646). Personality disorders include those that are categorized as antisocial, schizoid, obsessive-compulsive, avoidant, borderline, dependent, histrionic, narcissistic, and schizotypal. While there is continuing debate about the classification of these disorders, with some experts suggesting different groupings, the existence of these disorders is not disputed. The behavior pattern of each disorder must be markedly different from what is acceptable by the cultural environment of the individual. Inflexibility in personality disorders indicates that the behaviors can cause serious problems in functioning and impairment and that they are not easily subject to behavioral modification. The result is often depression and distress that leads to a person seeking treatment (worst-case scenario). Distress and impairment in social, occupational, and personal situations is a common feature of all personality disorders. On the streets, workers are more likely to encounter people with antisocial personalities, but workers will encounter all types of disorders. Those who are homeless are more likely to have a personality disorder because the behavior associated with personality disorders frequently leads to social dysfunctions, loss of employment and income, and resultant homelessness. However, not everyone who is homeless has a personality disorder, and many successful citizens can be described as having features of personality disorders without sufficient impairment to result in homelessness. Personality disorders are seen by professionals and researchers as an enduring pattern of inner experience and behavior that deviates markedly from the expectations of the culture of the individual who exhibits it. These patterns are inflexible and pervasive across many situations. The onset of the pattern can be traced back at least to the beginning of adulthood. To be diagnosed as someone with a personality disorder, a behavioral pattern must cause significant distress or impairment in personal, social, and/or occupational situations. Many people have some behavioral indicators but do not experience significant impairment. This diagnosis is not typically given until a person is into adulthood (age eighteen), and the behavior pattern has become established and is enduring.

Other Prevalent Disorders

There are several other disorders that are especially prevalent among homeless people. We briefly introduce them here and will explore them further in chapter 9. Recent studies have noted that there is an unusually higher incidence of some disorders in homeless persons that have serious consequences for functioning. Life experiences accounting for these disorders include trauma, alcoholism in one's birthmother, and serious head injury (Hopper, Bassuk, & Olivet, 2010). Most of these disorders have only recently come to the attention of those who work with homeless persons, and as yet there are minimal supports for those afflicted. A history of trauma, both before a person became homeless and as a result of the homelessness, is now recognized as a major contributor to emotional and behavioral problems among homeless people (Hopper et al., 2010). This history of trauma is also frequently a major concern for veterans returning from combat zones, for victims of domestic violence (Olson-Madden, Forster, Huggins, & Schneider, 2012), and homeless youths (Hwang et al., 2005). In addition, violence and resulting trauma are prevalent on the streets; there is the likelihood that a homeless person has been traumatized both before and after becoming homeless. There is thus a greater likelihood of traumatic stress and PTSD among the homeless.

Many people also report a history of brain injury caused by events such as automobile or sports accidents, major illness, or an incident that results in oxygen deprivation to the brain, and cerebral bleeding (Hopper et al., 2010). This kind of injury can result in both memory and behavioral impairments. These include cognitive problems such as slowness of thought, difficulty in concentration and attention, and problems with communication, reasoning, problem solving, judgment, reading, and writing. They also include emotional dysregulation (mood swings, depression, anxiety, anger management, excessive laughter or crying, agitation), inability to self-monitor behavior, difficulty relating to others, inappropriate social responses, abrupt behaviors including acts of violence, and delusions including paranoia (Christensen et al., 2005). It is important to recognize that the moods and behaviors of brain-injured individuals cannot be addressed in the same way as those with mental illnesses that are not organic in nature: the injury is inevitably permanent and is not the result neurochemical imbalances; treatment with medication can have limited effectiveness. Most often consistent behavioral therapies can help brain-injured persons to learn functional skills that help them to cope. Without a case manager or consistent family support, persons with a brain injury can find themselves in difficult and legal situations that they are unable to cope with. The most difficult situations are those where the injury creates limitations but does not meet the criteria necessary for a guardian to be assigned to that person. In these cases the person is left to her own resources and often becomes a victim of legal and social forces.

Fetal Alcohol Syndrome Disorders FASDs have recently become recognized as significant disorders that cause lifelong impairment (Clarren, Weinberg, & Jonsson, 2010). Persons with FASD have a developmental disorder that has many of the features of those with a brain injury. Behavioral indicators include hyperactivity, poor judgment and impulse control, lack of insight, and an inability to maintain focus on the consequences of behavior. Alcohol use, a frequent additional factor, aggravates these indicators. The complexities of care are impacted by the fact that although FASD impairs cognitive processing and behavioral controls in adults, it is not recognized as an adult disability. It can be difficult to achieve and maintain a supportive safety net for those afflicted. These adults also go on to have children of their own, and since most of these adults also abuse alcohol, their children are likewise impacted (May et al., 2009). Aboriginal people in Canada and the American Indian population in the United States are disproportionately represented among those affected with FASD, thus we are more likely to encounter Aboriginal people with FASD among the homeless.

WHAT CAUSES MENTAL DISORDERS AND WHAT ARE COMMON TREATMENTS?

There are a number of different explanations for what causes mental and behavioral disorders.

1. Genetics or heredity. Some mental and emotional disorders have a strong genetic component, such as depression, and often occur in multiple members of the same extended family.
2. Prenatal influences. The influences of nutrition and exposure to noxious environmental factors and illnesses have become more widely known (Bouchard & McGue, 2003; Weinstock, 2005).
3. Early developmental influences. The impact of illness on young children, as well as the effects of maternal deprivation, trauma, and lack of adequate nutrition has been documented (Streissguth, Barr, Kogan, & Bookstein, 1996; Wadsworth & Kuh, 1997).
4. Personality influences. Persons highly susceptible to neuroticism are more susceptible to a mental illness (Bouchard & McGue, 2003).
5. Environmental influences. Safe food, water, and neighborhoods; educational opportunities; and social networks all influence the stable emotional development of individuals.
6. Abuse of alcohol and drugs. Toxic factors of substance abuse also have an influence on the development of mental disorders.
7. The stress theory. Certain strong stressors can create or aggravate a mental disorder such as an anxiety or depressive disorder (Weinstock, 2005).
8. Experiences with trauma and abuse. Those exposed to trauma and abuse have a significantly higher risk of developing a diagnosable mental or substance-abuse disorder, or both.
9. Socioeconomic influences. Low socioeconomic status has been linked with higher rates of mental disorders (Lozoff, Jimenez, Hagen, Mollen, & Wolf, 2000).

Most professionals now accept the view of multicausation in many disorders. Some influences are greater with specific disorders such as depression, where there is a strong familial pattern, and bipolar disorder, where there is a strong hereditary link. However, usually no one factor is exclusively responsible for a specific disorder.

Descriptions of mental and behavioral abnormalities have been found in all parts of the world since the beginnings of recorded time. Depending on the cultural norms and beliefs, the causes of these symptoms were presented as aberrations of the spirit, the influx of evil spirits, the vengeance of an angry deity, the influences of witches and other magical creatures, imbalances of humors (blood, bile, phlegm within the body), the influences of ingested potions, and the secret powers of shamans; responses varied depending on the current social and political environment (Foucault, 1988). Treatments consisted of combinations of physical and spiritual ritualistic practices. People did not recognize the differences between spiritual afflictions and mental illnesses. Healers were often shamans who practiced both religious and healing rituals and used a variety of methods: prayer, incantations, medicines, and psychological and physical punishments, occasionally including torture. The advent of medicine as a recognized profession in the ancient Mediterranean world (Arabia, Egypt, Greece, and Rome), led to the recognition of systematic influences of body functions, as it was believed to be central to the treatment of moral and behavioral afflictions. This included such primitive treatments as drilling holes in a person's skull to let out the bad humors.

Eventually, the treatment of mental illness led first to the development of hospitals for the confinement of the mentally ill, and then to the application of moral treatments that emphasized humane, meaningful application of a positive, usually rural, environment to help heal the troubled soul. In the 1800s a number of influences led to greater urbanization and also greater need for psychiatric hospitals as poor country folk no longer were available to care at home for those afflicted with a mental illness (Grob, 1994). The result was that institutions established for moral treatment became custodial places for the mentally ill. This custodial focus, where there was little treatment and considerable mistreatment, continued until the mid-1900s. By 1960 considerable publicity of the miserable conditions of these institutions, public sympathy toward human rights in the United States, the availability of medicines to control the worst psychiatric symptoms, and Supreme Court rulings to provide the least restrictive level of care (for the mentally handicapped, which spilled over into the mental health population) resulted in massive closing of these institutions (Hudson, 2005). With deinstitutionalization, the mentally ill were back in the community. The lack of adequate recognition for their needs resulted in many being placed in large-scale boarding homes that provided little more than custodial care (Grob, 1994). Others were moved into SRO buildings—literally a room with a bed and a hot plate. Often bathroom facilities were shared and there was a lack of meeting rooms or recreation spaces. Facilities were insufficient for independent living, and unacceptable to most people placed there. They were generally squalid and in unsafe parts of town, and were infested with cockroaches and other vermin. The mentally ill released from large institutions found their quality of life greatly diminished and their sense of freedom not much improved because they lacked the personal and financial resources to find a place of their own. The most resourceful took to the streets.

What the preceding short description of the evolution of the care of the mentally ill fails to capture is that this was the common care for the poor, and not for the middle and upper classes. Historical accounts of the well-to-do indicate that treatment of mental disorders was usually home-based, with rooms and if necessary servants allocated to the care of the afflicted. Attics and spaces away from busy living areas were also used to confine mentally ill family members. In some extreme cases, afflicted persons were sent to a convent or priory where religious friars and their servants took care of the afflicted for a well-earned and considerable sum of money. By the 1800s the moral treatment movement was so popular in England that retreats for upper-crust gentry were found all over that country and were available to even aspiring middle-class individuals (Mechanic, 2007). In the United States the larger institutions that provided moral treatment underwent a transition to custodial care for the poor. When it was impossible for an individual to be kept at home, the well-to-do sought treatment in smaller private psychiatric establishments where they continued to receive upper-crust care. This separation of rich from poor continues to define psychiatric care in the United States. The homeless who have mental health problems continue, by and large, to come from lower socioeconomic backgrounds or from families who have abandoned the care of their sick loved ones. Many persons with mental illness who come from stable, well-off families continue to be supported by them in some fashion, be it basements converted into recreational rooms and then ancillary apartments, converted garages, or family-supplied apartment units.

In Canada the divisions between rich and poor in the reception of mental health services is not as clear. Private psychiatric clinics never became established, and those persons in need of asylum care who were financially well off presumably were sent by their relatives to American or European facilities. Publicly run psychiatric institutions were established in most provinces and received all those who required custodial care. In the 1960s, when Canada adopted universal health care, mental health was included; this led to the rapid deployment of psychiatric services to local general hospitals. Large asylums were abandoned. Unfortunately, as in the United States, funding for community-based programming and care did not follow patients into the community.

The movement of people out of asylums and into the community was a major social upheaval in the latter part of the twentieth century. It was a catastrophe for those who had spent much of their lives in institutions and who had become dependent on the services and shelter they provided. Neither financial resources nor adequate treatment followed these deinstitutionalized people into new homes. Community treatment resources were lacking, and thus "rehabilitation" was a sadly misapplied term for those unfortunate to have no supportive relatives to assist (Torrey, 1988). At the same time, there was another social movement that saw a rise in the use of recreational drugs and alcohol. This led to the development of a new cohort of dysfunctioning adults who were substance dependent. Some of those who became adults during this period developed a mental disorder either prior to, as a result of, or independent of substance use. These persons came to be identified in a number of ways: as dually diagnosed, chemically addicted mentally ill, and with co-occurring disorders. In chapter 9 we will take a look at drugs and how they both cause and are caused by emotional and behavioral disorders before a brief look at what happens when a person experiences a mental disorder combined with substance use and abuse.

BASIC INTERVENTION STRATEGIES IN UNFAMILIAR SITUATIONS

Safety First

1. Determine ability to communicate.
2. Assess for orientation, level of stress, and hypervigilance.
3. Determine ability to engage in continued conversation.
4. Engage in neutral, nonconfrontational conversation.
5. Ask how you can be of help.

Despite a desire to help, many people are hesitant to interact with those who appear to be in emotional or mental distress. This reluctance comes from several sources, some real and others not, such as those due to the stigma associated with mental illness. We looked at stigma and discussed that many people are worried that those with a mental illness are dangerous. Despite the extensive publicity given to those who have a mental illness diagnosis and who commit violent and horrific crimes, most people with a mental disorder are not violent and are more likely to be the victim than a perpetrator of a crime (Mechanic, 2007). However, the concurrent use of alcohol or other drugs make a person's behavior erratic and often hostile, thus caution is always warranted. There is the attendant concern that one could say the wrong thing and further aggravate an existing condition. A person who is struggling with symptoms of a mental disorder most often is aware that there is something wrong, that he is not functioning well, that feelings of sadness and hopelessness are not the norm, and that the struggle to function on a daily basis is not something everyone else is experiencing. This realization may lead to alienation, and then to increased depression. The alienation may also stem from a realization that the voices one is hearing or the beliefs one has may not be normal. All of these can quickly lead to fear and resultantly to a defensive posture in the hopes that no one can get close enough to detect the unusual experiences the individual is having. Whether there is a further withdrawal or a defensive posture, the basic phenomenon is the same: a fear of what is happening and a lack of control over one's thoughts and feelings.

The approaches to engagement in the helping relationship explored in chapters 2 and 3 are also fundamental aspects of sensitive, respectful, and helpful interactions with those who may have a mental illness. These approaches are based on fundamental principles of respect for the dignity and humanity of each person we encounter. But implicit in this respect is the understanding that when a person is in acute distress the helper must be prepared to take a gentle but firm lead in providing safety and securing additional help. Those on the frontline, working outside the security of agency walls, are often the first to be faced with situations where the physical, psychological, or emotional safety of one or more persons is at stake. It is up to these frontline workers to decide on the extent and nature of the outreach to a person who may be suffering from a mental disorder. Their job is complicated by several factors. First, there is no way of accurately assessing the situation on the streets. Second, the troubled individual may be under the influence of drugs and/or alcohol, thus making their reactions erratic and unpredictable. In figure 7.2 you can see how this interplay of thoughts, moods, emotions, behaviors, and drugs can swirl around inside a person's mind. To make this picture even more complex, the person may mask the desire for help under a cloak of denial, or may flatly refuse help.

For those who are working primarily inside an agency that serves homeless and high-risk persons, the challenges of intervening with a person who

Figure 7.2. Complex Interplay of Thoughts, Feelings, and Drugs

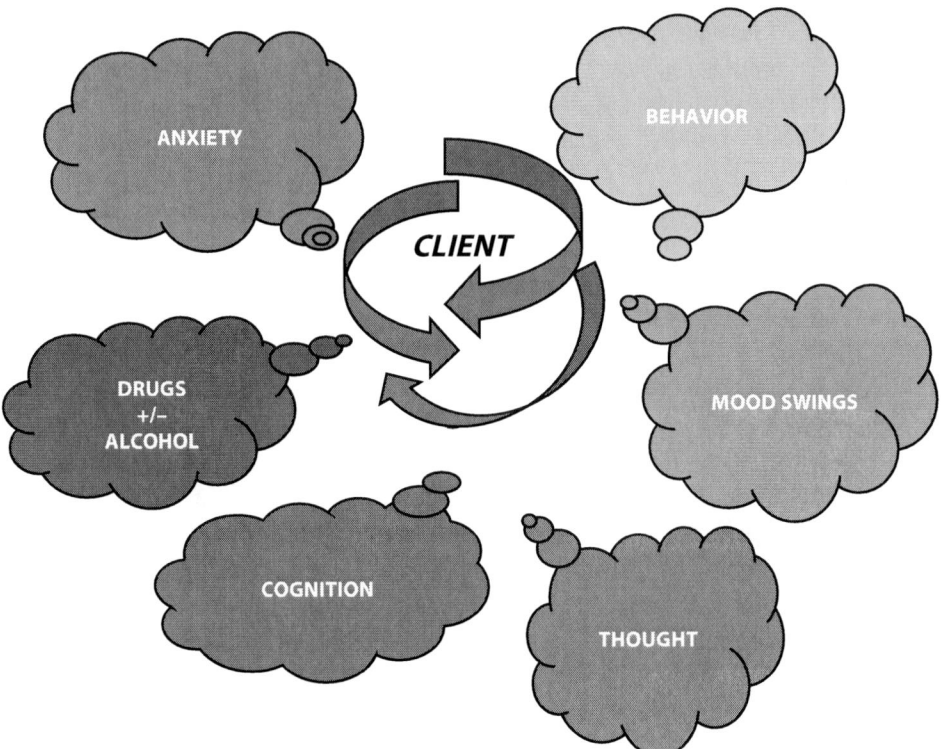

potentially has a mental illness and/or an addiction are challenging in different ways. In these situations the individual has usually become a client in some sense in that help has been sought or at least considered. Workers need to understand what has motivated a person to seek help and to determine what recently happened that may be the precipitant to looking for help *now* and to establish a clear motive of the person coming in to seek assistance. An important consideration is the extent of the person's motivation to get help because of a real desire to change or because of a need to play the system for financial or other benefits. In addition, the potential client may have a lot of indecision or ambivalence about the nature of this help and any conditions on which it is provided. There may concerns about trust and confidentiality and any substance-use issues may be minimized or denied in order to avoid being denied help.

EXERCISES

Some of these exercises are best done before the information discussed in this chapter is presented. This engages you in thinking about some of the complexities of mental disorders and your preconceived ideas about them.

Exercise 1. Stigma

Write brief answers to the following questions. If this is part of a class exercise, follow up with a discussion in small groups. Each group should select a spokesperson who can provide feedback to the rest of the class.

1. Your brother/sister/daughter/son has announced the intent to marry. The partner is lovely, but has a family full of alcohol (or drug) abusers. What is your response?
2. You find out that the person who you have started to date has been hospitalized and has a diagnosis of schizophrenia (or bipolar disorder or major depression). What do you do?
3. You have a good friend who has been traumatized and suffers from PTSD. He can sometimes be erratic and unpredictable in emotional reactions. You are planning a party. Do you include this friend?
4. Take any of the above scenarios and substitute a work or school situation.

Exercise 2. Common Beliefs about Mental Disorders

1. In groups of three (or four), discuss your view of the origins of mental disorders. What has your training and experience taught you?
2. How common do you believe mental illness is?
3. How do cultures other than Euro-Canadian or Euro-American have different ways of understanding and dealing with mental disorders?

Exercise 3. Group-Based Discussion about Common Misunderstandings

Divide the class into groups of four or five and give each group one or two of the following questions to discuss. Have a spokesperson report back to the entire group. Have the entire class discuss. This discussion focuses on common misunderstandings that people have about those with mental health or addiction problems.

Exercise 4. The Attribution Questionnaire (AQ-27)

Jean is a thirty-year-old single man with schizophrenia. Sometimes he hears voices and becomes upset. He lives alone in an apartment and works as a clerk at a large law firm. He has been hospitalized six times because of his illness. Keeping that person in mind, how would you personally respond in each of the following instances (table 7.2)? Please rate yourself from 1 = not at all, to 9 = very much.

Table 7.2. The Attribution Questionnaire: AQ-27

1. I would feel aggravated by Jean.	1 2 3 4 5 6 7 8 9	not at all very much
2. I would feel unsafe around Jean.	1 2 3 4 5 6 7 8 9	not at all very much
3. Jean would terrify me.	1 2 3 4 5 6 7 8 9	not at all very much
4. How angry would you feel at Jean?	1 2 3 4 5 6 7 8 9	not at all very much
5. If I were in charge of Jean's treatment, I would require him to take his medication.	1 2 3 4 5 6 7 8 9	not at all very much
6. I think Jean poses a risk to his neighbours unless he is hospitalized.	1 2 3 4 5 6 7 8 9	not at all very much
7. If I were an employer, I would interview Jean for a job.	1 2 3 4 5 6 7 8 9	not at all very much
8. I would be willing to talk to Jean about his problems.	1 2 3 4 5 6 7 8 9	not at all very much
9. I would feel pity for Jean.	1 2 3 4 5 6 7 8 9	not at all very much
10. I would think that it was Jean's own fault that he is in the present condition.	1 2 3 4 5 6 7 8 9	not at all very much

Table 7.2. (Continued)

11. How controllable, do you think, is the cause of Jean's present condition?	1 not at all	2	3	4	5	6	7	8	9 very much
12. How irritated would you feel by Jean?	1 not at all	2	3	4	5	6	7	8	9 very much
13. How dangerous would you feel Jean is?	1 not at all	2	3	4	5	6	7	8	9 very much
14. How much do you agree that Jean should be forced into treatment with his doctor even if he does not want to?	1 not at all	2	3	4	5	6	7	8	9 very much
15. I think it would be best for Jean's community if he were put away in a psychiatric hospital.	1 not at all	2	3	4	5	6	7	8	9 very much
16. I would share a car pool with Jean every day.	1 not at all	2	3	4	5	6	7	8	9 very much
17. How much do you think an asylum, where Jean can be kept away from his neighbours, is the best place for him?	1 not at all	2	3	4	5	6	7	8	9 very much
18. I would feel threatened by Jean.	1 not at all	2	3	4	5	6	7	8	9 very much
19. How scared of Jean would you feel?	1 not at all	2	3	4	5	6	7	8	9 very much
20. How likely is it that you would help Jean?	1 not at all	2	3	4	5	6	7	8	9 very much
21. How certain would you feel that you would help Jean?	1 not at all	2	3	4	5	6	7	8	9 very much
22. How much sympathy would you feel for Jean?	1 not at all	2	3	4	5	6	7	8	9 very much
23. How responsible do you think Jean is for his present condition?	1 not at all	2	3	4	5	6	7	8	9 very much
24. How frightened of Jean would you feel?	1 not at all	2	3	4	5	6	7	8	9 very much

Table 7.2. (Continued)

25. If I were in charge of Jean's treatment, I would force him to live in a group home.	1 not at all	2	3	4	5	6	7	8	9 very much
26. If I were a landlord, I probably would rent an apartment to Jean.	1 not at all	2	3	4	5	6	7	8	9 very much
27. How much concern would you feel for Jean?	1 not at all	2	3	4	5	6	7	8	9 very much

Source: Corrigan, Markowitz, et al. (2003).

1. For the previous questions, if the diagnosis was a bipolar illness, a major depression, or PTSD, would your ratings differ?
2. Consider Jean to be a woman. Rate your answers and see if you are more likely to apply stigma-related behavior to a man or woman, or if you may stigmatize some behaviors differently depending on the sex of the individual.

The AQ-27 Score Sheet

The AQ-27 consists of nine stereotype factors; scores for each factor are determined by summing the items as outlined below. Note: Items are reversed score prior to summing up for the avoidance scale. By reverse scoring we mean that the values are interchanged so that 1 = 9, 2 = 8, 3 = 7, 4 = 6, 5 = 5, 6 = 4, 7 = 3, 8 = 2, 9 = 1.

_____ Blame = AQ10 + AQ11 + AQ23
_____ Anger = AQ1 + AQ4 + AQ12
_____ Pity = AQ9 + AQ22 + AQ27
_____ Help = AQ8 + AQ20 + AQ21
_____ Dangerousness = AQ2 + AQ13 + AQ18
_____ Fear = AQ3 + AQ19 + AQ24
_____ Avoidance = AQ7 + AQ16 + AQ26 (Reverse score these three questions.)
_____ Segregation = AQ6 + AQ15 + AQ17
_____ Coercion = AQ5 + AQ14 + AQ25

The higher the score, the more that factor is being endorsed by the responder.

JOURNALING

1. Anger in men may be a sign of an underlying depression. Can you think of an example from your work that would indicate where it would be important to clarify if this issue was one of anger or depression?
2. Stigma is a major issue for persons with a mental health problem. Have you seen indications of stigma at work? On the streets?
3. Do you see this stigma in those with addictive disorders? Is it worse for men or women? Does the type of addiction make a difference?

CHAPTER 8

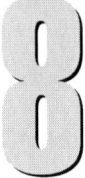

ADDICTIONS: MIND- AND MOOD-ALTERING SUBSTANCES AND BEHAVIORS

KEY ISSUES
- Understanding of the various levels of care and for whom they are most suitable
- Understanding of models of recovery
- Familiarity with precontemplation, and early intervention phases of the recovery process
- Introduction to appropriate interviewing skills to optimize recovery-seeking behaviors
- Awareness of treatment philosophies in mental health, addictions, and dual diagnosis
- Examination of concurrent addictions and what happens when one addiction is substituted for another

OVERVIEW

Various forms of alcohol and other mood- and mind-altering substances are used by a vast majority of North American people. Table 8.1 shows the reported use of various substances, both in the past year and over a person's lifetime. It does not include the abuse of prescription drugs that can also act as mood-altering drugs and are used by a substantial number of persons. The comparisons show that Canadians report more alcohol use but less use of other substances. While these percentages appear to be small, they translate into millions of users across both countries. The reported use of alcohol and substance-use disorders by persons who are

Table 8.1. Prevalence of Alcohol and Drug Use

	Lifetime	Past Year
United States (reported for those age 12 and over)		
Alcohol	82.2%	66.2%
Illicit drugs	47.0%	15.3%
Marijuana and hashish	41.9%	11.6%
Cocaine	14.3%	1.5%
Crack	3.2%	0.3%
Heroin	1.6%	0.2%
Hallucinogens	14.1%	1.6%
Ecstasy	5.7%	0.9%
Inhalants	8.0%	0.7%
Canada (reported for those age 15 and over)		
Alcohol	89.7%	78%
Cannabis	39.4%	9.1%
Cocaine/crack	n/a	0.9%
Hallucinogens	n/a	0.6%
Ecstasy	n/a	0.7%

Source: United States: National Institute on Drug Abuse (NIDA, 2013); Canada: Health Canada (2012). Note: NIDA is under the umbrella of the Substance Abuse and Mental Health Services Administration (SAMHSA).

homeless has been difficult to accurately measure because most of those participants available for research reside in shelters and thus these studies fail to include those who are doubled up or sleeping rough. However, some well-designed studies report rates of alcohol and drug use to be between 50 and 70 percent (Palepu et al., 2013). These studies focused on dependence on substances rather than on substance use, since use by itself would not signal a need for intervention.

In the past fifty years the substance-abuse and mental health fields have undergone several changes in the way problems with addictions are referred to. Previously used terms have included drugs, abused substances, addictive drugs, illegal drugs, addicts, and drug users. When a person had a mental illness and also used or abused substances, the label of "dually diagnosed" was originally applied. Current terminology favors "substance-use disorder" and "co-occurring disorders" when a person has a diagnosable mental disorder and uses nonprescribed drugs. We will use this terminology throughout this chapter and the rest of this book.

SUBSTANCE USE WORLDWIDE

Mood- and mind-altering substances—solid, liquid, and gas—are used for a variety of purposes, including as a part of religious rituals, to relieve pain, to enhance social occasions, and as a way to relieve feelings of depression, anxiety, and tension. You can readily see in figure 8.1 the cross-cutting effects of mood- and mind-altering substances (O'Connell, 1998). Some act as a mild influence on feelings and cognition, and others have powerful impacts that can also include damaging physical effects.

Alcohol is widely available in almost all jurisdictions, and is the most widely abused substance in both countries. It is also the most widely abused substance among homeless people. Table 8.1 illustrates that in the United States the past year use of alcohol was four and a half times higher than use of illicit substances; in Canada it was eight times higher. Substance use also includes a host of other drugs, legal and illegal, that can be absorbed through the skin, swallowed (ingested), injected, and inhaled. We will first look at

Figure 8.1. The Interplay of Moods, Cognitions, and Drugs

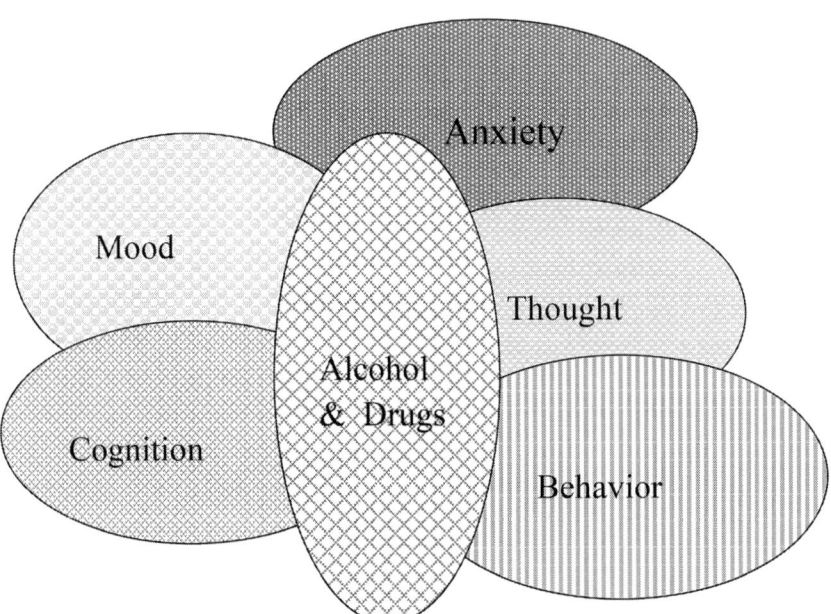

what these substances are, what they do, and what the implications of addiction and dependence are; then we will explore the effects that they have on people with preexisting mental health disorders.

Substances of abuse fall into several categories, primarily with respect to their primary or desired effect. Some have more than one effect. Broadly speaking, some act as stimulants, or depressants, or hallucinogens, and some have mixed effects. These substances can be naturally occurring, such as the psilocybin mushroom; processed from plants, such as alcohol, opium, and cocaine; and artificially created in laboratories, such as methamphetamines. Figure 8.2 gives a quick overview of the most commonly occurring substances of abuse in North America. In addition to these, new chemicals and new combinations continue to enter the illegal drug market. Those who work directly in the substance-abuse field find it necessary to keep in close contact with law enforcement personnel who are frequently the first to run across new "dope" (substances).

Figure 8.2. Substances of Abuse

Substances of Abuse

- Alcohol (beer, wine, hard liquor)
- Amphetamine (methamphetamine, Adderall, diet pills)
- Caffeine (coffee, soda, tea, energy drinks)
- Cannabis (marijuana, pot, hashish)
- Cocaine (crack, coke, freebase)
- Hallucinogens (LSD, MDMA/Ecstasy, mescaline)
- Inhalants (gasoline, paint thinner, glue)
- Nicotine (tobacco)
- Opioids (heroin, methadone, Vicodin, Oxycontin, Percoset)
- Phencyclidine (PCP, ketamine)
- Sedative/Hypnotic/Anxiolytic (Valium, Xanax, sleeping pills)
- Other/Unknown (e.g., nitrous oxide)
- "Polysubstance"

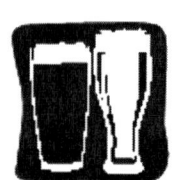
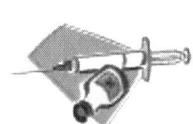
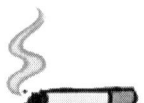

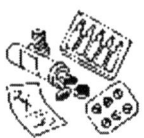

MOOD- AND MIND-ALTERING DRUGS: A BRIEF HISTORY

The history of alcohol and drug use puts into perspective some common human behaviors that have existed since early civilizations. Because drugs and drink have been used for social, religious, and war-related purposes since the earliest days of mankind, they are ingrained in the social and cultural fabric of many societies. Throughout time and across all of the continuously inhabited continents we find people modifying through natural and chemical processes a variety of substances that can then be used for their mood- and mind-altering abilities. Common plants such as hemp, poppies, some types of mushrooms, potatoes, barley, corn, grapes, other fruits, yak milk, whale blubber, and honey have all been converted into solids, liquids, and gases that are used for a variety of purposes. These include for religious rituals, to relieve pain, as an enhancer of social occasions, and as a way to relieve feelings of depression, anxiety, and tension (Gately, 2008). In the past two centuries, substances that are now illegal were sanctioned and promoted for medical benefits. Some, such as cocaine and heroin, did not receive the social and legal prohibitions that result in legal punishments until the twentieth century (Winick, 1992) as their addictive potential and ramifications to society became apparent. Marijuana was legally available until the beginning of the twentieth century, when many countries began to ban this substance, in apparent conjunction with limiting the opium trade and reducing competition between hemp and the cotton industry in the United States. Legalization of marijuana is gradually returning in some states and is the subject of considerable debate in Canada where it is available for medicinal purposes.

While there are hundreds of substances that have mind- and mood-altering effects, we are mainly concerned with those most commonly found in North America and most frequently available to people with limited opportunities to acquire drugs and with few financial means to do so. Most widely available is alcohol, which is legally obtained in almost all jurisdictions, and is the most widely abused substance (Musto, 1991). Mood-altering substances also include a host of other drugs, legal and illegal, that can be absorbed through the skin, swallowed, (ingested), injected, and inhaled. We will explore alcohol in a class by itself, and then examine other drugs. We will first look at what these substances are, what their physiological and psychological impacts are, and what the implications of addiction and dependence are. Then we will explore the effects that they have on people with preexisting mental health problems.

> **Textbox 8.1. The History of Alcohol**
>
> An excellent history on the production and use of alcohol can be found in *Drink, A Cultural History of Alcohol,* by Iain Gately (2008). Some of Gately's book is summarized in this section.

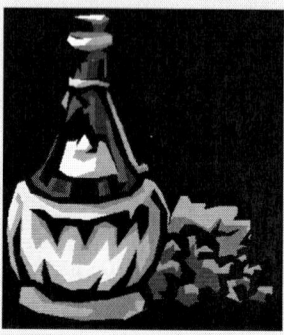

Historical Themes: Why Do People Use Psychoactive Substances?

Alcohol and other mood- and mind-altering drugs affect a whole constellation of thoughts and feelings. Human beings have recognized the emotional and physiological impact of mood- and mind-altering substances in efforts to cope with stressors of life and to achieve a change in mood and feeling for thousands of years. In fact, people were probably producing alcohol before they learned to write. There is evidence of the use of mood- and mind-altering chemicals in virtually every society. Through serendipitous events and experimentation, early human beings found that specific plants, in addition to having medicinal properties, reduced negative emotions such as fear and anxiety, reduced pain, enhanced positive emotions, and altered states of consciousness. In many early societies, and in some modern societies, these effects also had a strong spiritual dimension. A short tour through the history of alcohol and drug use will help to put current use in some context.

Prehistory and the Neolithic Period (8500 BC–4000 BC)

Alcohol has been the most popular psychoactive substance over the millennia. It has been found in residue of ancient crockery in China, India, Persia (Iran), Babylon, Egypt, Greece, and northern Europe. Plants were valued for their medicinal properties and were also used for their psychoactive properties. Today, approximately four thousand plants that yield psychoactive substances have been identified. Not all those used by non-Western cultures are known or documented. However, all cultures have found ways to mitigate pain and the discomforts of human ailments. Similarly, plants valued for medicinal and psychoactive use have been found in pottery fragments from the same places and times as alcohol. We have found evidence that hemp was used in China more than seven thousand years ago. The stems were used as fiber, the seeds for food, and later the leaves for psychoactive effects; its use spread throughout the East. Likewise opium, probably first cultivated in India, found widespread acceptance as a powerful reliever of physical pain and emotional distress.

Ancient Civilizations (4000 BC–AD 400)

Egyptian hieroglyphics recommended moderate consumption of beer, which may have implied a recognition of problematic inebriation by some. There is concurrent evidence from the Old Testament, where similar statements are found. Wine had become recognized as an important component of some religious ceremonies. Hippocrates recommended opium as a painkiller. By the time of Hippocrates in 400 BC, the use of hemp leaves (marijuana) and opium in liquid and powder form had found its way from the Middle Eastern countries surrounding Persia to the western Mediterranean region. During this time, beer and wine were the most common beverages in the Middle East and Europe.

Middle Ages (AD 400–1400)

By the Middle Ages, when Greek and Roman influences had spread throughout Europe and the British Isles, alcohol—ale, beer, wine, and mead—were basic food staples used at all meals. The beverage of choice was dictated by cost and social class, with ale being the common beverage of the poor in England. Mediterranean countries featured wine. During this time the recognition of differential effects of alcohol and drugs was discovered. That is, opium and other drugs can be medicinal at low doses, a psychoactive drug at a moderate dose, and a deadly poison at high doses. This was a critical development in the differential use of certain drugs. The refinement of certain chemical processes by Muslim scientists led to the discovery of the process of distillation in Spain. This meant that alcohol could be extracted from wine and used in its pure, concentrated form, and thus be used as a more concentrated and potent substance. Hashish was similarly refined from less potent marijuana. Although the use of alcohol was forbidden in the religious text of Islam, the Quran, hashish, a potent form of marijuana, was not expressly named; however it was considered forbidden because it is an intoxicant. Despite this prohibition it became a popular substitute in some Islamic societies.

Renaissance and Age of Discovery (1400–1700)

Development of distillation techniques led to alcohol with greater potency and greater ease of intoxication. Together with the increase of international trade this potency led to greater varieties of wine, such as sherry, port, and claret. Meanwhile the availability of large amounts of sugar from Caribbean plantations led to the development of rum. Thereafter came gin, developed in Holland around 1650 as a result of the distillation techniques discovered a few centuries earlier. Gin is a classic example of government-supported alcohol production and consumption in England. With few taxes, gin and rum were widely and cheaply available; this soon led to a crisis of overconsumption in England by the early 1700s. At the same time, in this Age of Discovery, global sailing voyages expanded trade to Africa, the Americas, and the Far East. Through trade and colonization European explorers, soldiers, merchants, traders, and missionaries carried their own culture's alcohol- and drug-using customs to the rest of the world. In return, opium and its by-products, including morphine and heroin, also introduced because of distillation techniques, were soon available in Western Europe.

Age of Enlightenment and Early Industrial Revolution (1700–1900)

It is safe to say that the Age of Enlightenment also became an age of widespread alcohol abuse. During the London gin epidemic, from 1710 to 1750, one in six public houses was a gin house. The production of gin in 1700, 1.23 million gallons, rose to 7 million gallons in 1751. This led to the first major government effort to curb alcohol use through control of consumption in England. The Tippling Act of 1751 prohibited distillers from selling gin; prices rose and consumption declined. Stiff taxes and strict regulation of sales brought the epidemic under control but created considerable public dissent. This was a prelude to similar reactions to the American Prohibition era 180 years later. In America, the first temperance movement (limiting drinking) was started in 1785 by Dr. Benjamin Rush, a prominent founder of mental health treatment.

Meanwhile the use of opium became fashionable among the upper classes and was most used in the form of laudanum. This era also saw, with scientific advancements, the discovery of psychoactive properties of gases such as nitrous oxide, commonly known as laughing gas. In 1804 morphine was first refined from opium. Morphine is ten times more powerful than opium, causing it to be a more effective pain reliever. By the mid-1850s the reusable hypodermic needle had been invented. Now drugs could be put directly into the bloodstream, creating more-immediate and more-intense effects. Within twenty years heroin was refined from morphine. While marketed as a remedy for coughs, chest pain, and tuberculosis, it quickly became widely used for its psychoactive properties. Soon thereafter, by the 1890s cocaine was being sold as an ingredient in beverages (Coca-Cola) and medicines (cough syrups). Nonetheless, alcohol remained the most prevalent form of psychoactive substance because it was easily created from local grains, fruits, and other fermentable products.

Twentieth Century and Beyond (1900–2012)

The beginning of the twentieth century saw an explosion of tobacco use, fueled by the development of the automatic cigarette-rolling machine (1884), a milder strain of tobacco enabling smokers to inhale deeply, advertising, and a more plentiful supply of tobacco leaf. Advertising had become popular in the nineteenth century and became an important vehicle for persuading people of the acceptability of smoking and the use of medicinal preparations that included ample amounts of cocaine. Throughout this time advances in drug development, manufacture, and administration led to the widespread use of an immense number and assortment of drugs, many with psychoactive properties. Thorazine, developed for anesthetic use, was quickly recognized for its antipsychotic properties and administered to people with psychosis. Amphetamines, synthesized and used as a decongestant, became widely known with regard to their mood- and energy-enhancing qualities, as well as their addictive potential. Prohibition (United States) led to massive illegal use of alcohol. By the middle of the century, drug manufacture, both legal and illegal, as well as drug transport of opium, heroin, cocaine, and synthetic drugs, had become widespread. What made this availability more problematic was that newer techniques allowed for the development and availability of more-concentrated, purer, and more-potent drugs. It also allowed drugs to be mixed with other substances, some of which enhanced addictive qualities and some of which were lethal.

Drug and alcohol control had been tried in America in the nineteenth century, and the temperance movement, which allowed for restrained use, gave way to absolute sobriety. Temperance movements were also found in some European countries and in Australia. The temperance movement did not succeed in establishing total sobriety, but it did lead the way for Prohibition in the 1920s. While American prohibition of alcohol was not repealed until 1933, it was removed from the legal books in Canada by the mid-1920s, which led to the well-known smuggling of alcohol across a casually guarded international border.

Recognition of Addiction Treatment (1925 and Beyond)

By 1925, nearly a hundred years ago, addiction was recognized as a problem that required formal treatment. Narcotic maintenance clinics were established in the United States and alcoholism was listed as a mental disorder. The resistance by many to the notion of alcohol as a mental disorder was fueled by the association of mental disorder and insanity, which many people rejected. This resistance led to the self-help recovery movement in 1934: Alcoholics Anonymous (AA), founded by two alcoholics, Bill Wilson and Dr. Bob Smith. Later, spin-off models focused on narcotics addiction (Narcotics Anonymous) and families of alcoholics (Al-Anon). This peer support, nonmedical intervention has proven to be highly effective in helping many substance abusers and has found its way into recovery plans for eaters (Overeaters Anonymous) and gamblers (Gamblers Anonymous).

The introduction of the war on drugs (1972) led to forty years of pursuit of illegal manufacturing, processing, and distribution of drugs. The increased criminalization of drug use in other countries was largely influenced by US drug policies. The war on drugs expanded the underground economy in illicit substances and did little to curb use. It has recently been recognized as failing to have met its objectives (Musto, 2002). In the meantime, the emergence of harm reduction models in Canada and Europe has provided a different and somewhat effective way for some users to reduce their addictive behaviors. Finally, in a reversal of trends in the United States, the

US federal election saw the decriminalization of marijuana and its authorized use for medicinal purposes become a reality in Oregon and Washington state. There is some movement in other regions to follow suit. In Canada, marijuana can be used legally for medicinal purposes, and possession of a small amount of marijuana has not been punished for many years; public opinion for its legalization continues in a positive trend.

Why Is This Historical Background Important?

This brief glimpse at the history of alcohol and substance use provides some perspective on its universality and the reality that abuse has accompanied use since the earliest of times. A summary of the key historical themes includes these facts:

- Psychoactive substances are found in all societies.
- Psychoactive substances have been used for over 10,000 years.
- Some potential problem behaviors associated with some substances have always been recognized. These include dependency, and the lethargy and diminished productivity often observed in chronic abusers.
- Drugs increased in potency and availability as scientists learned how to refine and manufacture drugs and to extract the psychoactive chemicals from plants.
- Modern transportation increased the availability of drugs from other parts of the world.
- Developments in medicine made it possible to more quickly and easily get drugs into the body. The faster the administration, the quicker the effect.
- Modern drugs are more potent and provide a faster impact than those previously available. This makes them potentially more quickly addictive.
- It is now possible to manufacture drugs with minimal technical equipment. The synthetic drugs, often manufactured illegally, provide a cheap and quick market for traffickers; their addictive potential is much higher than legal substances. (Gately, 2008)

Out in most communities one now finds a multitude of substances called by different names. Some names, such as dope, pot, hash, and horse, are transnational, while others receive a local name. They may be the same or different from drugs by the same name in another community. The current drugs of choice out on the streets may be determined by availability and price, with cheaper drugs most often used by the poor. Given that each drug, and each combination of drugs, has its own profile of how it impacts a user's mood and behavior, it is important for service providers to keep up to date on their knowledge of currently available and popular substances and their effects. The lack of supply of one drug may lead users to other substances, often with unknown effects. Because there is no control of quality, purity, and composition, what is offered may not necessarily be what is advertised. When it comes to drugs, you can't be certain of what someone has taken.

> **Textbox 8.2. Methamphetamines: Cheap and Deadly**
> A good example of drug availability, toxicity, and lethality is the use of methamphetamines, also known as crystal meth. An inexpensive version can be made quickly and cheaply using common home chemicals. However, the purity and toxicity are usually unknown and can be physically hazardous. Addiction is rapid and its negative physiological effects are almost immediate. It tends to become more available at times when supplies of other drugs are scarce because it can be readily produced with locally available ingredients.

USE, INTOXICATION, ABUSE, AND DEPENDENCY

While many people safely use some substances, their use can become problematic both because of the effects that the substance has on the individual during one episode of use (substance induced) and the effects the individual experiences from frequent and excessive use, which varies from abuse to dependence (Munson, 2001, p. 147). The effects of one-time overuse include intoxication and withdrawal. Intoxication involves the maladaptive behavior and psychological and physiological effects that are the direct result of substance use. It is a reversible syndrome that is characterized by the unique characteristic effects of the drug(s) used. Withdrawal is substance-specific in its presentation. It involves the maladaptive physical, psychological, and behavioral changes that a person experiences in the process of discontinuing excessive and prolonged substance use, and causes significant distress and impairment. Some withdrawal syndromes, such as withdrawal from alcohol, can be life-threatening.

Substance abuse and dependency result from prolonged use of one or more substances despite the negative consequences—relational, social, performance (work or school), and legal—associated with prolonged excessive use. While the demarcation between abuse and dependence is not precisely defined, it is commonly accepted that dependence involves development of tolerance (more substance is used to achieve the same effect), a withdrawal syndrome when the individual attempts to stop using, and preoccupation with getting and using the substance (DSM-5). Most persons who are homeless and who are using drugs are abusing these substances and generally experience a withdrawal syndrome in attempts to become and remain sober. Appendix 5 provides a list of common intoxication and withdrawal effects.

DRUG PATHWAYS AND BODY REACTIONS

The way that a drug enters the body has considerable influence over how fast the user feels the effects. Since the chemical needs to reach the centers of the brain that control feeling, thought, and emotion, the faster the route, the more immediate and usually the stronger the impact. The central passage of chemicals to the brain is through the flow of blood, which is pumped by the heart to the lungs, and then sent to the brain. Thus the fastest way to get a drug to the brain is through inhalation. This is why ether is such a fast and powerful anesthetic. It is also the reason that crack cocaine, which is smoked, starts with a rush of euphoria within ten to twenty seconds following inhalation. By contrast, cocaine that is injected must first travel to the heart before reaching the brain, which delays its effect and the extent of its impact.

We can trace the impact and effect of other drugs the same way. In nicotine patches, the drug is absorbed through the skin, travels through small capillaries to reach larger veins, before reaching the heart and then the brain. Drugs that are swallowed first have to be broken down by the stomach and absorbed into the circulatory system through the intestinal walls before hitting the blood superhighway and eventually getting to the brain. This is one reason why smoking and injecting drugs are favored by those highly addicted and in need of an immediate high.

Although alcohol is typically swallowed and needs to be broken into different chemical parts before being absorbed into the bloodstream, it has historically been the favored mood-altering substance of many cultural groups around the world. One constant has been the abundant use and overuse of alcohol socially, as a part of recreational activities, and as an effective way to calm the nerves, ease the jitters, dull the senses, and forget, among others. Because of its ease of availability and its social acceptance, alcohol has also become the most widely abused substance. Even when the availability of other drugs on the street is scarce, alcohol is usually available. It can easily be made at home; homebrew can be both potent and toxic. Thus frontline workers will be exposed to alcohol use—and abuse—on a daily basis. Alcohol has serious side effects, during both the intoxication and withdrawal stages, which is why we first turn to look at its effects. It is also frequently used in combination with other substances that either intensify the effects of the drugs, such as anti-depressants, or are used to counteract some of the unpleasant effects of other drugs, such as a depressant after use of a stimulant (cocaine is a good example of such a stimulant which is used in combination with alcohol as a depressant). For these reasons we focus first on alcohol and its pervasive effects.

Alcohol: Major Effects

One quick and simple way to classify alcohol and drugs is by the immediate effect they have on the body and the mind. It is the immediate effect that most users seek, preferring to deal with negative or adverse effects after experiencing the immediate relief that the drug offers. Alcohol is first and foremost a depressant and initially slows physiological responses. In a rebound effect it may also increase other responses. Alcohol is given its own special attention for several important reasons:

1. It is the most frequently abused substance among those who are homeless.
2. Its effects are pervasive on the body and the mind.
3. Withdrawal from alcohol is a critical health issue and potentially life-threatening

The frontline worker will frequently encounter people who are under the influence or are sobering up. Not all need medical intervention, but

> **Textbox 8.3. The Rebound Effect**
>
> A human body tries to maintain a state of physiological balance called homeostasis. The intake of alcohol or drugs throws off this equilibrium. As alcohol is a depressant, it will slow down physical responses such as heart rate and blood pressure. In an effort to compensate for the slowdown, the body accelerates its responses, resulting in faster heart rate, higher blood pressure, anxiety, and other symptoms. This is called a rebound effect. The more severe the rebound, the more dangerous and life-threatening it can be. Not all substances have a serious physical rebound effect, but those that do require immediate medical attention for the user.

some do and it is usually the first person on the scene who will need to make a judgment call. Given the fact that alcohol may also be taken with other drugs, it is not always apparent whether the interaction of the two may aggravate or diminish the withdrawal response. It is always wise to err on the side of caution and request a medical evaluation if withdrawal is present and any serious signs emerge.

Alcohol is typically swallowed and thus travels to the stomach and intestines, where it is absorbed into the circulatory system and makes its way to all vital organs in the body. As a result, extensive alcohol use causes damage to all major body organs that attempt to cope with the biochemical responses to alcohol. The result is a vast array of physical and mental problems (table 8.2).

> **Textbox 8.4. Withdrawal Signs: The Opposite of Intoxication**
>
> A rule of thumb in the detection and treatment of withdrawal from any mood- and mind-altering substance is that the withdrawal signs and symptoms will be the opposite of the intoxication symptoms. For example, if a drug's immediate effect is sedation, its rebound effect will be agitation.

In addition, alcohol intoxication and withdrawal can cause significant physiological responses, some of which may be life-threatening (table 8.3):

Alcohol Withdrawal Syndrome

An outreach worker or a shelter worker can encounter alcohol withdrawal syndrome any hour of the day and any day of the week, on the streets and

Table 8.2. Physical and Mental Effects of Alcohol Abuse

Physical	Mental
Bleeding in the digestive tract	Depression and suicide
Pancreatitis	Memory loss
Liver disease, including cirrhosis	Dementia
High blood pressure	Anxiety and agitation
Sleep dysfunction	Sleep dysfunction increases depression and lack of concentration
Cancer of the esophagus, liver, colon, and other areas	Irreversible brain disorder (Wernicke-Korsakoff syndrome) caused by chronic alcoholism
Erectile dysfunction	
Menstrual cycle changes	
Heart damage	

in shelters. It is most common in the morning hours when the shelters have closed intake for the night and those with withdrawal tremors seek a place to sleep. Safety is not usually a concern—just a place to sleep it off. Late afternoon is another time when withdrawal symptoms are frequent, especially during a heat wave, when the effects of the alcohol still left in the body are amplified and plenty of water may be hard to access.

Alcohol withdrawal typically begins within twelve to twenty-four hours after the last drink and can last up to five days. Major symptoms typically begin within forty-eight hours and peak at seventy-two hours. They can be life threatening. They require immediate medical attention. In addition to the above signs, more-serious complications include the following:

- Delirium tremens (DTs): DTs are a combination of agitation, anorexia (not eating), severe memory disturbance, and hallucinations. They usually begin within one day and stop after five days but may not occur until the second week after a person stops drinking.
- Alcoholic hallucinosis: Found in persons with serious alcohol dependence, this refers to auditory hallucinations reported two or more days after the last drink. They can be frightening and confusing.

Table 8.3. Physiological and Psychological Signs of Intoxication and Withdrawal

Physical signs of intoxication	Psychological signs of intoxication	Signs of withdrawal
Slurred speech	Irritability	Nausea or vomiting*
Lack of coordination	Mood swings	Anxiety*
Unsteady gait	Short attention span	Depressed mood or irritability
Blackouts	Decreased judgment	
Loud and frequent talking	Decreased inhibitions	Malaise or weakness*
	Interference with memory	Hyperactivity
Nystagmus (involuntary eye movements)		Sweating/increased blood pressure*
Flushed face		Tachycardia (heart palpitations)*
Slowness of movement		Tremor of the hands, tongue, or eyelids*
		Orthostatic hypotension: dizzy spell on standing suddenly*

* = Evaluate for medical intervention.

- Generalized seizures: These may occur two or three days after a person stops drinking.
- *Note:* Concurrent drug use may change the time and duration of the withdrawal complications.

A vicious cycle of alcohol overuse can be amplified as illustrated in the following scenario. As the individual starts to experience withdrawal through tremors and agitation, headache, and thirst, she experiences a stronger craving for booze. This starts a quest for alcohol at any price; when she obtains the booze, she will have an immediate urge to gorge—that is, to drink too much too fast. This overloads the body with too much alcohol, which both increases tolerance for its effects and further damages the liver with alcohol overload. Breaking the cycle is difficult because of the body's strong demand for relief from painful withdrawal symptoms. Detox facilities and sobering-up stations are the most supportive and helpful ways to provide supervised withdrawal.

Challenges in remote and rural communities where alcohol—legal, illegal, and home-brewed—is often abused include the fact that sobering-up places may consist of the local jail, and that breaking the law through commission of petty infractions such as loitering may be the only way that someone can get a start on the sobering-up process. In these rural communities abuse has been reported at ages twelve and below. When kids do not get access to alcohol they often turn to inhalants such as gas and glue, which are legally available. We will speak more of this later in this chapter.

OTHER COMMON TYPES OF MIND- AND MOOD-ALTERING DRUGS

The substance abuse treatment community classifies drugs, regardless of whether they are legally or illegally obtained, according to the kind of effect they have on the body (table 8.4). The major groupings and types in North America are alcohol, barbiturates and similar sedative-hypnotics, opioids derived from the poppy plant and its synthetic partners, amphetamines and similar synthetics that stimulate the adrenal system, cannabis (marijuana and hashish), powdered and crack cocaine, hallucinogens (LSD, PCP, psilocybin), and inhalants (gas, glue, paints, aerosols). We will quickly look at their primary effects, the dangers of use and overdose, and the problems of withdrawal and dependency.

Barbiturates and other sedative-hypnotics have been available as legal, controlled drugs, and also illegally for over a century. They are usually taken orally or intravenously and are often used pre- and postoperatively to combat pain and anxiety. Physically they depress the central nervous system, creating sleepiness, relaxation, increased talkativeness, and euphoria. Symptoms of intoxication may include impaired attention, irritability, anxiety, aggressiveness, and mood lability. Barbiturates, as depressants, are life-threatening both as overdoses and during withdrawal from use. They slow down the central nervous system, thus decreasing respiration and heart rate. Their use concurrently with alcohol is both potent and dangerous because of the combined depressant effects of both substances. Seizures during withdrawal, in addition to anxiety, insomnia, and agitation, can lead to life-threatening medical emergencies. Withdrawal can be equally medically problematic, which

Table 8.4. Drugs, Their Effects, and Their Appeal

Class of Substance	Some Examples	Specific Effects	Appeal
Alcohol: CNS depressant	Wine, beer, spirits (hard liquor)	Sedation Impaired coordination Impaired concentration Rapidly fluctuating moods Disinhibition	Reduced anxiety Social lubricant Disinhibition
Other CNS depressants: sedatives, hypnotics, anxiolytics	Hypnotics, sedatives, minor tranquilizers including barbiturates and benzodiazepines	Sedation Reduction of anxiety Decreased muscle tone and coordination	Sedation Reduced anxiety
CNS stimulants	Amphetamines Dexedrine Ephedrine Cocaine (powdered and crack) Ritalin	CNS arousal Anesthesia Increased energy Decreased appetite Improved mood Euphoria Agitation, belligerence, paranoia, hallucinations (high doses/prolonged use)	Perceived sense of competence Euphoria Sexual arousal Sense of increased energy and alertness
Narcotics and opioids	Opium, heroin, morphine, methadone, analgesics (all pain killers)	Sedation Reduced anxiety Euphoria Apathy Reduced sensitivity to physical and emotional pain CNS depression of breathing, coughing, circulation	Reduced sensitivity to emotional and physical pain Reduced anxiety Initial rush of euphoric feelings

Table 8.4. (Continued)

Class of Substance	Some Examples	Specific Effects	Appeal
Cannabinols	Marijuana, hashish	Decreases anxiety Produces shift in concentration and dissociative reaction Alters perception of time and space Alters judgment of speed and distance Decreases motivation and concentration At high concentrations, produces hallucinations	Dispels boredom Narrow focus of concentration Exaggeration of senses and emotions Anxiety reduction Dissociative effects
Hallucinogens or psychedelics	LSD, mescaline, psilocybin (mushrooms), MDMA (ecstasy), designer drugs	Visual illusions Perceptual changes Dissociative Altered sense of time Hallucinations, depersonalization, derealization Euphoria	Alters sensory input Accentuates mood Creates illusions Synesthesia (crossover from one sense to another) Sense of affiliation and bonding (MMDA)
Inhalants/Solvents	Glue, paint, paint thinners, cleaning agents, aerosol propellants, other petroleum products	Mild intoxication Hallucinations Loss of memory, confusion Visual disturbances Decreased appetite	Immediate effect of an intoxicated state Readily available legally
Phencyclidine (PCP)	PCP (angel dust) Note: This drug can be stored in the body, unmetabolized, for days or weeks. The drug effect can be reexperienced as though the drug had just been ingested, even months after last use.	Characteristics of depressants and stimulants In high doses: hallucinations, paranoid delusions Depression Disorientation and confusion	Relaxation Euphoria Dissociation Sensory distortion Blocks physical pain

CNS = central nervous system.

is why detoxification should occur under strict medical supervision. Inhalants, such as gases and liquids that turn quickly to vapors, are often inhaled by those with limited or no access to alcohol, such as youths and alcoholics with no funds for regular booze. Inhalants are universally obtainable, and many have no restrictions on their sales to minors.

ADDICTIVE MECHANISMS AND PATHWAYS

There are several ways to examine and understand addiction (figure 8.3). The first way looks at the different factors that influence the development of an addictive disorder. They include biological factors of heredity; individual factors of personality, talents, and abilities, and physical, psychological, and emotional capacities; and environmental influences of family, friends, home life, peers, the community we live in, socioeconomic status, and the culture that we belong to (and many others).

The classical pattern of progressive alcohol use and consequent performance dysfunction in individuals is depicted by the Jellinek Curve (figure 8.4). Based on a concept of disease progression of alcoholism developed by Jellinek (1960), this curve was developed to help those suffering from alcoholism and treatment providers to identify various stages in the progression of the disease.

The curve consists of a slope downward that highlights the kinds of behavior that indicate progressively more substance dependence with one behavior usually preceding the next:

- Occasional relief drinking that leads to constant relief drinking
- Development of tolerance to alcohol
- Surreptitious drinking and urgency of first drink
- Feelings of guilt and inability to discuss the problem
- Decreased ability to stop drinking, even when others do so
- Excuses for drinking, leading to remorse over drinking
- Neglect of other interests
- Family and friends avoided, or attempts at a geographical cure (move away to try new beginnings)
- Work and money problems

Figure 8.3. Interplay of Factors That Lead to Addictions

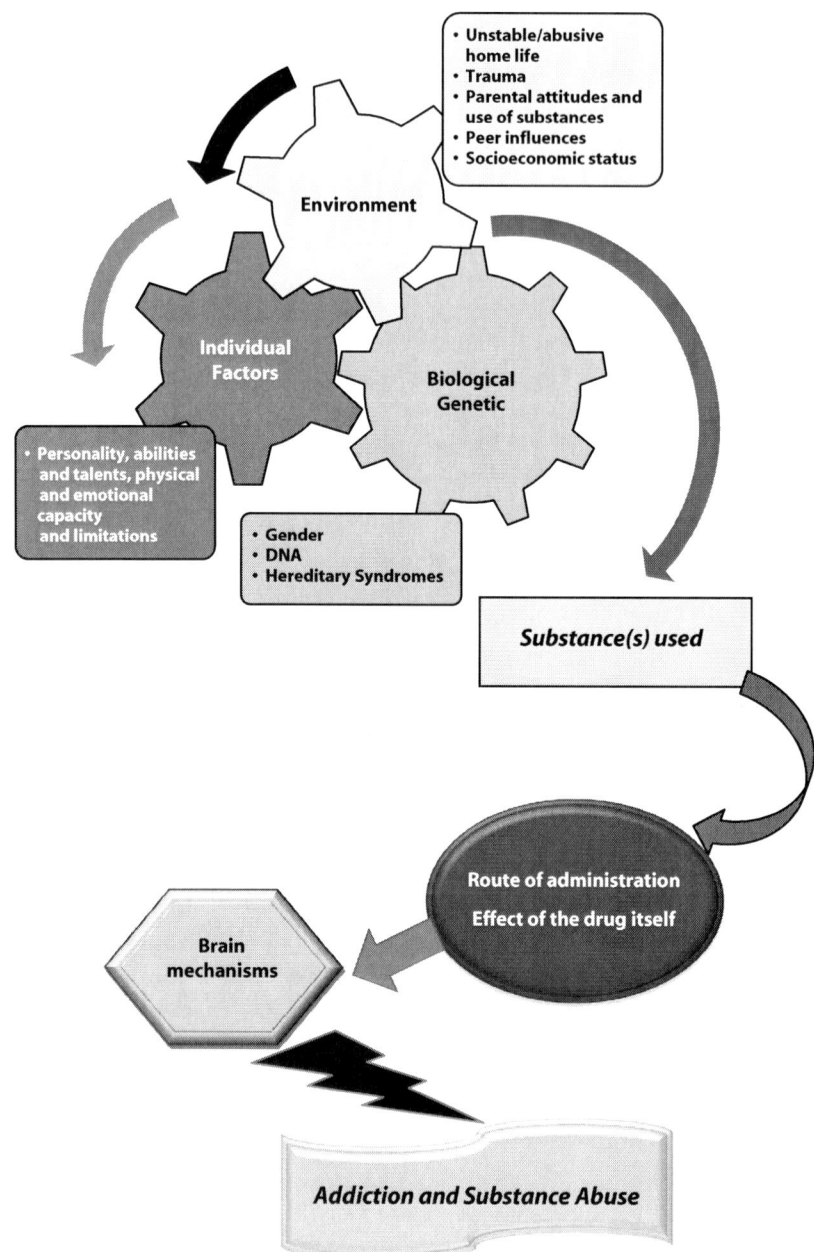

Figure 8.4. Addiction and Recovery: The Jellinek Curve

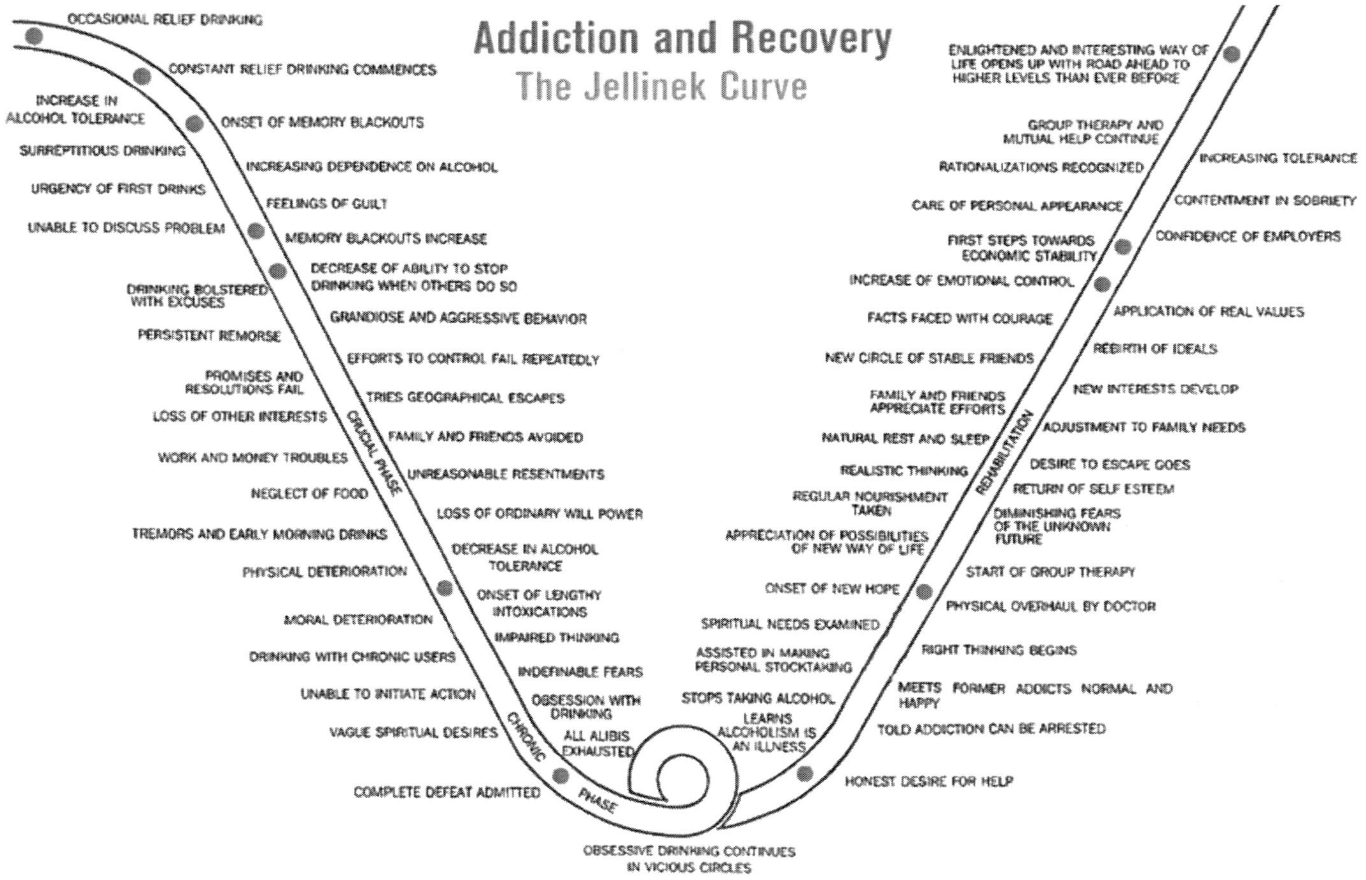

- Neglect of food
- Physical deterioration: morning tremors, decreased tolerance for alcohol
- Moral deterioration and impaired thinking
- Onset of lengthy intoxications
- All alibis exhausted and defeat admitted

At this stage a person has hit rock bottom and the only choices are recovery or death from chronic alcoholism. Interventions may happen at any point along this path. They consist of the following and are modified to account for the extent (how long) and the chronicity (how much physical and mental damage) of the alcoholism on the individual. These steps generally are in progressive order, as follows:

- Accepts that there is a problem and begins to learn about alcoholism as a disease.
- Starts to think about quitting and contemplates treatment (move from pre-contemplation to contemplation).
- Agrees to seek help.
- Stops drinking and begins treatment (inpatient or outpatient, depending on need).
- Meets others in treatment and the recovery process.
- Learns more about the progressive nature of alcoholism and enters group therapy.
- Joins a self-help group.
- Improves self-care and starts a healthy diet; appearance begins to improve.
- Evaluates the impact and damages to self and others as a result of the alcohol abuse.
- Recognizes the need to stay away from substance-using people and places; mourns this loss.
- Evaluates the moral and emotional damages caused by drinking and incorporates a spiritual element in recovery thinking.
- Examines and addresses relationships with family and friends damaged by the drinking behaviors.

- Changes social and recreational habits, seeking new, nonusing friends.
- Develops new ways of coping emotionally.
- Develops new employment and work behaviors.
- Recognizes that relapse is a continuing threat and makes contingency plans to address relapse warning signs.

Although there has been some dispute about the accuracy of the curve, and its applicability for those who have not experienced the extremes of chronic alcohol abuse, it continues to be a model used in treatment. For many persons in addiction recovery this curve hits home and provides a clear and specific outline of behaviors that most can relate to. It provides some indication of the level of severity of the addiction but does not indicate what the appropriate interventions should be at any specific stage of the addictive cycle. A simplified version of the Jellinek model shown in figure 8.5 indicates the critical points along the path to addiction.

The Jellinek model does indicate that treatment cannot truly be effective until there is an honest acceptance of the disease. It provides a road map to sobriety and recovery from abuse and dependence on alcohol and other abused substances. In the light of what we currently know about alcohol and other addictions, most treatment specialists would add, at the right side of the bottom of the curve, a slot to indicate that detoxification from alcohol and other substances is the first step to sobriety.

Today substance-abuse specialists also refer to the stages of change model developed by Prochaska and DiClemente (1986). This model describes the mileposts that an individual needs to reach in order to move to a substance-free lifestyle. It is used to define the intensity and focus of treatment for an individual and thus to wisely prevent entrance into treatment when motivation is not present, and discharge when recovery and abstinence have not been fully achieved. While the Jellinek curve details specific destructive behaviors during the critical phase of alcohol abuse, the Prochaska and DiClemente model focuses on identifying thoughts and behaviors that indicate an awareness of an abuse problem, the indicators for a readiness for change, the commitment to actively change behaviors, and the acquisition of a changed lifestyle. The Jellinek model may help substance abusers to specify destructive behaviors and their consequences, but it does not specify when someone is ready to change, be it in the critical or chronic stage of addiction. The stages of change (figure 8.6) indicate the readiness

Figure 8.5. Stages of Addiction

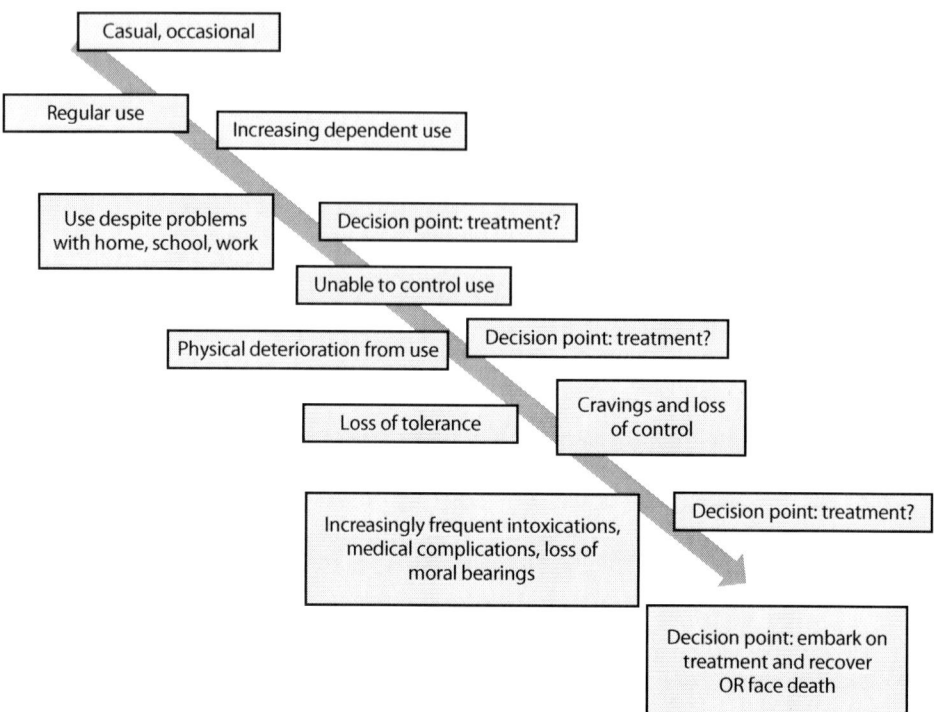

for treatment and help frontline workers to concentrate with clients on precontemplation and contemplation phases, which is where most persons encountered will be struggling.

SUBSTANCE-ABUSE TREATMENT

Detoxification, Intensive Treatment, and Levels of Care

For many people who lose their housing, drinking is initially part of a social level of interacting with others in the same situation. It then often progresses to selectively drinking with a special cohort of like-minded individuals, and then moves on to protecting one's stash. Group drinking then becomes less of a social affair. The drinking behavior of the main characters in *Ragged Company* is illustrative of these behaviors.

Figure 8.6. Stages of Change

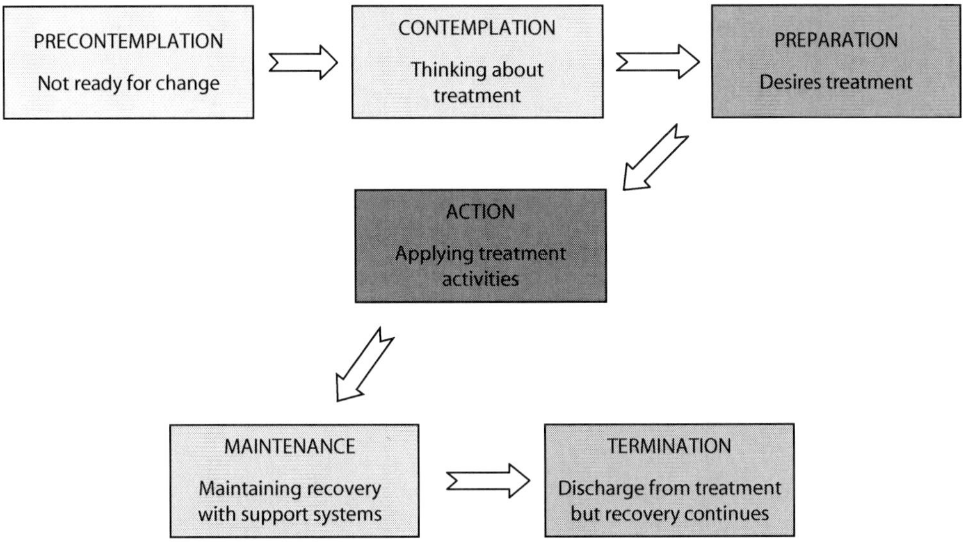

```
┌─────────────────────┐      ┌─────────────────────┐      ┌─────────────────────┐
│   PRECONTEMPLATION  │  ⇒   │    CONTEMPLATION    │  ⇒   │     PREPARATION     │
│  Not ready for change│      │  Thinking about     │      │  Desires treatment  │
│                     │      │     treatment       │      │                     │
└─────────────────────┘      └─────────────────────┘      └─────────────────────┘
                                                                    ⇓
                              ┌─────────────────────┐
                              │       ACTION        │
                              │  Applying treatment │
                              │      activities     │
                              └─────────────────────┘
                                       ⇓
┌─────────────────────┐      ┌─────────────────────┐
│     MAINTENANCE     │  ⇒   │     TERMINATION     │
│ Maintaining recovery│      │ Discharge from treatment│
│ with support systems│      │ but recovery continues │
└─────────────────────┘      └─────────────────────┘
```

Source: Prochaska & DiClemente (1986).

With the Jellinek Curve in mind, we can turn to looking at what interventions are necessary to help a person become and remain sober. These interventions fall into three well-defined stages of treatment for addictive disorders: detox, intensive treatment, and after-care. Detoxification, the first essential step to recovery, involves the withdrawal or elimination of the abused substance from the body. Thereafter intensive treatment focuses on helping the individual to understand substance abuse, its impact, the personal reasons for using, and identification of the personal and life changes essential for continued abstinence. The final phase is ongoing personal self-care and supportive help to continue abstinence and follow a substance-free lifestyle. Table 8.5 gives an overview of the different treatment options, both in the community and in residential settings that are available. It also provides details on the criteria that are normally used to determine what level of treatment is indicated, and the intensity of service that each type of treatment program generally provides.

The withdrawal from alcohol and some other substances, such as barbiturates, can be complex, a serious medical issue, and potentially life-threatening, especially when use has been chronic. As the body has adapted

Table 8.5. Substance Abuse Levels and Locations of Care

Level of care	Treatment Modality Name	Clinical Needs and Examples of Treatment Settings	Level of Intensity by Number of Hours
Level I	Outpatient	No medical problems that may complicate treatment Low severity of problems Low-intensity outpatient	Minimum of four hours and less than nine hours weekly
Level I-D (detox)	Outpatient detoxification without extended onsite monitoring	Medically supervised, in office or clinic setting or treatment facility	One hour, two to three times weekly
Level II	Intensive outpatient Day treatment/partial hospitalization	Intensive outpatient treatment, structured day or evening program, or clinically managed structured day program	Range from nine to forty hours weekly
Level III-D (detox)	Clinically managed detox	Residential detoxification	Twenty-four hours daily for two to seven days
Level III	Residential	Residential treatment, structured therapeutic community	Twenty-four hours daily for twenty days or longer
Level IV	Full medically managed intensive inpatient treatment, hospital setting	Withdrawal symptoms or potential of withdrawal severe enough to require inpatient care, physician management, concurrent serious medical problems, hospital	Twenty-four hours, emergency services, one to five days

to the repeated ingestion of substances it has physically attempted to accommodate to the substances. This is one reason why a heavy user will develop a tolerance to the effects of the substance, and seek increasingly more of the substance in order to feel the same mood- and mind-altering effects. When the substance is no longer available the body attempts to develop a physiological balance, known as homeostasis. Textbox 8.3 discusses the need for this homeostatic balance. In human terms, the lack of balance means feelings and reactions previously suppressed or controlled by drugs now are felt to a greater extreme. Anxiety and depression are two of the most common that surface in intense form when drugs and alcohol are withdrawn. Other physical responses such as heart rate, blood pressure, rapidity of breathing, feelings of irritability and excitement, and many more are likely to become more intense during withdrawal from alcohol and drug use. While in some medically prescribed instances withdrawal may be gradual in order to avoid an extreme medical crisis, in most instances the discontinuation of use is sudden and the days immediately following can be acutely distressful for the individual.

The timing and place of the detoxification can often be chosen by the individual, depending on motivation and the availability of a safe place with support and supervision. In many instances where a person is incarcerated or hospitalized the withdrawal can be unplanned and often unmotivated. In these instances the medical personnel in the facility should be alerted to the possibility of medical complications from certain life-threatening withdrawal syndromes.

Levels of Care

When speaking of levels of care, mental health and substance-abuse professionals refer to the location of treatment and also the intensity, type, and duration of treatment required to help a person achieve a level of sobriety that can be maintained with regular and consistent maintenance. Treatment can occur in a residential setting or on an outpatient basis. It can be as short as fourteen days or last several months. Unfortunately, the length of residential stay for optimal treatment results has no support in research. Rather, in almost all situations the length of stay is determined by what the individual's health benefit plan will pay, and the practice of length of stay predicated on insurance coverage has become ingrained in the residential treatment community as accepted fact, albeit without proof. People with independent wealth who can and will pay privately can find programs whose length of stay is more individually determined. For those who are homeless and dependent on publicly paid programs (United States) and the guidelines of provincial health-care plans (Canada), residential treatment is generally capped at twenty-eight days. Outpatient treatment can consist of frequencies ranging from daily (a day treatment program) to several times a week (intensive weekly), and decreasing to weekly and less frequently depending on need, progress, and the amount of service provided under the payment plan. Maintenance usually consists of a support group meeting on a weekly or individually determined basis.

The availability of an array of treatment options is most likely to occur in cities and larger towns that can support these types of services. This means that those living in small towns and rural locations have to opt for residential care away from home and have few continuing treatment options when they return; they are often thrust back into the lifestyle that originally supported the addictive behaviors. In addition to the availability of treatment options, there is, when all options are present, a need to further identify which persons will achieve sobriety at a specific level of treatment intensity. The rule of thumb is to offer no more intense services than required but to not expect treatment success if sufficient treatment supports are not available.

The American Society of Addiction Medicine has developed a COC model that addresses treatment need along several dimensions: (1) medical risk associated with acute intoxication or withdrawal; (2) concurrent medical conditions that present medical risk during detoxification and intensive treatment; (3) psychological and behavioral conditions that present treatment risks during detoxification and early treatment, including the concurrent need for psychotropic (generally referred to as psychiatric) medication; (4) acceptance of the abuse and motivation or readiness for change; (5) extent of the possibility of relapse and degree of medical consequences of relapse; and (6) the recovery environment's support of relapse prevention. The greater the risk in each of these areas, the greater the necessity for more intensive supervision and support in detox and early intensive treatment. A matrix chart that uses these six American Society of Addiction Medicine criteria to match treatment need with treatment intensity was presented in table 8.5. This chart presents levels of care as least intensive at level I and suggests incremental implementation of increased care so that greatest need for medical intervention and inpatient care is provided at level IV. Although this staging system has good face validity—that is, it appears to be appropriate—it is important to remember that this matrix has not been completely tested for validity and reliability, and thus remains a medical "best opinion."

The need for medical supervision should always take priority when a person withdraws from substance abuse. Detoxification (often called detox) and intensive treatment can take place in either hospital or residential treatment settings. The difference between these two is the amount of medical supervision and life-support equipment available in case of acute crisis or complications. Hospitals provide the most specialized medical care, important for those with concurrent medical conditions that require constant monitoring while the body experiences withdrawal from toxic substances. Residential treatment facilities for substance abuse usually have medically trained staff but do not have the intensity of medical specialists or the facilities for specialized care. In situations where there is a concurrent psychiatric condition, monitoring is best conducted in an inpatient unit where the medications can be adjusted according to the changing reactions of a person experiencing detoxification.

While detox rids the body of the noxious effects of alcohol and drugs, it does not address the mental and emotional issues that interplay in addictions, not does it deal with the devastating social and lifestyle issues that usually create additional problems. While it is possible to evaluate some of the factors that will determine ongoing intensive treatment, such as lifestyle, the existence of concurrent medical and psychiatric disorders, and the extent of support in the individual's community upon discharge, it is not possible to accurately evaluate the degree of motivation to change or the relapse potential. In addition, the long-term emotional effects of substance use do not dissipate as quickly as the physical withdrawal rids the body of toxicity. Simply put, the emotional withdrawal and behavioral changes needed for continued sobriety and substance-free living take considerably longer to deal with than the detoxification period.

Dealing with the additional emotional and behavioral changes required for continued sobriety is the immediate goal of treatment. Intensive treatment consists of a combination of activities that address the acceptance of the addiction; the need for fundamental changes; the recognition of the impact of the addiction personally and on close relationships; learning about alcohol, drugs, and the addictive process (see figure 8.6); the assessment of individual strengths, weaknesses, and problem areas of functioning; the development of alternative behaviors and lifestyles to replace addictive behaviors; and the restoration of damaged relationships (where possible). This is a large list of goals, not easily accomplished in the limited few weeks most addiction treatment programs have for intensive treatment.

AA, NA, and Other Peer Support Programs

The treatment interventions and levels of care do not include AA and related self-help groups, primarily because they are outside the professional treatment continuum. Nonetheless, their existence for seventy-five years, widespread acceptance, and numerous testaments of effectiveness make these groups a fundamental component of recovery from alcohol and other drugs. Because of the AA community's historical refusal to engage in research, there is no evidence as to how many people have been helped to begin a path of sobriety, to use AA as the primary means of achieving an abstinence-free life, or to support continued sobriety. But people speak most loudly with their actions, and AA has been attended as a support program of choice for millions of persons who have been challenged by addictions. It is also routinely recommended by professionals for those who are in and continuing recovery.

MOTIVATIONAL INTERVIEWING AND THE NEED FOR CHANGE

The frontline worker is most frequently presented with the challenge of the uncommitted abuser of alcohol and other drugs, who may not necessarily admit to an addictive behavior. Confronting a person with the problem has been shown to be rather ineffective in many instances, and often leads to greater resistance to engage in any meaningful dialogue around change. Motivational interviewing has been shown to be an effective way of helping an individual to move from denial through the stages of change to active treatment. The effectiveness of motivational interviewing comes from the fact that it avoids confrontation of the abuse with all of its negative implications. Instead, it uses a positive view of the individual as able to change and a process of reflection of the person's behavior as separate from his inherent worth.

Motivational interviewing has several important aspects that differentiate it from other interviewing and counseling techniques. Fundamental to motivational interviewing is the recognition that a person has inherent

> **Textbox 8.5. Fundamentals of Motivational Interviewing**
> Use a positive, empathic approach.
> Establish trust—slowly.
> Focus the conversation on the individual's expressed goals.
> Gently explore discrepancies between goals and behaviors.
> Avoid judgment of discrepancies.
> Avoid conflict and confrontation that may spark a power struggle.

worth and that while their actions may be unacceptable, as a person they are likeable. This is the basis for establishing a positive relationship based on empathetic understanding, mutual trust, and acceptance of the other person and his worldview. The distinction of acceptance of the person without acceptance of destructive and addictive behaviors is thus fundamental to the establishment of this relationship. Within the framework of this relationship, the worker and the counselor can begin to sensitively approach the goal of having the individual recognize, accept, and determine to change maladaptive and destructive behaviors. The process includes some basic elements that use a cognitive behavioral format.

The path to change begins with a positive, empathic, mutually trusting relationship, and this must be the first goal. Within this context there are several important cautions. The conversation should ideally emerge from learning about a person's expressed goals, regardless of how great or insignificant they may appear. These goals become the foundation for establishing a plan of action and exploring how it can be achieved. This is also the place in the developing relationship for noting the discrepancies between what is said and the realities of how a person currently behaves, and how these align with or contradict the action plan. Within this context, avoiding argumentation is essential to maintaining a level and mutually respectful relationship that avoids a power struggle and the denial that often follows a confrontation. As arguments are among the various ways that people resist accepting the truth, you need to learn to roll with the resistance and understand that it is part of the process. Throughout all interactions, support the person's efforts, remembering for both of you that self-efficacy is fundamental to change; that everyone can, in time, make the changes; and that change is within the person's own control and not that of anyone else. Based on the work by Donovan and O'Leary (1978), table 8.6 presents some attitudes held by many people who have problems controlling their alcohol use. These

Table 8.6. Drinking Related Internal/External Locus of Control

1. I feel so helpless in some situations that I need a drink.
2. Trouble at work or at home drives me to drink.
3. Without the right breaks one cannot stay sober.
4. Many times there are circumstances that force me to drink.
5. I get so upset over small arguments that they cause me to drink.
6. Staying sober depends mainly on things going right for me.
7. Oftentimes, other people drive me to drink.
8. It is impossible for me to resist taking a drink if I am at a party where others are drinking.
9. I cannot feel good unless I am drinking.
10. Sometimes I cannot understand how people can control their drinking.
11. Once I start to drink I can't stop.
12. Drinking is my favorite form of entertainment.

elements emphasize behaviors and consequences while avoiding the most common features of direct confrontation: resistance and denial.

RELAPSE AND RELAPSE PREVENTION

Most addiction specialists accept the reality that addictive disorders are not cured in the sense that they will never again pose problems for the individual who has been through treatment. To the contrary, most persons who have dealt with a substance-abuse disorder continue to deal all their lives with prevention of relapse into use of any addictive substance as this use usually and eventually leads to a return to abuse. Thus alcohol and other addictive substances are viewed as having a high potential for relapse and prevention has to be both a focus of active treatment and a lifelong strategy.

There are risk and preventative factors that predispose a person to relapse or help to prevent return to problem use. Some of these factors include those internal to the individual and some depend on the environment into which the person returns after inpatient rehabilitation (Brown, Vik, Patterson, Grant, & Schuckit, 1995). Individual protective factors include a higher socioeconomic status, a stable childhood, and a sense of self-efficacy (Marlatt, Larimer, & Witkiewitz, 2011). Risks for relapse include the level of commitment to sobriety, the individual's personal goals for sobriety, basic attitudes about substance use and abuse, the extent to which alcohol and other substances are used to regulate a person's mood, and whether the individual had plans to relapse. Protective factors to relapse prevention include level of commitment to continued counseling and/or supports such as AA, support from family, an alcohol-free living environment (no drinking cues readily available), and planned substance-free recreational and social activities (Donovan & O'Leary, 1978, p. 767). McKiernan and colleagues (McKiernan, Cloud, Patterson, Golder, & Besel, 2011) developed a short questionnaire that helps to determine the extent to which a person feels that he has control over thoughts, feelings, and behaviors around drinking and using drugs (see appendix 3). Modeled after previous work by DiClemente and colleagues (DiClemente, Hansen, & Ponton, 1996) that looked at four categories of high risk for relapse (negative affect, physical and other concerns, urges to use, and positive states and social interactions), the present measure is both short and focused and divides self-efficacy into two main areas: issues around the extent to which a person may be tempted to use, and the same scenarios with a focus on the confidence a person has to not use in specific situations. Frontline workers may find this useful in discussing relapse prevention strategies with clients.

HARM REDUCTION

Many substance users may not be ready to contemplate a drug-free lifestyle. However, they often will respond to suggestions of alternatives that may reduce the harmful effects on themselves and society of their substance-abusing behaviors. This approach is most often referred to as "harm reduction." It can best be described as a "set of compassionate and pragmatic approaches for reducing harm associated with high risk behaviors and improving the quality of life" (Lowinson, Ruiz, Millman, & Langrod, 2004, p. 5). When referring to addictive substance use, it incorporates a range of behaviors from safer use, to managed use, to reduced use. There are a number of strategies that fall under the umbrella of harm reduction: needle exchange programs, safe injection sites, methadone maintenance, safe driving or designated driving programs, condom use and availability, and tolerance of sex trade workers in certain locations. Canada and the United States have different levels of acceptance of harm reduction. Harm reduction programs have an important role in the care of homeless and those at high risk for homelessness. Because of the high rates of substance use in this population, and the attendant risk of contracting STDs, including HIV/AIDS, strategies that lower the probability of transmission are an important personal and public health issue. These strategies are discussed in more detail in chapter 3 on health-related issues. One important consideration in this discussion on harm reduction is the recognition and acceptance that substance abstinence may not be a realistic or acceptable goal for everyone and reducing risk is preferable to the consequences of continued dangerous behaviors.

EXERCISES

1. Attend an open AA or NA meeting of your choice. Write up your experiences and impressions as part of your journal.
2. Reflect on whether you disclosed that you were a student, or whether you avoided that issue. What were your reasons?
3. Attend a different self-help meeting. Reflect on the differences between the groups. How is this important for supporting a person to go to a twelve-step meeting?
4. Did you disclose your student status the second time? Reflect on the issue of self-disclosure in substance-treatment programs.
5. If you have previously attended an AA or other twelve-step group, how was this experience similar? How was it different?
6. Attend a mental health self-help group and reflect on that experience.

JOURNALING

1. Anger in men may be a sign of an underlying depression. Can you think of an example from your work that would indicate this depression hidden underneath anger may be an issue?
2. Stigma is a major issue for persons with a mental health disorder. Have you seen indications of this at work? On the streets?
3. Do you see this stigma in those with addictive disorders? Is it worse for men or women? Does the type of addiction make a difference?

CHAPTER 9

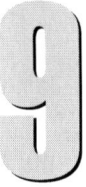

CO-OCCURRING DISORDERS AND TRAUMA-INFORMED CARE

KEY ISSUES	Co-occurring disorders
	Intervention challenges for those with co-occurring disorders
	Trauma
	How organizations can create a trauma-informed service environment
	Traumatic responses
	Consequences of trauma
	What trauma-informed care indicates for the service provider
	Issues of FASD and TBI for homeless persons

OVERVIEW

The recognition of substance-abuse and mental disorder as two distinct but co-occurring disorders first came into use in the early 1980s when mental health practitioners began to observe increasing numbers of mentally ill young adults using marijuana and other illicit drugs along with (sometimes instead of) their psychotropic medications (McKiernan et al., 2011). The concept of two simultaneously diagnosable disorders, one a mental illness and the other a substance-use disorder, was given different labels over the years, among which were the dually diagnosed, mentally ill chemical abuser, substance abuser/mentally ill, co-occurring mental disorder and addictions, and co-occurring disorders. The current trend is to use the "co-occurring disorders" title to indicate specifically which disorders and substances are the focus of discussion. This also helps to distinguish those disorders where mental illness is involved with addictions from medical conditions or developmental disorders that occur along with either a mental health disorder or an addictive one. In this chapter we will first address the challenges of working with those who have both a substance-abuse problem as well as a psychiatric diagnosis of a major mental disorder (i.e., in the areas of depression, bipolar disorder, schizophrenia, and severe anxiety). We will then examine the conundrums in identification and treatment caused by three other frequently co-occurring problems that are prevalent among homeless persons: trauma, traumatic brain injury (TBI), and fetal alcohol spectrum disorder (FASD).

CO-OCCURRING DISORDERS

Many persons who use alcohol and drugs also have one or more mental health problems, some of which are significant mental disorders. When these problems are serious enough to warrant a diagnosis, we speak of persons who have co-occurring disorders consisting of substance use/abuse and a mental illness. In addition, many persons with dual disorders are challenged by low incomes and homelessness (DiClemente, Carbonari, Montgomery, & Hughes, 1994).

Mental disorders and substance-use problems often overlap in several ways.

1. Each affects a person's mood and behavior.
2. Almost all of the behavioral and emotional signs and symptoms of a mental disorder can also be indicative of the influence of mind- and mood-altering substances.
3. Alcohol or drugs can worsen or improve a person's emotions and thoughts/cognitions.
4. Substance use, even without addiction, can disrupt the fragile emotional and behavioral balance experienced by those with a mental illness.

When a mental disorder and addictive substance use are both present, it is most often impossible to determine which disorder is primary, that is which occurred first, which is dominant (is the greater problem), or if the co-occurrence is coincidental. In addition, many persons who have a mental illness may have more than one psychiatric disorder. The existence of additional medical conditions may further complicate the diagnostic and treatment picture. An example would be an individual with a substance-abuse history, a diagnosis of bipolar disorder, a medical condition of multiple sclerosis, and a history of (several) heart attacks. The only effective way to understand the emotional and behavioral complexities of this scenario is to have the individual in a stable environment free of illegal substances and alcohol so that he can be observed and evaluated for mental and emotional issues brought on by the overlapping of these conditions, without the influence of nonprescribed drugs. These evaluations may be difficult to obtain as it is only feasible in a controlled hospital environment where there is less easy access to nonprescribed drugs, and greater availability of trained staff who understand the interplay of the biological, medical, and psychosocial issues. Most persons resist this approach as they see it as confining and a deprivation of personal freedoms, and thus a comprehensive evaluation usually occurs only when a person is hospitalized involuntarily. Even then, it is not always possible to ensure that illegal drugs are kept away from the individual: an ongoing problem is that visitors bring contraband drugs into psychiatric and other medical facilities.

There are several ways that the challenges of co-occurring disorders present themselves. For example, anxiety and depressive disorders are the most common mental disorders people experience, and they are also the ones most often self-medicated by people trying to feel better. There are several reasons why people drink alcohol beyond social sharing of beverages: to relax, as a social lubricant (reduce anxiety), and to feel better (relieve depression). They use cocaine and amphetamines to stimulate or energize themselves (relieve depression), and barbiturates to calm themselves (relieve depression). When people stop abusing alcohol and drugs, the underlying emotional distress reappears and may be felt more acutely because of the lack of anything to relieve this distress (a rebound effect). Unless addictions treatment professionals are able to recognize this distress, the individual may relapse or, in extreme cases, look to end his life. Thus substance-abuse treatment requires knowledge of how mental illness complicates rehabilitation and recovery from substance use/abuse (Marlatt et al., 2011).

Another challenge for those with co-occurring disorders and their treatment providers is the impact that street drugs and nonprescribed medications may have on a person who is already taking medication for a mental disorder. We need to take an additional look at the impact of drugs on human physiology in order to fully appreciate the diagnostic and treatment problems that co-occurring disorders present. As a rule, any substance that enters the body through any route will have a physiological and possible psychological impact. When two or more substances are taken together, the result may be one of the following effects:

1. Two (or more) drugs interact to increase the effect of one or both (potentiate the chemical effect). This synergy may be additive (has a simple additional effect), exponential (one greatly increases the effect of the other), and/or cumulative (the effects amount over time).
2. Two drugs interact and (a) decrease the effect of one or both, (b) decrease the effect of one but not the other, (c) increase the effects of one while decreasing the effects of the other, (d) produce unintended side effects of one or both, or (e) decrease the effect of either or both to a greater extent with continued use.
3. Two drugs interact and each neutralizes the effect of the other.
4. Drugs may have effects that affect concentration and logical thinking or increase psychiatric symptoms such as hallucinations or delusions.
5. Street drugs may be adulterated with other, unknown substances and may also be of higher or lower potency than claimed. This can affect intended and unintended effects of the drugs.

The dangers of mixing different drugs without medical supervision (as happens on the street and with those prone to using illegal drugs) is that any one or more of the above synergistic or interactional effects may be consequences of drug use. The individual may not be using large quantities of illegal substances but may be highly sensitive to interactive effects. The person may decompensate (have an acute increase of psychiatric symptom) and require hospitalization. There is often no clear way to determine which is the cause and which the effect until a person has been clean and sober—that is, not under the influence of alcohol or drugs—for a considerable period of time, usually at least thirty days, depending on the drugs that may be involved.

Research has found that the presence of a substance-use disorder among those with a serious mental illness increases the risk of treatment noncompliance, violence, incarceration, and HIV infection (Drake & Wallach, 2000).

The co-occurrence of major mental disorder and substance-abuse disorders among homeless persons is estimated to be around 70 percent (Drake, Yovetich, Bebout, Harris, & McHugo, 1997). As we explore later in this chapter, these numbers do not include those who are also impacted by TBI or FASD. Some persons may have multiple disabilities. When examined together, these disabilities impact many homeless persons and present significant challenges to frontline workers since it is often not obvious upon casual greeting that a person is impaired.

Co-occurring mental illness and substance-use disorders are especially problematic for a number of reasons. The previous chapters on mental disorders and substance use discussed the various behavioral and cognitive ways in which a person can be affected. One of the major challenges is that signs and symptoms can be related to each, or both, areas. Figure 9.1 provides an illustration of this.

The behavioral and cognitive presentation of a person under the influence of alcohol or drugs may mimic many of the signs of mental illness, including labile emotions, difficulty in cognitive functioning, irritability, and so on. For example, a person who has a psychotic illness may find marijuana to have a pleasant, relaxing effect. However, pot smoking often is associated

Figure 9.1. The Interplay of Drugs and Various Mental and Emotional States

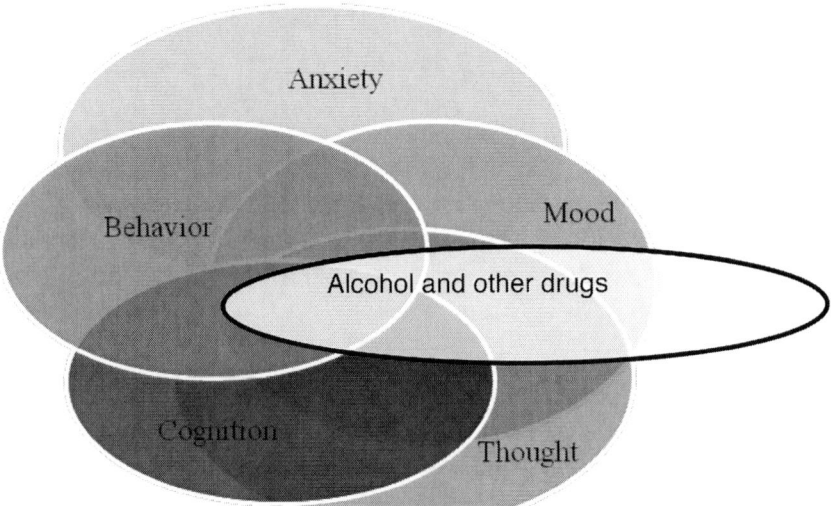

with loosening of cognitive processes, especially in someone who is predisposed to a psychotic illness. In this instance, the user may feel more relaxed but at the same time have increased difficulty with processing information and reality testing. When alcohol has recently been used it will be relatively easy to detect with a Breathalyzer. Other drugs require a toxicology screening that will take hours or even days and is thus not practical in an outpatient setting or emergency situation. Other confounding factors include the fact that withdrawal from alcohol and street drugs can mimic psychiatric symptoms. The drug dose may also be problematic.

The concept of a therapeutic window for drugs is illustrated in figure 9.2. It is a simple model that points out that every drug has a safety and effectiveness range of the amount of the drug that is in the body at any given period of time. This is known as bioavailability and is affected by the type of drug and the route of administration. The time from ingestion, absorption, or inhalation until the impact of the drug is felt may range from seconds to minutes. When too little of the drug is used there will not be an adequate therapeutic effect; when too much is used, the effect can be toxic. The dangers of taking too much of a substance is that it becomes toxic in the body and will create adverse reactions, some of which can be life-threatening. This applies to all drugs, not just prescribed ones. Added to this

Figure 9.2. The Therapeutic Window

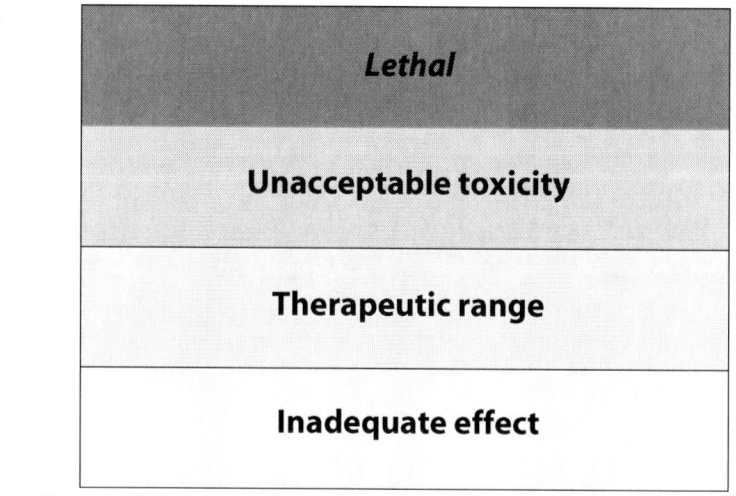

Drug concentration
(low to high)

is the serious issue that in the case of street drugs there is no accurate measure of the amount of the drug in any single dose and thus the dangers of toxicity are much greater. Street drugs are also often adulterated with unknown or undeclared substances that may pose additional hazards as their decomposition in the body may interfere with other ingested substances. Another factor involves the body's biochemical actions that break down a drug into its chemical components, after which the drug becomes nontherapeutic and is eliminated from the body. This biodegradability depends on age, general health, and other physical factors. The result is that the variation in the psychoactive effects of a drug in the body changes over time as a drug is biochemically processed, broken down into smaller parts which may not be psychoactive, and the psychoactive parts of the drug gradually become less concentrated.

There are also synergistic and interactional effects of multiple drug and alcohol use. If an individual is taking medication for a mental disorder, the alcohol and/or street drugs may interfere with the therapeutic action of the prescribed medication in one of several ways:

1. The drugs could enhance the action of the prescribed medications, raising them to toxic levels (synergistic effect).
2. The drug would not interfere with the prescribed medication (no effect).
3. One drug would reduce the effectiveness of the other (problematic when a person is expected to take a certain amount of a medication for its therapeutic effect and the other drug used reduces this effect below that of the therapeutic window).
4. The interaction of the drug could create additional unpleasant side effects (interactional effect). Some interactional effects can be life-threatening.

People with a mental disorder may find that there are desirable benefits to using substances such as peer acceptance for drinking socially or using marijuana. There may also be temporary minimizing of unpleasant effects of prescribed medication for mental illness. These are in addition to the relief sought for the initial symptoms. Thus a depressed person may want to take amphetamines or cocaine, which are stimulants. A manic person may look for the relaxant properties of marijuana, and an anxious person may seek benzodiazepines to calm down.

Not all drugs are absorbed and broken down into components at the same rate. The bioavailability of a drug—that is, the amount of the drug that is active in the body at any given moment—will differ depending on the substance used, in some cases ranging over many hours or days. In some instances, such as crack, the bioavailability of the cocaine is short, whereas in other cases, such as marijuana, the bioavailability lasts longer and traces can be detected days later. This bioavailability will affect mood and behavior for an indeterminate period. Even small amounts of alcohol or a drug may disturb the mental health of a person with a major illness. The problem is often that the individual is unaware of this disruption, especially if it is in areas of perceiving reality and thinking abstractly. That is, a person may become paranoid with no self-awareness thereof. If the individual experiences a positive change in mood, there may be less inclination to accept the concurrent negative consequences. In addition, the amount taken may not be sufficient for a person to be labeled an abuser, but even minimal use may upset a fragile mental health balance.

TREATMENT OF THOSE WITH CO-OCCURRING DISORDERS

One of the major challenges in the treatment of persons with a mental illness and substance-use disorder is that most professionals in one area, such as mental illness, are not trained in the other area, such as substance-use disorder. As a result, many signs and behaviors in one area are not addressed in treatment in the other. Furthermore, since many substance-abuse treatment programs believe in being drug free, psychotropic medications, which are an essential part of treating some mental illnesses, are often not included, or their importance is underrecognized. The frequent result is that a person may receive psychiatric treatment and then return to substance use when discharged from the hospital. Even more problematic is the frequency with which inpatients are able to access alcohol and/or drugs, thereby interfering with their psychiatric treatment.

Since the onset of the recognition of dual disorders in the 1980s, there has been a consistent message that those who have difficulty with concurrent alcohol and substance use along with a mental disorder need to have an integrated approach to treatment that includes addressing both disorders at the same time by the same clinician and treatment team (Drake & Wallach, 2000). Treatment also needs to consider the psychosocial dimension of care such as case management services, housing, rehabilitation, and ongoing support. One promising approach that integrates mental health and addiction treatment approaches uses an ACT team that employs the model of behavior change described by Prochaska and Norcross (2003) (and discussed in chapter 8) to motivate adults with serious mental illnesses into treatment for mental health and addiction problems. Since this approach can be used on an outpatient basis, although its uptake is long term (a year or more) it appears to have an impact without the use of prolonged inpatient treatment. Use of this approach also has implications for frontline workers who are challenged with how best to approach and interact with people who have dual disorders.

Co-occurring mental illnesses and substance-use disorders can be thought of as two overlapping conditions, with each varying in severity from mild to severe and with the greatest challenge in treatment being for those who have severe impairments in both domains.

TRAUMA AND TRAUMA-INFORMED CARE

The term "trauma" has come to be widely used to describe events that may have been upsetting to witnesses and participants. We stand in danger of having this description overused, which would lead to it losing its full meaning. The traumatic events that we refer to in this section are those that overwhelm a person's ability to cope or that present a real threat to life, bodily integrity, or sanity. The aftermath of traumatic experiences includes a wide range of physical, emotional, and interpersonal responses that, if observed without knowledge of the precipitating events, may appear as abnormal behaviors. Taken in the context of trauma, they are perfectly understandable as ways in which the victim has attempted to cope with unendurable situations (Drake & Mueser, 2000). Within the homeless sector, there are many events that occur on a daily basis that are also traumatizing or retraumatizing, and that can evoke extreme upset, fear, and at times terror in participants and observers.

Trauma-informed services are those where all staff, including administrators, organize and provide services in ways that acknowledge the impact that trauma and abuse have on the development and behavior of survivors, especially children. This does not imply that staff provide specific trauma therapy. That is an area reserved for those trained and qualified in trauma-related therapies. However, it does mean that all persons in the organization understand that the emotional and behavioral reactions of those who have experienced trauma and abuse need to be understood in this context and that services need to be presented in ways that will enhance the empowerment and recovery of these persons. Trauma-informed services respect the need for control by survivors. Staff understands that survivors need to feel empowered and reestablish self-efficacy through such basics as always being included in service planning and decision making about matters that concern them. It means providing an environment that is calming, with minimal tension, and it means helping clients to find ways in which they can reestablish patterns of non-trauma-based behavior and identify places where they can feel safe. In working with homeless persons, this means understanding that shelters that lack any form of privacy are perceived as inherently dangerous and result in people being on constant watch for signs of danger of further abuse or trauma.

> **Textbox 9.1. Self-efficacy**
>
> "Self-efficacy" was a term first used by Albert Bandura (1993) to describe a person's ability to succeed. An expanded use of this term includes a person's sense of self-control, ability to manage, and sense of competence. We use this wider term to explain the importance of regaining personal power and sense of self-competence (Prochaska & Norcross, 2003).

> **Textbox 9.2. Current Trauma Care Related Information**
>
> In recognition of the importance of trauma-informed care, SAMHSA has a National Center for Trauma Informed Care and Trauma Services that provides up-to-date information for service providers and those seeking help on best practices in trauma care. http://beta.samhsa.gov/nctic/about

From victim to survivor, terminology matters to most of those who have lived through horrible situations. Trauma involves having one's sense of self-efficacy, self-control, and/or self-determination destroyed. When it originates in childhood and involves caregivers, it destroys one's sense of safety (Kortrijk et al., 2013). When in the midst of a trauma people are usually called "victims," and when the trauma has passed, they are called "survivors." But surviving is more than escaping death—it also entails recovering from the aftereffects of the experience(s), effects that can be complex and multifold. Recovery implies addressing a host of emotional and behavioral issues that can lead to thriving—when survivors have moved on to use the wisdom gained from the trauma to enhance their lives and those of others.

TRAUMA AND HOMELESSNESS: WHAT IS THE CONNECTION?

Most homeless persons have experienced trauma in their lives, and many were traumatized as children (Herman, 1992). The experience of a trauma evokes a number of different reactions in people, many of which can be misunderstood as to their nature and cause. For example, a heightened startle response and hypervigilance are frequently experienced by those who have experienced traumatic events. In addition, trauma is associated with a host of significant behavioral and emotional responses, including depression, anxiety, dissociation, hypervigilance, avoidance, difficulty trusting others, and alcohol and substance abuse (Briere & Scott, 2006). The prevalence of traumatic experiences among those who are homeless makes it imperative that frontline workers and the organizations that employ them understand the nature of traumatic experiences, how traumatic reactions are manifested by victims, and the ways they influence the behavior and coping skills of those affected. In recognition of the importance of trauma-informed care, both SAMHSA and the Centre for Addiction and Mental Health have excellent resources for best practices in trauma-informed care.

An upsetting event, whether it is witnessed or experienced directly, is not necessarily a trauma. There are several different ways of defining trauma, most common of which is the description used by the American Psychiatric Association in its diagnostic manual. The DSM-5 describes a traumatic event as events that include exposure to war as a combatant or civilian, threatened or actual violent personal assaults (e.g., sexual violence, physical attack, active combat, mugging, childhood physical and/or sexual violence, being kidnapped, being taken hostage, terrorist attack, torture), natural and human-made disasters (e.g., earthquake, hurricane, airplane crash), and severe accident (e.g., severe motor vehicle or industrial accident). For children, sexually traumatic events may include inappropriate sexual experiences without violence or injury. A life-threatening illness or debilitating medical condition is not necessarily considered a traumatic event (American

Psychiatric Association, 2013, p. 274). Some traumatologists would add the additional descriptor: A traumatic event "is extremely upsetting and at least temporarily overwhelms the individual's internal resources," as this reflects the fact that people who experience major threats to their psychological integrity can be as traumatically injured as those who have their life threatened or who have a serious physical injury (Hopper et al., 2010). Witnessing death or serious injury in these events or in serious automobile accidents, assaults, and murder is also considered to be traumatic. Physical, emotional, and psychological damage caused by domestic violence and perpetrated by persons known to the victim and bystanders are also considered to be traumatic as they include violent personal assaults.

The incidence of exposure to trauma hovers around 61 percent for men and 51 percent for women, with women reporting greater incidents of rape, sexual abuse, and childhood physical abuse, and men reporting more-frequent exposure to accidents and violence. These American figures approximate a similar study of trauma in Australia (Briere & Scott, 2006, p. 82). Children who experience physical, emotional, or sexual abuse require specialized trauma services because the impact on their development can be profound. Trauma can and often does affect the ways in which the child relates to adults and those perceived as threatening to the child's integrity. Adaptations by children developed in order to safeguard the (child) victim from further physical and psychological hurt can have profound impact on the ways in which the adult survivor of childhood abuse struggles with many aspects of life including abusive close relationships; feelings of lack of self-worth that lead to poor educational and job performance; difficulty managing healthy, nonexploitative relationships; difficulty with controlling feelings (affect regulation) that leads to poor anger control and substance use to cope; difficulty parenting in the absence of a healthy role model; inappropriate sexual behaviors with few or no boundary controls; and alienation from family members who do not recognize or accept the severity of the abuse. The abused and traumatized child often feels like "damaged goods that no one wants."

What Are Traumatic Reactions?

Current practice calls for symptoms of traumatic stress to be categorized into four groups: symptoms of (a) intrusion, (b) avoidance, (c) reactivity/arousal and anxiety, and (d) negative mood and cognitions. Many adults exposed to a trauma will experience symptoms in one or more of these groups, but only about a third will go on to develop a stress reaction or a PTSD that meets the diagnostic criteria for a psychiatric disorder (Norris & Slone, 2007). In children the response is often different and requires a separate description. The most common thoughts and feelings associated with trauma include anxiety, fear, confusion, a sense of loss, grief, sadness, shock, disbelief, denial and minimization of the event, shame or blame, irritability, and anger. For many victims who have experienced violence and abuse, especially as children, dissociation—a detachment from the world that may extend to losing a sense of self, time, and current surroundings—is not uncommon. Traumatic memories, stored in visual, auditory (hearing), and olfactory (smell) centers in the brain can be awakened by similar sights, sounds, and smells in daily life. These restimulations are usually referred to as "triggers." They can be especially disconcerting if the victim is either not consciously aware of the trauma (repressed memory) or has not yet connected past events with present-day happenings. Traumatic symptoms are technically grouped in the following categories:

- Symptoms of intrusion that involve reexperiencing the traumatic event through thoughts, dreams, recurring images, nightmares, flashbacks, or a sense of reliving the experience or distress when exposed to reminders of the traumatic event.
- Symptoms of avoidance that include images, words, conversations, people, places, and activities that remind the individual of the event.
- Symptoms of reactivity/arousal and anxiety that are exhibited in difficulty sleeping (falling asleep, staying asleep), irritability, hypervigilance, poor concentration, restlessness, and exaggerated startle response.
- Symptoms of negative mood and cognitions that include signs of depression, and dissociative symptoms such as
  - A reported sense of numbing, detachment, or reduction in emotional responsiveness;
  - Reduced awareness of one's surroundings;
  - Derealization, or the subjective experience of the diminished or lack of reality of the outside world;
  - Depersonalization, or the subjective experience of the sense of unreality of one's self; and

- Amnesia, or dissociative amnesia where one is unable to recall the trauma or an important aspect of the trauma, even though one was consciously present at the time (that is, not due to head injury that would reduce awareness).

Traumatic reactions are most likely to be severe and long lasting, and to cause serious disruption in personal functioning and interpersonal relationships, if the trauma has one or more of the following characteristics:

1. It is caused by a human rather than an act of nature.
2. It is repeated (occurs more than once).
3. Its occurrence is not predictable.
4. The trauma involves more than one of the following: physical, psychological/mental, or intrusive components.
5. The trauma is sadistic in nature.
6. The trauma or traumatic events occur in childhood.
7. It is perpetrated by a caregiver—parent, relative, teacher, coach, or someone in authority such as a religious leader.

Those who have experienced childhood trauma of both a physical and sexual nature present with complex trauma, which is thought to arise because of the (usually) prolonged severe and repeated nature of the trauma and its interpersonal origins (those caused by another human rather than by an act of nature) (Briere & Scott, 2006; Norris & Slone, 2007). Prisoners of war, concentration camp internees, and victims of prolonged domestic violence are also believed to have complex posttraumatic experiences. The complexity arises from the prolonged, interpersonal, and often developmental aspects of the experiences. These traumatic experiences result in problems involving interpersonal boundaries, relationships, personal self-awareness, and affect regulation (behaviors that reduce tension). They can also include compulsive or indiscriminate sexual behaviors, eating disorders, substance abuse, self-mutilation, and suicidalilty (Norris & Slone, 2007). Victims often lack ability in the following areas: seeing the world as a safe place; trusting others, especially adults; self-soothing strategies (used to calm oneself); avoiding exploitation; and having organized thinking for making decisions.

Textbox 9.3. Using the Terms "Sexual Assault" and "Rape"
In Canada all sexual abuse is referred to under the term "sexual abuse and assault." In the United States the term "rape" specifically denotes sexual assault with intrusion into the physical body of the victim, and is considered a separate offense. We have not distinguished rape from sexual assault in this chapter consider both to be traumatic offenses and can range in intensity and severity.

Homeless women and youths are especially likely to report a history of childhood abuse, including sexual abuse (D'Andrea, Ford, Stolbach, Joseph Spinazzola, & van der Kolk, 2012). This helps to explain some of the causes of seemingly self-destructive relationships and extreme behavioral and emotional reactions that can result for these victims. The behavioral consequences unfortunately often lead to increased negative outcomes for these victims. While appropriate therapy can help them recognize and begin to overcome these negative behaviors, it is a long-term process that must start with efforts directed at affect regulation before any substantial therapy can address the traumatic bases of the dysfunctional behavior.

Multigenerational Trauma

War, natural disasters, and genocides are among the major traumatic events that affect people around the world. Researchers have documented that survivors transmit the emotional, psychological, and behavioral effects of trauma down through generations. Trauma is transmitted through spoken and written words, attitudes, body language, and at times by silence. Much has been written about the multigenerational effects of the Holocaust, and some on the transmission of trauma behaviors and responses by World War II veterans to their children (van der Kolk, Roth, Pelcovitz, Sunday, & Spinazzola, 2005). Less is known about traumatic effects of other wars and atrocities. Recent attention has grown around the traumatic effects of colonization and residential school experiences and abuses targeted at Native Americans and Aboriginal Canadians. Physical and sexual abuse and deprivation of native language and cultural identity have left a lasting mark on subsequent generations of Native American and Canadian Aboriginal people. This in turn has been a significant contributor to dysfunctional behaviors and relationships that Aboriginal people continue to struggle with. Their overrepresentation among the homeless, especially in Canada, is a legacy of colonial oppression and trauma. Interventions with Aboriginal persons need to thus be sensitive to the retraumatizing effects of the abuse of power and lack of cultural awareness of the importance of traditional ceremonies and healing practices.

MISIDENTIFICATION AND MISDIAGNOSIS

Homeless people are recognized as having past traumatic experiences more frequently than those who have always been housed. Additionally, life on the streets leads to further traumatic experiences. The personal attempts that victims make to deal with the multiple effects of trauma can easily be misidentified or misdiagnosed. The responses can lead to multiple problems in interpersonal functioning, affect regulation, and self-destructive behaviors, especially among victims of child abuse. Without using a trauma-informed lens, agitation is frequently not recognized as disrupted self-soothing. What appears to be paranoia or a distrust of others may be the result of an inability to see the world, or many parts of it, as a safe place. Behavior that appears on first glance to be self-sabotaging can in fact be an avoidance or a preemptive step to avoid exploitation, even though it may sometimes be an overreaction. Likewise, what appears to be a paranoid distrust of others may in fact be based on experience. The overwhelming emotions that result in distorted thinking and perceiving may be misunderstood as psychotic experiences and result in the false labeling of a person as psychotic. Likewise, the disorganized thinking that can arise during the extreme stress of trauma may also be inaccurately labeled as psychotic whereas it may be part of an acute stress reaction. The reality may be that this was a protective measure to remain, in some sense, safe.

Dissociation has often been mislabeled because it does not fit neatly into commonly categorized symptoms and becomes classified with psychotic behaviors when it may be a protective reaction to the trauma and triggers that remind a person of the trauma. Dissociation ranges from momentary lapses in attention all the way to feeling as though there are, in hind-sight, large periods of time when the individual doesn't know what happened. As a result, a person may find himself in a place with no memory of how he got there; he may not remember what has happened for the past few hours (or days). He may find evidence of having engaged in some activity such as shopping with no recall of having done so. He may wake up and not remember the previous evening, with no intake of alcohol or drugs to account for the memory gap. Others may insist that they met the person, but he might have no memory of any such meeting.

> **Textbox 9.4. Vignette**
>
> The following is a scenario reported by the victim of multiple childhood abuse.
>
> Consider me a bastard child, my mother Native, my father black, conceived in the back of a Chevy and raised by my grandparents. Nobody wanted me. My mother was unexpected and wasn't wanted either. She was also abused. She was sixteen when she gave birth to me, and by the time she was twenty-five she had four more children, all with different men. Those kids got even worse treatment than I got from my grandparents. I was in protective custody with Child Welfare for the first two weeks of my life. But my grandmother had what some would describe as a religious awakening about family duty and blood ties, so she brought me home and insisted that my grandfather agree to keep me. I wish she had just left me there; the orphanage could never have been worse than what I went through. I was abused as a kid and was sent to a school where I didn't know the rules for fitting in and how to behave. The kids bullied me at school and my grandparents beat me at home, all because I was not good enough. So my childhood was more complicated because my grandparents beat each other and me, and my uncle sexually molested me. I don't want to go into those details. When my mother found out about the sexual stuff, and my cutting myself, she tried take me away . . . etc. etc. But that didn't work, and besides I would not have been better off with her and her latest pack of kids. Beatings, abuse, lies, and secrets were my life at home and school was no place of safety. No surprise, then, that alcohol and drugs began to be the only ways for me to feel good. I left the house when I was fifteen and spent most of the next five years living on the streets and getting into trouble. I don't think I was attempting to be self-destructive. I just didn't care.

The results of the behavioral and emotional dysregulation that occurs in someone who has suffered multiple abuse may be that a person is labeled with one or more psychiatric diagnoses that do not actually apply: a chronic PTSD may be a more accurate description. Some of these labels may describe a current emotional state such as depression or anxiety, dissociation, or substance abuse, and may include acute stress and PTSD. Other diagnostic labels are stigmatizing and may further damage an already fragile ego. Among these are the personality disorders, especially borderline personality disorder, and the psychotic disorders such as schizophrenia. These labels are then prescriptive of specific psychiatric treatment protocols, including certain psychological and psychopharmacological (drug) therapies that may further aggravate the initial symptoms. Most importantly, these labels frequently fail to recognize and honor the need for victims to regain control of their lives, become empowered, and develop ways to regulate their emotions so that healing can begin. Victims of trauma can be retraumatized and further traumatized by people and processes that fail to recognize trauma-related behavior as adaptation to extreme stressors.

Trauma-Induced Cognitive Distortions

Trauma and abuse alter the way a victim perceives the world and interpersonal relationships and the type of traumatic experience(s) will have a marked influence on the nature and extent of those cognitive alterations. For example, a person who is a survivor of a plane crash where most were killed will be commonly troubled with the question of, "Why did I survive?," whereas the victim of childhood abuse would be apt to ask "Why did it happen to me?" For those who have suffered severe and repetitive abuse, especially as children, a host of questions related to personal safety, the ability to trust, and views of adults and intimate relationships are all (mis)shaped by the abusive experiences. The following are some of the common cognitive distortions voiced by victims of childhood abuse, sexual abuse, and domestic violence.

Trauma-Induced Victims' Thoughts and Emotions: Safety, Trust, Self-Esteem, Power and Control, Intimacy and Connection

Safety

- The world is not a safe place.
- Others, especially adults, will hurt me.
- I must always be watchful of the possibility of being hurt.
- To keep myself safe I must always be on guard, even when sleeping.
- I am afraid that no one will protect me when I am in danger.

Trust

- As a child I could not depend on others to take care of me.
- I will be betrayed by others.

- If people see me as vulnerable, they will make fun of me.
- I cannot depend on others to take care of me.

Self-Esteem
- I don't deserve happiness.
- No matter how hard I try, I will never be good enough.
- I am damaged or evil.
- I deserve the bad things that happen to me.

Power and Control
- I am afraid to lose control over people and events.
- If I lose control I will be hurt.
- I am afraid in relationships where I am not in control *or* I am afraid to be in relationships where I control.
- Power is about dominating others or being dominated.

Intimacy and Connection
- I am afraid to let others know who I am.
- People will not like me if they really know what I have experienced.
- I will always be alone.
- I am different from other people.
- I will always be alone and alienated from others.

Given the multiple ways in which trauma influences the emotional, cognitive, and behavioral aspects of a person's coping, it is not surprising that these indications present themselves in people who are housed in emergency shelters and who seek assistance in housing. Hopper and colleagues (2010) created a list of examples of typical behavior that may be trauma induced (table 9.1).

WORKER REACTIONS AND INTERVENTIONS

Workers who have had training in understanding what trauma is and how it may be displayed by persons recovering from traumatic experiences are in

Table 9.1. How Common Trauma Reactions May Explain Some "Difficult" Behaviors or Reactions within Homeless Service Settings

Traumatic Response	Common Indicators of Traumatically Induced Behavior
Is easily triggered	Has traumatic reactions to sights, sounds, certain behaviors, or mannerisms. Finds busy or noisy areas of the shelter to be uncomfortable or upsetting.
Heightened anxiety	Expresses worry and apprehension over many things.
Hypervigilance	Always appears to be on guard, always watching others. Note: Hypervigilance needs to be distinguished from a more extreme psychotic paranoia.
Heightened startle response	Startles easily, seems jumpy much of the time, and overresponds to sudden noises.
Dissociation	Seems to be emotionally disconnected from ongoing events, appears unreactive, may not remember being some place recently, loses track of time.
Difficulties concentrating	Seems distracted, unable to focus on tasks or conversations. This is especially observable in training or educational and vocational settings.
Emotional dysregulation	Has wild mood swings and difficulty controlling emotions; goes from laughing to crying. Staff and residents have difficulty predicting emotional outbursts.
Flashbacks	Reports sensory (visual, auditory, taste, olfactory, or tactile) reexperiences of the trauma, or parts of it. This may be observed as a sudden change of behavior.
Nightmares and insomnia	Is unable to sleep, and wanders around the shelter; complains of bad dreams.
Distrustful	Is extremely wary of engaging in conversation, appears suspicious of others at all times, and tends to isolate from others in the shelter.
Poor control of anger	Is easily provoked to anger, even in seemingly benign situations.
Emotional numbing	Has diminished emotional reaction to events, both positive and negative, and appears to be emotionally cold or unreactive.

Table 9.1. (Continued)

Traumatic Response	Common Indicators of Traumatically Induced Behavior
Difficulties with boundary issues in interpersonal interactions	Exhibits either inappropriate closeness or self-disclosure of personal information *or* extreme distancing and suspicion of others. Is too quick to make friends.
Avoidance	Avoids persons, places, or things that may be a reminder of the trauma. This includes avoiding meetings with counselors, where emotionally upsetting issues may be discussed, as well as places and things that serve as reminders of trauma.
Excessive use of alcohol or drugs	Uses drugs and/or alcohol to cope with anxiety and stress.
Psychosomatic symptoms/ frequent complaints of malaise	Has frequent headaches, digestive upsets, and fatigue not explained by other physical conditions.
Risk-seeking behavior	Repeatedly does things that involve high degrees of risk: has unprotected sex, shares needles, goes places where there is known danger, drives recklessly.
Feelings of shame	Continually expresses feeling of shame for behavior.
Self-blame	Blames self for negative events and apologizes or makes amends where blame clearly belongs elsewhere.
Learned helplessness	Presents self as less capable or able to do something than is really the case; does not follow through on suggestions or plan for self-improvement. This is often seen in women where learned helplessness has a related gender bias as well.
Loss of sense of fairness or sense of order in the world	Expresses feelings that life is always unfair, that there is no justice or order in the world, that the system is against him.
Overdetermined need for control	Needs to be in charge over others, and to control the conversation or group dynamic. This usually masks a deep fear of loss of control.
Sees self as victim	Remains in situations and relationships where she is taken advantage of or abused. This is often seen in domestic violence shelters.
Difficulty following rules	Is triggered by those in authority, and has difficulty with shelter guidelines and rules.
Irritability, sudden emotional outbursts	Has problems getting along with shelter residents and staff.

a better position to respond to clients in ways that do not further traumatize them than are workers who have not had that training. They are also able to use approaches that emphasize understanding that traumatic reactions are coping behaviors and not just pathological problems. The need for physical and emotional safety and the importance of empowerment in recovery are better understood by workers who are trained in trauma-informed care. At times a client may mention that he has been exposed to trauma and abuse previously. The worker should be able to acknowledge that this must have been horrible, but refrain from deeper exploration of the incident(s) or issues involved. If a client denies a history of trauma and abuse, even though you suspect that it may be present, it is important that you do not probe for further information, and you respect that some people have, for various reasons, suppressed memory of unpleasant events. These memories will surface if and when a person is able to emotionally deal with them. If a client is in distress, access to specialized help from a trauma-informed and trained therapist is important. Workers are not expected to be trauma therapists or to explore issues of trauma with clients. Clients whose distress is marked by uncontrollable feelings of anger or self-destruction (suicide) should be seen by crisis specialists as soon as possible and provided with one-on-one support in the interim. When clients have been able to address trauma issues therapeutically, there may come a time when workers can advocate and support them in moving forward, but that should be done in coordination with the counselor who has been working on trauma-related issues.

At the same time it is important to recognize that workers may have their own history of trauma and/or abuse. To the extent that a worker is aware of this history and has taken efforts to deal with this legacy, he is well equipped to understand and deal empathetically with a client who has similar issues. This does not mean that the worker will share detailed personal information, but it does mean that the worker is able to convey the "been there, done that" understanding of lived experience. It also implies that the worker will have sufficient self-awareness to recognize when another person's story will trigger personal trauma feelings and responses. In these instances it is imperative that the worker be able to ask someone else who is not triggered to step in and handle the current situation. A more difficult dilemma occurs when the worker has not previously recognized or dealt with past trauma and is now faced with trying to help someone else. We cannot help someone to walk a road that is a minefield of memories for us. The usual response will be to deny the other person's reality in order to protect ourselves from similar painful personal issues. In other words, the worker needs to step away and deal with his personal issues and allow another person to provide the direct interaction with the trauma survivor.

In an organization that has adopted a trauma-informed approach to delivering services and interventions, the understanding of trauma and its results changes in the ways that clients are understood. These interactions with clients should be evident to all levels of staff and administration. This not only reduces the possibility of retraumatizing clients, but it also increases the opportunities for those clients to be readily referred to specifically trauma-trained helpers. In addition, the organization may be able to provide trauma-informed special services such as support and psycho-education groups. Ten principles that span the work and concern of workers and management have been identified as important to trauma-informed services. Initially developed to address the issues of women survivors of childhood abuse, including sexual abuse and domestic violence, which often have precedents in childhood abuse, these principles have been recognized as applicable to a large number of trauma survivors. Some are more broadly applicable to all client-oriented services, but are especially important when trauma experiences influence clients. These ten principles follow:

1. Workers recognize the impact that the experiences of being a victim have on personal development and coping strategies.
2. The primary goal of services is recovery.
3. Services employ a recovery model that values a person's participation and respects self-efficacy.
4. The person's (victim's) choices and control over the recovery process are maximized.
5. Helping relationships emphasize safety and trust. They are consistent and predictable, and not shaming or blaming.
6. The service environment respects survivors' needs for an atmosphere that is safe, nonviolent, respectful, and accepting of the individual.
7. Services emphasize a person's strength, adaptation, and resilience.
8. Services avoid traumatization that may occur through confrontational approaches and other reminders of the trauma.

9. Services strive to be culturally competent and understand experiences in this context.
10. Services seek consumer survivor input in organizing and evaluating services. (Norris & Slone, 2007)

TRAUMATIC BRAIN INJURY: BEHAVIORAL AND PSYCHOSOCIAL IMPLICATIONS

A brain injury that happens after birth and that is the result of a sudden trauma such as a violent blow to the head, rapid acceleration or deceleration as the brain moves rapidly inside the skull, or an object piercing the skull is considered a traumatic brain injury (TBI). The severity of the injury depends on the extent of damage to the brain and ranges from mild to severe. The extent of injury and impairment has led to the classification of TBI into three areas: severe, moderate, and mild TBI, with the most severe resulting in loss of consciousness of more than twenty-four hours and mild injury resulting in loss of consciousness of less than one hour. Mild injuries may result in temporary—less than a minute—loss of consciousness and may leave the injured person with a headache, dizziness, mild confusion, vision problems, tiredness, difficulty concentrating, or difficulty sleeping. The immediate effects may diminish within days or residual symptoms may last weeks. Moderate to severe trauma results in loss of consciousness for minutes to hours or even days. In those who are not unconscious, a headache may get progressively more severe, and there may be nausea, significant mental confusion, and seizures. Massive trauma, with brain tissue destruction and/or bruising of the tissue, often results in impairments in many areas of functioning including activities of daily living, regulation of behavior, and regulation of feelings. Because the destruction can affect physical and mental health, TBI can be described as a co-occurring disorder of physical, emotional, and behavioral components.

TBI occurs in about 12 percent of the population and is primarily caused by automobile accidents, falls, sport/recreational injuries, and assaults, with accidents and assaults being the main causes in youths, and accidents and falls the main causes in the elderly. Approximately 43 percent of those hospitalized for TBI will be disabled (Corrigan, Selassie, & Orman, 2010). Many persons will experience more than one lifetime TBI; studies of TBI among the homeless indicate that they are more likely than the general population to experience multiple TBIs.

Studies indicate that it is also a co-occurring disorder with substance-use disorders. A history of substance-use disorders is found in one-third to one-half of persons with TBI; in those receiving substance-abuse treatment about the same fraction (one-third to one-half) have a co-occurring TBI. Furthermore, of those who are receiving substance-abuse treatment, many have had multiple TBIs. The high incidence of alcohol abuse among many who are homeless leads to an increase in the number of falls when a person is highly intoxicated. Intoxicated persons are less likely to fall in a safe manner or try to prevent the fall. Head impact can thus be sudden and serious (Langlois, Rutland-Brown, & Wald, 2006).

TBI is most frequently discussed in terms of the physical disabilities that may result. Less is known about those who seek trauma-informed services as a result of the emotional and behavioral difficulties that the TBI may produce. Indeed, it is problematic to sort out the physical impact of a TBI incident from that which is attributable to the emotional consequences of the trauma. Several important facts have been examined, of which one major consideration is the TBI experiences and residual impact of veterans of overseas conflicts. These men and women make up a significant portion of homeless persons, especially in the United States; their war-related physical and emotional traumas have become a significant concern for the Department of Veterans Affairs. What is also known is that homeless men experience TBI at a rate double that of the general population (Hopper et al., 2010) and that the primary reasons for their injuries are automobile accidents, violence, and combat-related injuries. Persons with TBI are more likely to experience major depression, anxiety, PTSD, and substance abuse. These same problems appear among those who have encountered trauma without brain injury.

The challenge for services that help those who have experienced trauma and TBI is that the organic (physical) aspects of the TBI are frequently diffuse and impact various parts of the brain that influence behavior, personality, judgment, problem-solving abilities, and emotional control. It is difficult to determine to what extent these features are due to the traumatic event, the brain injury itself (which may not be reparable), or to the victim's predisposing personality (Elliott, Bjelajac, Fallot, Markoff, & Reed, 2005). Persons challenged with TBI may lack impulse control or judgment in nonspecified areas, may have lost some reading or math ability, and may have lost other skills that cross a large range of inherent and acquired abilities. Similar to those who have a trauma history without TBI, these individuals will respond best in an environment that emphasizes a calm atmosphere, and nondemanding and nonjudgmental approaches. Persons with TBI need clear expectations, consistency, a dependable structure, and routine that does not overwhelm their sense of coping. Unexpected events, a change in routine, or a variation from previous experiences can be upsetting and anxiety provoking.

The number of homeless persons who report recent or previous brain trauma makes this an issue that should receive additional attention in both assessment of life challenges and potential behavioral problems. Long-term physical complaints with a neurological origin (TBI) are reported along with problematic behaviors that include irritability, depression, mania, anxiety, anger, impaired memory, attention and judgment, aggressiveness, impulsivity, and hyperactivity (Frost, Farrer, Primosch, & Hedges, 2012). All of these interfere with normal human relationships and stable functioning. Many persons are mislabeled as "difficult," "resistant to change," and "hard to engage," and are not provided with the medical assessment and behaviorally oriented interventions that may temper some of the dysfunctional behavior. The frequent result is loss of employment income and housing, involvement with criminal activities (lack of judgment in some), and incarceration. Recent reports indicate that an unusually high proportion of the prison population has TBI (Corrigan et al., 2010; Topolovec-Vranic et al., 2012).

The presence of substance use and abuse creates numerous challenges for the frontline staff. As a disinhibitor, alcohol may loosen the fragile grip on behavior control that some persons with TBI have. The most troublesome behavior is increased irritability and anger that is difficult to manage while someone is under the influence of an intoxicant. The person with TBI may already be less able to modulate his emotions and will not respond positively to any interaction that heightens tension. A calming approach, which may take time to be effective, is least likely to cause further upset or increased disturbance.

FETAL ALCOHOL SPECTRUM DISORDERS (FASDs)

FASD consists of a set of alcohol-related neurodevelopmental disorders that have severe neurological impact on the brain of developing fetuses and neonates. FASDs have recently become recognized as a group of conditions that affect fetal development as a result of maternal alcohol use. These disorders are described as a complex pattern of physical, behavioral, and cognitive abnormalities inconsistent with an individual's developmental level that cannot be attributable to genetic predisposition or family background (Ulloa, Marx, Vanderploeg, & Vasterling, 2012). While a person with a full FASD diagnosis has distinctive facial features in addition to multiple cognitive and behavioral deficits, there are many people who have significant neurological and behavioral deficits that are identified as an alcohol-related neurodevelopmental disorder. Difficulties in identification of FASD include the requirement that maternal alcohol abuse during pregnancy be confirmed and are complicated by the reality that there are no definitive biological markers or psychological tests. This lack of definitive diagnosis results in underreporting of this syndrome, but it is estimated to affect between 1 and 7 percent of the population, to be overrepresented among Aboriginal and Native American persons in North America, and overrepresented among homeless individuals (Dombovy, 2011). Persons with FASD have neurological impairments that have many of the features of those with a brain injury. They often have low cognitive abilities and poor decision making, in addition to a host of behavioral problems. Behavioral indicators include hyperactivity, poor judgment and impulse control, lack of inhibitions, lack of insight, and an inability to maintain focus on the consequences of behavior. Alcohol use, a frequent additional factor, aggravates these behaviors. Adults with FASD frequently run into trouble with the law and end up in correctional facilities where their unique problems are usually not recognized or understood.

> **Textbox 9.5. Fetal Alcohol Spectrum Disorder in Fiction**
>
> In the book *Ragged Company* one of the main characters, Digger, presents with a classic history of FASD, and possible TBI, including having an alcoholic mother and early childhood alcohol use. He relies on others to structure his life and provide fundamental supports so that he is not revictimized by other homeless persons. Digger also presents with classic indicators of trauma. Throughout the book his challenges with these two major issues are sensitively and poignantly depicted.

The complexities of care are impacted by the fact that although FASD impairs cognitive processing and behavioral controls in adults, it is not recognized as an adult disability. Many adults are not able to establish maternal alcoholism during pregnancy and remain undiagnosed, which also means that they have extreme difficulty in establishing disability that prevents them from competitive employment. Acquiring job skills, and securing and maintaining employment are real challenges for those impaired by FASD and alcohol-related neurodevelopmental disorders. They frequently become homeless and do not qualify for disability benefits, which means that their subsistence income is insufficient for independent living in most localities. It can be difficult to achieve and maintain a supportive safety net for those afflicted. These adults also go on to have children of their own, and since most of these adults with FASD also abuse alcohol, their children are likewise impacted (Chudley, Kilgour, Cranston, & Edwards, 2007).

EXERCISES

Case Example: Multigenerational Fetal Alcohol Spectrum Disorders

Tina is a single mother in her late forties who works episodically in the construction industry as a roofer. She is of Aboriginal descent but was placed in permanent guardianship with child welfare services as a toddler. Both her parents had substance-abuse problems and were unable to provide adequate care. No extended family member was able to take her into care. She was adopted at age five by a well-to-do couple of British descent and raised as a white Anglo-Saxon of British heritage. Her adoptive parents did not acknowledge her Indian heritage until Tina was twenty-two. She displayed numerous difficulties while growing up, constantly testing limits of acceptable behavior. By age fifteen Tina had developed a practice of regular alcohol consumption, absenteeism from school, highly sexualized behavior, and defiance of curfews set by her parents. By age seventeen she was pregnant and married the putative father. She continued to consume alcohol and her son was born with FASD indicators. The marriage lasted until her son, Cary, was nine, at which point Tina became a single parent. She has maintained contact with Cary's father.

Tina has some surprising strengths. She has always maintained contact with her adoptive parents. She sought information about her Aboriginal background so that she could understand her identity and then began to participate in culturally significant ceremonies. She has been exceptionally generous with family and friends in sharing her resources when she has them. She initially completed a certificate as a beautician and was employed, mostly part-time, for several years in this profession. She grew bored with this profession and returned to school for training as a licensed practical nurse. She worked as a nurse's aide both in retirement homes and privately for the next ten years but had her employment interrupted by charges of alcohol abuse and impaired driving. Despite these charges she continued to operate a motor vehicle. Tina maintained a home for Cary but often gave daily care over to Cary's father for extended periods of time during which she partied, used drugs, and was sexually active with multiple partners. When Cary was seventeen he lost his license for driving under the influence. At this time, Tina became less erratic in her behavior, sought training as a roofer in the construction industry, and settled into a relationship with one man. She continues to have binge drinking episodes, but has managed to remain self-sufficient. She couch surfs when not employed and has maintained a group of friends who also support this lifestyle.

1. Identify behavior and challenges that Tina faces.
2. Are there any events that can be described as both a strength and a challenge?
3. What would Tina need to remain stable in the future?

Group task (can also be an individual task in a smaller community)

1. List all trauma-related resources available to people in your community.
2. Are there separate resources for men? Women? Veterans? Youths? Victims of domestic violence?
3. Do any treatment providers and facilities in your community have trauma-informed services?
4. How can you advocate for trauma-informed services with local providers?
5. Is it possible to establish a support group for trauma survivors in your organization? In a related organization?

JOURNALING

Complete the trauma self-assessment scale in appendix 4.

1. Reflect on any potential traumatic experiences that you may have had. What reactions did you have at the time? What reactions do you have now?

2. What resiliencies do you have to help handle potentially traumatic experiences?
3. Identify a person you know who has had a traumatic experience. What helps that person to cope? Does that person have signs or symptoms of PTSD? How do you interact with that person when these signs or symptoms are evident?

CHAPTER 10

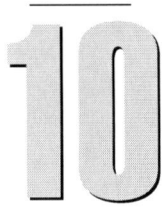

CULTURAL COMPETENCE WITH DIVERSE PEOPLE

KEY ISSUES
- Similarities and differences between cultural sensitivity and cultural competence
- How cultural differences may be expressed
- One's personal cultural background and the privileges and liabilities it may entail
- Mapping out plans for engaging people in culturally sensitive ways

OVERVIEW

There are more than two hundred languages spoken throughout North America in the twenty-first century. Fifty years ago there were fewer than one hundred languages spoken here. This increase reflects the rapid diversification of peoples and cultures that has created a multicultural society where there is no longer one dominant and preferred (Western European) worldview. As members of an ethnically and culturally diverse society, we have a responsibility to be aware of and sensitive to the various cultures and lifestyles that are part of the fabric of modern life. Race, country of origin, and indigenous status are some of the many issues of diversity that we encounter in daily life. Lifestyles also encompass, among other factors, a variety of religiously and spiritually based lifestyles, and sexual orientations and preferences. Culture is generally expressed in a shared worldview, as well as in the values, ethics, habits, and practices of the group, and may also include the accumulation of generations of learned behaviors and attitudes. In the following pages, we explore the meaning of cultural competence and cultural sensitivity. We examine some of the basic forms in which culture may express itself in some representative groups. We then invite you to examine your own cultural sensitivity toward your culture of origin and that of other cultures in your community. Finally, we look at how awareness of different lifestyles, worldviews, and values impacts your work with persons of diverse backgrounds. We are all members of at least one group and our membership helps us to define the meaning of the world around us and to shape our behavior. These worldviews and behaviors are part of our cultural heritage.

WHAT DOES CULTURE INCLUDE?

Culture is described in various ways, but has as a common meaning shared ways of thinking, feeling, and reacting; and shared values and worldview as evidenced in art, language, music, ways of governance, and psychosocial interactions. The "who we are," "what we do," "how we view ourselves and others," and what we consider as "normal," "acceptable," and "appropriate," are all influenced by the cultures that we belong to. It may be very visible culture, defined by our dress and mannerisms, or it may be more subtle and discovered only during prolonged conversation and interaction. It may be a widespread culture with local (tribal and First Nations) variations, such as that of Native American or Aboriginal Canadian peoples, or a very localized culture as practiced by Amish or Hutterite people. In addition to dominant cultures defined by heritage and ethnic affiliations, we often also incorporate subcultures into our worldview, attitudes, behavior, and lifestyles. These subcultures may involve the use of various languages, dialects, or specific vocabulary, as found in professional cultures such as law and medicine, and street cultures such as gangs. Culture may also demark a subgroup of a larger group, such as LGBT (lesbian, gay, bisexual, and transgender). LGBT people self-identify as a specific group, but are also part of a larger culture, be it European-based North American, African American, Chinese, Japanese, Indian, and so on. Culture contributes to a sense of belonging, most poignantly experienced when we are thrown into a foreign society with no local language skills and no understanding of customary and acceptable ways of behaving. Most of us may not have the opportunity to experience the alienation of being alone in a different society. In this chapter we hope to bring some of those areas of sensitivity to your awareness, as table

10.1 illustrates. This awareness leads to the difference between sensitivity and competence.

> **Textbox 10.1. What Is Culture?**
>
> Culture is an integrated system of learned behavior patterns that are characteristic of the members of any given society. Culture refers to the total way of life for a particular group of people. It includes [what] a group of people thinks, says, does, and makes—its customs, language, material artifacts, and shared systems of attitudes and feelings.
>
> (Matsumoto & Juang, 2012)

CULTURAL SENSITIVITY AND CULTURAL COMPETENCE

The influences that shape our behavior, values, attitudes, perception of the world, meaning of life, and context of social relationships are affected by the culture(s) that we belong to. We speak of multiple cultures because an individual may simultaneously identify with a specific ethnic group and with other groups that share distinct similarities in perspective, thoughts, and behavior, such as those who identify with sexual and gender minorities, those who have functional limitations such as the physically handicapped, those with hearing or vision loss, and persons in recovery from addictions. Similarly, those from backgrounds different from our own are shaped by influences that reflect their culture of origin. Culture awareness is the ability to take these considerations into account when we encounter people from backgrounds that are different from our own. What are various aspects of cultural competence? Cultural competence can be categorized along a continuum from awareness to sensitivity to competence:

- Cultural awareness: recognizing basic differences based on ethnic dress and language
- Cultural sensitivity: knowing that cultural differences and similarities exist without assigning values—i.e., better or worse, right or wrong—to those cultural differences
- Cultural competence: interacting with people of different backgrounds in a respectful and knowledgeable way using a set of acquired skills

Table 10.1. Stages of Cultural Awareness

Stage of Cultural Awareness	Description	Examples
Minimization	Recognizes basic, observable differences in areas of food, clothing, and language, but has little awareness or acknowledgment of the deeper expressions of culture in attitude, life philosophy, etc. or Describing all people in universal terms.	Culture seen only in terms of the food people eat, the language used, and distinctive clothing worn. or "All people are basically the same." "We all belong to the human race."
Polarization	Has a judgmental view of other cultures that sees cultural differences in terms of "us" versus "them." Sees own culture as "better." or Sees the other culture as preferable.	"Why can't they just shake hands when greeting you?" "Those people are just not sophisticated." "They have a much better way of viewing friendships."
Recognition	Realizes that there are cultural differences but does not understand that they extend into fundamental worldviews.	They have a different idea of time and what it means to be "on time." but "We all worship the same god."
Sensitization	Is aware of differences in worldviews, the importance of relationships, and the place of individual versus collective needs and rights.	"Family comes before everything else." or "We need to respect the importance of our society and place it before our individual needs and wants."

Table 10.1. (Continued)

Stage of Cultural Awareness	Description	Examples
Acceptance	Is able to be comfortable with cultural differences and is sensitive to differences as manifest in all aspects of living. Does not place values of good or bad, right or wrong, on differences.	"I am sensitive to differences and see them as expressions of ways of living."
Integration	Is able to be comfortable in different cultural settings, adapting to the ways of the current situation with acceptance. Is able to shift between cultures. Is able to discuss cultural differences and practices in nonjudgmental ways.	"I can be comfortable at a Native pow-wow, a Jewish wedding, or a Mexican fiesta, and enjoy them all equally."

This continuum can be further described using examples of behavior found in table 10.2, which details common reactions to cultural differences and stages of acceptance of these differences.

Cultural competence is developed through the awareness of cultural norms, language differences, acculturation, and the ability to differentiate between individual and culturally linked attributes. It includes the willingness to seek out the required information so that interventions are not based on personal biases. In assessment of individual needs and strengths, cultural competence also involves the skill to distinguish between attributes possessed by an individual and those characteristic of the person's culture (Clarren et al., 2010).

Basic to the development of any competence is your self-assessment and recognition of your attitudes toward differences in behavior, values, and attitudes, and your own biases in these areas. Since everyone is the product of his or her own culture, we need to increase both self-awareness and cross-cultural awareness. There are books and Web sites with instructions to deal with cultural diversity, but all acknowledge that while there is no recipe to follow, certain attitudes help to develop awareness, respect, and understanding. The following are some basic guidelines:

Table 10.2. Levels of Cultural Awareness

Level of Awareness	Description	Example
Minimal	Recognizes differences in clothing where this is obvious, but not in how clothing influences attitudes toward other aspects of life.	"They dress differently but are just the same as us underneath." "He goes to temple on Saturday and I go to church on Sunday. It's all the same."
Partial-cognitive	An intellectual understanding of basic differences in language, status of women, importance of family.	"We use the same words, they just sound different. When I say that something is spiritual we both know what that means."
Partial-experiential	Emotional/affective awareness of how important tradition is to family and community life.	"When that family gets together, which they do very often, there is so much laughter, talking, bantering, and singing. In my family we are more formal and watch what we say and to whom we say it. Our music comes from the stereo."
Moderate awareness of various aspects of cultural differences	Awareness of how language, tradition, views of spirituality, understanding of nature, etc. sculpt the way we think and how this understanding is not readily translated.	"We stand together at the river and he hears the songs of the ancestors and sometimes sees an ancient one. I see the blue sky and the birds and hear the river gurgle, but it doesn't carry the same messages."
Comprehensive: Accepted by those of other cultures as sensitive to and respectful of differences without trying to "become one of them"	Comfort with differences. Interest in learning about cultural differences and participating, when invited, in cultural activities and practices.	"There are so many things to learn from other people who have lived with other ways of looking at the world and who do things differently from how I do them. It is like hearing an orchestra: I can appreciate the music in a different way when I hear each instrument and how it sounds, what it contributes to the concert."

- Admit what you don't know. Knowing that we don't know everything, that a situation does not make sense, that our assumptions may be wrong, are part of the process of becoming culturally aware. Assume differences, not similarities.
- Suspend judgments. Collect as much information as possible so you can describe the situation accurately before evaluating it.
- Enhance your empathy. The emotional understanding of the experiences, feelings, and needs of others is vital to having true empathy for someone from another culture. In order to understand another person, we need to try walking in his shoes. Through empathy we learn how other people would like to be treated by us.
- Systematically check your assumptions. Ask your colleagues for feedback and constantly check your assumptions to make sure that you clearly understand the situation.
- Become comfortable with ambiguity. The more complicated and uncertain life is, the more we tend to seek control. Assume that other people are as resourceful as we are and that their way will add to what we know. "If we always do what we've always done, we will always get what we always got."
- Celebrate diversity. As a person and within your organization, find ways of sharing the cultures of your diverse clientele and workforce.
- Cherish the opportunity to enlarge your worldviews and understandings of humankind. The differing ways of seeing the world and its peoples can open new horizons of intellectual, emotional, and spiritual experiences and deepen our personal lives.

Awareness of who you are, what cultures are part of your background and lifestyle, and what awareness you have of other cultures forms the basis for cultural sensitivity. When we speak of cultural sensitivity, we refer primarily to the development of an awareness of differences among people from different backgrounds. When we speak of competence, we refer not to someone who knows differences in all cultures, but one who has acquired the ability to appreciate the multiple dimensions of these differences and to seek out whether the individual whom they are trying to help is different because of individual idiosyncrasies or because of cultural differences in specific areas.

The extent to which an individual, family, or group of people has assimilated the culture of another group is known as acculturation. The process of acculturation includes the incorporation of values, attitudes, beliefs, behaviors, worldview, and religion or spiritual expression into the original culture. This also includes the ability to resolve differences that may be fundamental, or to find a way to compartmentalize those differences so that they are expressed only within the culture that is dominant in a specific situation. An excellent example of acculturation is found within American Native communities. Some Native people dress for and practice a traditional lifestyle, espousing primarily traditional values and behaviors while others present as Anglicized, acting like and identifying primarily as Caucasian people of European extraction, and some Native (Aboriginal) people combine aspects of both worlds. Walking in both worlds is important to healthy living for those from other cultures. Research has shown that both native and immigrant youths who have been able to acculturate and feel comfortable in both their traditional culture and the dominant culture have the most stable and positive lives (Hawkins, Cummins, & Marlatt, 2004; Kohls, 1984). Thus acculturation is an extremely important component of life for those who need to deal with more than one cultural influence on their lives. For workers, this may be a critical component to helping a client to cope, and may be an especially important aspect for clients with recent immigrant backgrounds and those whose primary affiliation is with their culture of origin.

PERSONAL CULTURAL AWARENESS: WHO ARE YOU?

Where were you born? Where did you grow up? Were your parents born in the same country as you? Is that the country you now live in? Did you grow up in a community where the same language was spoken at home and at school? If not, how did this affect the way you met and kept friends? Was your home of a different culture in dress or religion or rituals than that of your classmates? How did that make you feel? Are you proud of differences or uncomfortable about them? How would you describe the culture that you belong to? Is there any other group—sexual preferences, professional, spiritual, or recreational—that further defines who you are? How much does your family history define your culture and who you are? Are there any missing pieces that would make this picture more complete?

With these questions we begin a search for our personal self-identity, based both on what we grew up with and what we assimilated from the world around us. In table 10.3 we can evaluate some of our own cultural experiences with those that may be different for others.

As a result of the prolific and frequent coverage of different groups by the popular press, we live in a society that has become aware of some of the most visible differences among groups of people. In a broad sense, most of us can identify differences between people from countries whose language and appearance are different from our own. However, these outward signs barely scratch the surface of differences that are rooted in fundamental values and beliefs. Culture is the intermingling of worldviews, values, attitudes, beliefs, and practices that shape the acceptable norms and behaviors of a group of people. We can view culture as whatever defines a society of persons, often demarked by a specific region or country, such as Japan; or as specific groups within a region, such as the peoples of southern and northern China; the Flemish of northern Belgium and southern Holland; or tribal groups such as the Sioux, Arapoho, Algonquin, Mi'Mac, Cree, Blackfoot, and Salish of North America; the Maya, Mixtec, and Zapotec indigenous peoples of Mexico; and so on. We also speak of culture as defined by an occupational group such as a music culture, a health-care culture, and of the legal or medical culture. Culture is used to denote the behaviors, beliefs, and lifestyles of persons of alternative sexual lifestyles, such as LGBT cultures. Recognition of the reality of differences across groups is a beginning toward the sensitivity needed to respond respectfully and effectively when providing services to those who are not from our own background.

> **Textbox 10.2. Cultures Are Not Homogenous**
>
> There are over four hundred different Native (indigenous) groups in northern North America alone, each with distinct cultural attributes. Thus it is imperative that we not overgeneralize and thereby miss the individuality and unique contributions of each group.

In all aspects of work with others, as we discussed in chapter 2, awareness of who we are, and how we speak and interact with others is fundamental to establishing mutually respectful relationships. Culture pervades our interactions with and understanding of people. Similarly, cultural awareness begins with self-awareness, of where we came from, what group(s) we belong to, and what our values, attitudes, and beliefs are. From that point

Table 10.3. Cultural Sensitivities

Behaviors, Attitudes, Values	My Culture	Another Culture
Eye contact: Consistent, infrequent, or not acceptable		
Hand shake: The norm regardless of sex, the norm for men only, not the norm for women Alternative: A kiss on each cheek expected among acquaintances or avoided, acceptable for women, or acceptable for both sexes		
Timeliness for business appointments: Early, right on time, measured interval of lateness (minutes or hours)		
Timeliness for social engagements: Early, on time, a bit late		
Dress for women: Carefully defined or relaxed Dress for men: Carefully defined or relaxed		
Interaction between sexes: Liberally allowed, limited, carefully proscribed		
Worldview: Cognitive, platonic, or existential and spiritual		
Importance of religion: Strongly connected to daily rituals and specific celebrations, or religion not a strong factor in daily life		
Importance of family in daily life: Independent lifestyles the norm, the family is the center of one's life		
View of disability: Accepted part of differences, or treated with shame and as a stigma		
Importance of material goods and possessions: Essential for personal success or to be shared with others; seen as symbols of class and social differences and distinctions, variable in importance: specific goods confer status		

of departure, we can begin to observe and appreciate the small and large differences between ourselves and other groups, and recognize them as different, not in any way implying that one is preferable or better than another—just different. To start, we need a personal reflection using the cultural behaviors, attitudes, and values listed in table 10.3 as a guide. Don't skip any: those for which you have no answers may provide important clues about you and your personal culture.

CULTURES, SUBCULTURES, AND MINGLING OF CULTURES

We generally do not have much difficulty in recognizing that there are differences between people of Western European descent and those from, for example, the Middle East, India, China, Mexico, Guatemala, Bolivia, and so on. While we may, in North America, refer to those whose appearance is different as belonging to a "visible minority," this sidesteps the reality that in their homelands we become the visible minority. People whose background is different but who "all look the same" are often grouped together despite the fact that they may come from very different backgrounds and lifestyles. Table 10.4 gives some examples of misconceptions about a person's origins and culture.

How do these differences matter? The life stories of people from different areas of the globe speak to historical events that date back hundreds of years and have, in many instances, created some degree of assimilation with the host country. While we can readily appreciate the fact that those who come from Caribbean countries share a heritage with African Americans and have seen similar oppression, in many instances there are pronounced levels of assimilation with the indigenous people of the islands. At the same time, world trade brought merchants from India who also settled in the Caribbean Islands, together with their Muslim customs, and have remained a clear presence on the islands. Their worldview is shaped by an assimilation of African, British, and Indian orientations. China is an example of a country of multiple cultures and languages that does not have a singular cultural expression. While there may be numerous generalities, there remain significant differences among various regions, and those again are different from persons coming from Vietnam, Thailand, or Laos. The basic issue here is the importance of accepting differences, and in being sensitive to the nuances that

Table 10.4. Cultural Misconceptions Based on Appearances

Appearance: Skin Tone	Assumption	Other Possibilities
Dark brown (also mislabeled as black)	African American	Caribbean
		Canadian
		African from various countries such as Ghana, Uganda, Kenya, South Africa, etc.
Olive complexion	Italian	Spanish
		Portuguese
		Greek
		Slavic/Serbian
		Israeli
Medium brown, with Arabic head dress	Saudi Arabia	Any of the Middle Eastern countries, each with its own tradition
Medium to dark brown	India	One of the African or Caribbean countries
	American Indian	
	Canadian Aboriginal	A person from the Caribbean or Africa whose ancestors migrated from the Indian subcontinent

make up these differences. All of these variations may be found among those who are homeless.

In a similar manner, there are also subcultures among homeless people that a worker should be sensitive to. Some of these subcultures refer to sexual preferences and lifestyles and can be overrepresented among some sectors of the homeless. One clear example is that of LGBT youths among homeless adolescents (Cochran, Stewart, Ginzler, & Cauce, 2002). Some of these subcultures have to do with the reasons for lack of stable housing: those with addictions, those with mental illness, those whose families live on the financial and emotional edge, those who share similar life histories of abuse, and those with ethnic or cultural communalities. In a reverse fashion, and as a caution, we note that understanding subcultures can influence a new worker's view on the main culture. In this instance, workers believing that they know a culture already without keeping their observation and listening skills viable can develop a false sense of familiarity and presume that what they experience represents the main culture rather than a subgroup of that culture.

Areas of Consideration in Applying a Cultural Lens

The lenses that we apply to considerations of culture and cultural differences are often colored by the discipline or profession that is applying the lens. That is, anthropologists, sociologists, psychologists, social workers, nurses, and other professionals bring their values and attitudes to which aspects of culture they emphasize and how they understand their importance. There is no single way of examining culture, but our interest is in respecting differences while attempting to help people from various backgrounds. People who emigrate and those who settle elsewhere as refugees carry their cultural heritage with them. In most instances they will initially settle near or within ethnic enclaves in the city or town receiving them. These enclaves are widely seen in New York, Los Angeles, Miami, Toronto, Vancouver, and, to a lesser extent, Montreal. While there are, for various reasons, lower rates of absolute homelessness among recent immigrants, some are roofless, many are housing vulnerable, and all need supports to remain independent. Thus the following areas may require the service provider's attention.

> **Textbox 10.3. Homeless Immigrants and Refugees**
>
> Obtaining accurate counts of homeless and housing vulnerable immigrants and refugees is challenging. Many are fearful of deportation if their inability to be self-sustaining comes to the attention of the authorities. However, inability to obtain jobs comparable to those the immigrants had in their country of origin force considerable numbers to take low-wage jobs that frequently are insufficient to meet escalating housing costs. This is a reality in both the United States and in Canada.
>
> (Berry, Phinney, Sam, & Vedder, 2006)

Family and Gender Constructions

To which differences and nuances should a frontline worker have a basic sensitivity? One cultural characteristic that immediately arises for many people begins with a culture's attitude toward the different roles and responsibilities of men and women. Despite Western values of equality between the sexes, there are many places in the world where this is not a reality. In North American society there are also subcultures that maintain different roles and responsibilities for women, many of them ingrained in religious beliefs. Among these subcultures are Orthodox and Hassidic Jewish, Amish, Hutterite, fundamentalist Christian, Muslim, Sikh, and those from many subcultures within the group of Asian countries. With these differences we may need to respect what we cannot always accept: that men and women are not necessarily treated the same way in all cultures.

The extent to which women are given equality with male counterparts is one of the most immediate and pervasive cultural differences across societies. While most Western (generally considered to be European and North American, as well as New Zealand and Australian) societies now proclaim equality between men and women, this is not the situation in many Middle Eastern, South American, and African countries where male dominance prevails. In Asian societies and many groups from the East that also have interwoven religious components, such as Muslim and Hindu cultures, any issues that involve family must be addressed to the men of that family. Would a female worker be open to not speaking to the women? A challenge may also be that of being open to a male-dominated perspective and attitudes toward a female worker. A question that this raises is if refusing to speak with a female worker is showing her disrespect or whether it is basically a cultural norm for that man.

Cultural Norms That Vary across Societies

1. Equality may be more explicit in law than in practice in countries where paternalism is still a prevailing family construct. These variations create vast differences in the degree to which women are free to make independent decisions and the extent to which they may be ostracized from their cultural communities for making independent decisions and choosing a lifestyle not dictated by male relatives.

2. Freedom of thought and expression is valued in North America, where children are taught less by rote than in many other countries. The development of critical thinking skills, creativity, and unique problem solving accompanies this support of independent thought. In many paternalistic societies rote learning continues to be the valued approach. Teachers are viewed as enforcers of society's paternalistic values where the father figure and the community leaders are

viewed as the source of all wisdom and are to be respected in all matters. Elders are respected as having wisdom, and it is disrespectful to question those senior in age. Questioning authority is forbidden.

3. The group is the main form of identification in many cultures. Unlike American and Canadian Western-oriented culture where individualism is valued and an individual is expected to internalize social rules, in group- or community-oriented cultures an individual is more likely to be shamed, ostracized, or sanctioned by the community for behavior that violates group norms (Al-Krenawi & Graham, 2000). The group provides the norms and sets the boundaries for behavior, and individual identity is bound to the group's identity. Within this framework it is understandable that education by rote learning and following prescribed rules is the expected behavior.

4. Fundamental cultural rules and norms are woven into the accepted ways of communication. Those cultures that are male or patriarchal in orientation will expect that all communication with those outside of the group (and outside of the family group) will be channeled through the male leader, authority figure, or patriarch. Male contact with women is strictly defined and limited to those within the family. Women may have contact and relationships with other women outside of the household, but not with men in other families. Communication, verbal and nonverbal, also follows cultural norms. Eye contact and the use of direct (a preferred North American cultural norm) and indirect ways of speaking differentiate cultures. North American Indian people (First Nations, Aboriginal, Inuit, etc.) are more likely to speak in indirect ways and to use stories and metaphors to convey meaning. In Canada this indirectness has seeped into the mainstream culture and thus Canadians are more likely to be muted and less direct than their American counterparts. However, in the multicultural society that has emerged in the past fifty years, acculturation still varies in its pervasiveness among different communities (Cochran et al., 2002). While many people on both sides of the border between Canada and the United States are also likely to carry over the attitudes from their parents and grandparents who migrated years ago, for some this has been minimal while for others the parental culture continues to dominate. Thus, as an example, people whose parents were born in India may continue to communicate in their

language of origin, which may also be more deferential to their elders. In this immigrant world, an example of language miscommunication occurs when a word in one language, or even a language from a different region, such as American, British, and Australian English, can have the same word convey a different meaning. One such example is the use of the word "bloke," which can range from reference to an ordinary man or regular guy, to refer to a not very bright person, to derogatory reference to a man.

> **Textbox 10.4. Fiction Can Sensitize Us to Other Cultures**
>
> The book *Wild Swans* provides a graphic and detailed portrayal of the role of a group-oriented culture and the impact any personal deficiency has had on the entire (extended) family in China.
>
> (Chang, 2003)

> **Textbox 10.5. Words with the Same Meaning**
>
> One example of a word that sounds the same but has a different meaning in different cultures is the word "wife," which connotes a female spouse in English; the word "wijf," pronounced the same as the English, can be a pejorative, disrespectful word for a woman in the Dutch language, however. Many cultures have also adopted words from other languages and countries but given them different meanings or nuances. Pop in Canada is synonymous with a soda in parts of the United States, where the word "pop" can refer to a father. To add to the confusion, the streets have their own language where common words have uncommon meanings, and are specific to that city or locale and not to the entire homeless population.

FURTHER CULTURAL DIFFERENCES

1. The role and meaning of food and drink as part of communication, establishment of relationships, both formal and informal, and components of ceremony and ritual.
2. Personal problems (mental health issues, family dysfunction, substance abuse) and stigma. It is never easy to acknowledge personal or family difficulties, but in some societies this is tantamount to an

admission of family insufficiency or deficiency. Especially in group- and communal-oriented cultures, the problems of the individual are those of the family and reflect the family. Thus someone who experiences depression brings shame on the entire clan, which in turn damages a family member's opportunities for a good marriage or a promising career. Children inherit the family shame and continue to be distanced from social and educational opportunities. Problems that range from genetic defects that cause physical and mental handicaps, to conditions such as epilepsy are all cause for shame, as are rifts in the social structure of the family, rebellious adolescents, marital breakup, extramarital relationships, and so on. The worker needs to be very sensitive to the difficulty that a person from a group culture may have in expressing personal problems and the self-felt shame that is inherent in such an admission.

3. Understanding of health and illness, its origins, and means to address disease. The origins of physical illnesses, their meanings, and the ways in which these are addressed vary among cultures. The extent to which some illnesses are considered to be of a spiritual origin or connected to a force such as yin/yang in Chinese medicine is an excellent example of this difference.

4. Role of traditional healers and helpers. All cultures have had persons who occupied helping or healing roles. In many cultures these persons continue to be respected and involved in attending to physical and mental, emotional, or spiritual illnesses. Healing plants and ceremonies continue to be part of these traditions and are an integral part of culture. An excellent example is within North American Native traditional communities in Canada, Mexico, and the United States where sacred ceremonies continue to be held and where many traditional healing plants are still used for healing. Traditional medicine is also valued by people from African, Asian, Indian, and South American communities. People from these communities may use the services of both Western medicine and native medicine. Likewise, acupuncture and traditional Chinese medicines proliferate and are widely used and respected by non-Chinese people. The role of traditional medicine is, for many, profound and many have experienced healing. The worker needs to be careful to respect these practices, and to be supportive of their use (Cohen, 1998).

5. Process of acculturation. Acculturation, the process of adopting and integrating the initial culture with a new culture, varies among cultures; how quickly this process occurs is influenced by several factors. The most obvious influence is the extent of similarity between the initial and new culture, as the values and attitudes, beliefs, and behaviors that are similar are easier to adopt than those that require major shifts in ways of being. A person from a patriarchal society will not assimilate values of equality and freedom of expression as quickly as someone from a country that gives equality to the sexes. Acculturation also involves the comfortable use of language and its idioms. The closer two cultures are to modes of expression, the easier the shift. Thus learning Chinese or Arabic is a challenge for those used to the Roman alphabet—and the reverse applies equally.
6. Time and its dimensions. Depending on the culture involved, being on time may mean showing up today rather than tomorrow. It may offend someone if you are late for a prearranged meeting. Time may also be an expectation of how long it will take for a targeted change to occur or for government officials to approve an application. Time may be viewed as today stretched out rather than a progression from past to future. That is, being in the moment may be the most valued action and any move toward futuristic plans is not as easily comprehended or accepted. The above are all variations of what time implies in different cultures. As helpers, we need to be aware of the expectations of time that others may have, as it sets the stage for how the helping relationship may unfold.

The above list is not exhaustive, and there is no intent to minimize the importance of one culture over another. We have deliberately chosen some examples because they represent clear alternatives to American and Canadian Caucasian-oriented culture(s). Given the immense number of cultures that have found a place in North America, it is impossible to mention all of them. Any omission is not intended as a slight, but is perhaps an opportunity and invitation for the student and reader to take a closer look at a specific culture in the light of some of the dimensions listed above.

CULTURE AND OPPRESSION

The twentieth century was witness to large-scale efforts to annihilate large groups of people and cultures. The Jewish, Roma, and other peoples during the Nazi Holocaust; the Armenians in the genocide that began in 1915; people embodying old customs and culture during the Cultural Revolution in China (Totten & Bartrop, 2008, p. 89); and the Tutsi and moderate Hutu people in Rwanda are all examples of the atrocities committed in the past one hundred years. Cultural genocide has been in existence for long before that: the nineteenth century was witness to clearly articulated efforts to wipe out Native American, Australian Aboriginal, and New Zealand Maori peoples by British and other English-speaking people who believed that Caucasian cultures were superior and indigenous people "savages," "illiterate," and "idolatrous." This false notion of racial superiority (for, after all, the targets were persons of visibly different racial backgrounds), failed to eliminate Aboriginal people, although decimation of the population nearly accomplished that. When efforts to annihilate the indigenous people failed, a process of assimilation, the forcible removal of children and placement into residential school in order to teach them Anglo Saxon–based ideologies, language, and customs, resulted in further reduction of native languages, customs, and lifestyles. This process of cultural suppression of traditional lifestyles is known in Canada and Australia as colonization. In the latter part of the twentieth century, with the repeal of some of the most egregious discriminatory and repressive laws in Canada and the United States, there has been a substantial revival in Native (Aboriginal) culture and practices in both countries.

> **Textbox 10.6. Aboriginal Experiences with Residential Schools**
> The film *Rabbit Proof Fence* (Noyce, Olsen, Winter, & Noyce, 2002) is a vivid portrayal of the plight of three Aboriginal (Australian) girls who are removed from their homes and sent to residential school. It is a highly moving film that dramatically portrays colonial attitudes toward the Aboriginal people of Australia and the Aboriginal desire to retain autonomy and traditional life.

Colonialism and the residential school era have left enormous damage on native communities, families, and individuals in both Canada and the United States. In addition to the destruction of family lifestyles by the forcible removal of children to English-only schools, where contact between siblings was forbidden, cultural and religious practices were banned both in these schools and on the reservations. The result was that multiple generations did not learn of the language, customs, and beliefs of their parents and ancestors. More importantly, they learned that their heritage was "inferior" and that the religion, language, and practices of the "white man" were "superior" in every way. Finally, they did not learn how to live in families, how to be children with parents or siblings or members of extended families. They were deprived of essential tools for family making in their own adulthood. The effects continue to be experienced through the process of multigenerational trauma (Berry, 2010).

The repression and attempted annihilation of indigenous North American cultures was made immensely worse by the physical and sexual abuses committed by many adults toward children in these schools. Childhood abuse, especially physical and sexual abuse, traumatizes children and leaves lasting scars. Many of those abused suffered PTSD, and some continue to suffer PTSD, as a result of those experiences (Evans-Campbell, 2008; Shelley, Sussman, Williams, Segal, & Crabtree, 2009). We discuss trauma and trauma responses in chapter 9, and explore some of the ways in which it is manifested in Native/Aboriginal people. It is important to be aware that those trauma-related reactions that Native people have may have been as a result of their own residential experiences or responses learned from parents who had those experiences.

> **Textbox 10.7. Traditional Medicines**
>
> In many Native American and Aboriginal cultures, sage, sweetgrass, or cedar, considered sacred medicines, are used in ceremonies. They are traditionally burned and wafted much like incense is used in some Christian rituals. One such ritual is a traditional house welcoming to a new home that begins with purifying the house with burning sage. Native people who follow traditional beliefs view this as an important ceremony. In one instance a young man of Canadian First Nations heritage was moving into a "smoke-free" apartment building. Arrangements were made to turn off the smoke detectors, which included warning the fire department, so that the ceremony could be conducted in an uninterrupted fashion. This is now a standing procedure in the agency. Workers should become sensitive to house moving-in rituals that are important in many cultures.

THE CULTURE OF HOMELESSNESS

There is a culture among those who sleep rough, just as there was a culture among the hobos of the 1930s. In the Great Depression that lifestyle was complete with signs of safe places, houses that would provide some food and/or shelter and those to avoid, and a distinct vocabulary referring to the essentials of life on the tracks (railroads) and avoidance of the law. Those who sleep rough in this generation have also developed their own culture, some of it reminiscent of the hobo era and some with modern overtones. It may vary somewhat across different locations, cities, towns, and rural areas, but it is still distinct in the attitudes and behaviors that are part of this lifestyle.

> **Textbox 10.8. Living Rough: One Aspect of Homeless Culture**
>
> The first two chapters of the book *Ragged Company* provide graphic details of what this homeless culture may look like. It provides details about how people relate to each other, what is defined as private space in public areas, what personal information is shared with others, and how intrusions are handled. There are variations among different communities, but the basics of the behaviors, lifestyle, and attitudes of those who sleep rough is clearly captured by the author.
>
> (Wagamese, 2008).

Many people who live on the edge, in the rough, and who seek a formal shelter only in the most extreme weather conditions, prefer privacy and seek sleeping space away from others. There are some who would rather settle with others in an encampment, whose needs for group support are greater than the urge for privacy. Some are fearful of authorities, others turn a cold shoulder, but in all, the tendency is to avoid contact with officials and to have a controlled amount of contact with others. Eye contact is minimal, conversations are carried on with adequate space between people, clothing is usually in layers, and there is a pervasive attitude that Main Street will not accept them and will avoid them, fearful of personal safety. Workers need to be respectful of the personal space a rough sleeper may desire. The willingness to speak with someone who is from Main Street, even someone who is a helper, may be limited or nonexistent. Introductions may need to be made with the help of another street person whom they trust. The language used will probably be blunt, direct, and to the point, and the person may be wary, vigilant, and hesitant to speak. All of these are within norms and do not, of themselves, indicate anything other than normal street vigilance. This is especially important to remember when you, as the worker, are trying to determine if there are also some mental health issues. (See chapter 7 for greater detail on indications of mental disorders.) All of these behavioral and communication indicators may also be filtered through the additional cultural lens of an immigrant, migrant, or Native American or Aboriginal person.

ORGANIZATIONAL CULTURE

Sociologists and organizational psychologists describe organizations as having their own cultures. By this term they refer to the values, attitudes, behaviors, norms, and beliefs that shape an organization, its purpose, and how it conducts its business (Schein, 2006). Much of what has been explored about this concept of culture began in the business world and has only more recently come into the forefront of human service organizations (Waegemakers Schiff, 2009). What might this concept have to do with helping homeless persons?

Homelessness has become a field of work and it has evolved into one that is laden with values: the rights of individuals, their emotional struggles, the ethics of doing good, and avoiding the pitfalls of competing interests all contribute to the daily encounters that workers face in advocating for clients. As we discussed earlier, burnout is a serious occupational hazard for those who must do their jobs with feeling and empathy. In this climate workers need to be able to function with the understanding and support of managers and leaders who recognize that human service work is demanding and does not respond to traditional corporate world values of production and economy of action. Thus organizational values that empower individuals, honor the caring and compassion of workers, and allow for the processing of feelings as an important work-related activity are paramount.

Organizations that acknowledge and respect diversity present themselves in ways that demonstrate their sensitivity to the strong moral and emotional components of working with homeless people. The décor of buildings and office spaces will reflect the cultures of the clients served. Brochures explaining services will be available in the language of the clients, and waiting rooms will have reading material in those languages. Staff will receive awareness training, and thus be knowledgeable about the traditions, practices, and ways of communicating of the clients who come. Translation and interpretation services are recognized as essential and are accessed as needed. The agency will also be sensitive to the double-bind imposed by having family members or close friends act as translators/interpreters. These agencies will also be aware of important holidays, rituals, and rites of passage for clients of specific cultures, and will make provision for them (Waegemakers Schiff, 2009).

In order to use a *housing first* philosophy in providing permanent shelter, organizations also need to have developed values of interagency collaboration, a respect for individual empowerment of clients served, a recognition of the importance of a harm-reduction approach to helping people, and a willingness to provide individualized supports for as long as necessary without viewing this as a negative dependency. The attitudes that service providers convey to vulnerable individuals will have an immediate and lasting impact on their efforts to get people stabilized in housing.

EXERCISES

1. In a classroom setting, ask each group of four or five students to identify ten different cultural groups within the local community. If the community is large, assign each group a particular geographic area of the world such as South America, Africa, or East Asia. Alternatively, ask each group to identify different indigenous groups or religious groups, or different sexualities. After identifying the groups, have students list what they know—and do not know—about three of the identified groups. How would they get more detail about these different cultures? Is there any way they could have direct contact to increase their awareness?

2. Present each group of students with a case scenario (family recently homeless), and ask them to determine a plan of action to help the family. Change the demographics of the family for each group in the class. For example: have a family of four—two young children and two adults, or perhaps six children, a grandparent, and an aunt or cousin, all in the same household. Family background can be varied as by the following (or find local examples): African American, Metis (Canadian Indian and French heritage), Native American or Canadian Aboriginal living off reserve, Mexican Hispanic, Caribbean Hispanic, Iranian immigrants who are Muslim, or Ugandan refugees. Have the parents as partners in either a same-sex marriage or living common-law. Have a class discussion around how differences influence our engagement and planning decisions, both positively and negatively.

3. Plan a cultural awareness class. Have students from different ethnic backgrounds present, and have them include in their presentations examples of dress, food, music, dance, art, or whatever they wish to illustrate. Have them speak about their ways of adapting to a different culture, if applicable.

JOURNALING

1. How do you define and describe your own cultural orientation? Are you also part of a subculture?
2. Examine your own cultural background. What are the values, attitudes, and beliefs of your culture? Are there any specific groups that your ethnic group holds negative stereotypes about? Do you share these?
3. What privileges does your cultural orientation include? What are the best parts of your culture? What are the least desirable?
4. Would you prefer to belong to a different culture? Why? Can you identify some aspects of the subculture of homelessness? How is belonging to a different culture than your clients challenging for worker interactions with your clients?

CHAPTER 11

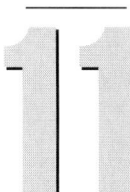

Ethics in Practice

> **KEY ISSUES**
>
> Ethics, values, and morals
> Overview of ethical guidelines related to mental health, addictions, and medical treatment
> Confidentiality and consent to treatment
> Proper boundaries with clients and how to avoid ethical pitfalls and slippery slopes
> Conflicts of interest not just about money
> Common ethical conflicts in the field
> Ethical standards related to documentation and report writing
> Skills to write effective case notes, assessments, and discharge summaries

OVERVIEW

Working with people is interlaced with our values, and with the values of the people we work with and of society. In order to work respectfully with others we need to be aware of the many ways that value systems influence what we do and how we do things. A discussion about the rights and wrongs of how we behave is important because our individual value system and ethical beliefs influence everything that we do. While ethics deals with what is good and bad about behavior, it is also about human respect—one person's respect for another. Ethics is about our self-awareness of the rightness and wrongness of our behavior and is based on values of the dignity and worth of human beings. Right and wrong are not universal absolutes—that is, they are not precisely the same in all countries and cultures. They are influenced by religious and philosophical beliefs as well as by whether a society has a group or individual orientation towards its worldview and lifestyle. But we concentrate here on what is considered as the norm within North American society, which has primarily an individual orientation: the rights of the individual are the first order of consideration.

In society, ethical behavior encompasses respect for the individual, a person's right of self-determination, and the sacredness of life. These values should always be at the forefront of any interactions we have with those we want to help. To be aware of and sensitive to the importance of values in our work we need to look once again at what life's struggles and challenges are like for a person who is homeless. Being homeless places a person in a very vulnerable position—disadvantaged, and often disparaged and misunderstood. Most have few resources to handle many of the financial, legal, and practical life challenges they face. Working with vulnerable people thus demands that we take care to ensure their safety and respect their human rights, that we not abuse the power that we have as a result of our jobs, and that we seek to empower them. Working with homeless people also often means being at the edges of the law (for both worker and client) and having our basic morals, values, and ethical practices challenged on a daily basis.

We first explore why and how ethical issues became important in services delivery and, although there may be similarities, we distinguish between ethical issues of the workplace and ethical issues with clients. Then we explore the major ethical principles that underlie the way most decisions are made. Through case examples we look at common ethical dilemmas and the importance of developing an agency culture that understands and accommodates both personal and professional issues. The case examples also look at common ethical dilemmas faced by service providers and by homeless persons, and ways to address those dilemmas.

WHAT ARE SOME ETHICAL ISSUES IN WORKING WITH HOMELESS PERSONS?

The first and most obvious questions are these:

- Is it ethical to tolerate anyone being homeless?
- Does everyone have a right to housing?

- Are homeless shelters an acceptable way to house people who have no income?
- Are homeless shelters any better than the poorhouses of the eighteenth century?
- In what way do these questions look at respect of individuals and a person's right to self-determination?
- As a worker there are some important considerations: What is your reaction when you come across a homeless person panhandling on a busy street?
- Are you offended by this behavior, or uncomfortable in crossing paths with someone who needs to beg for food?
- Do you condemn the woman who prostitutes herself in order to pay for shelter and food for her kids? Her behavior may in many places be illegal, but is it unethical?
- How do you react to words often used to describe homeless people: shiftless, irresponsible, dope fiends, bums, vagrants, street workers, hookers, derelicts, bag ladies, homeless waifs?
- Do some of these words evoke your compassion, discomfort, disgust, or pity?
- Are any of these reactions not ethical?
- Are you proud of your work because you are helping "some poor unfortunate soul" to get a better life, even if you have to tell her what to do?
- Is your attitude and way of helping ethical?
- Do you worry about buying a homeless person a Big Mac, or do you not want to spend the extra money on a sandwich?
- Do you ask what the person would like to eat, or not?
- Do you think that all sex trade workers stay on the streets because they like the money, or because it lets them get drugs?
- Is it ethical to arrest someone for loitering or vagrancy because he looks as if he is homeless?
- Is it ethical to discharge a patient from the hospital to the shelter system, knowing that there is no adequate follow up, care, and diet for their condition?

The above questions are but a small fraction of the numerous ethical and moral dilemmas that workers and their clients face on a daily basis. They raise a host of issues about what we consider to be fair, appropriate, acceptable, and morally just ways of addressing the lifestyles and behaviors of those who are unhoused or marginally housed. Behind each question lies the issue of what is ethical behavior and to what extent we tolerate rather than confront the amoral and unethical aspects of these lives. Before addressing these questions we will take a quick look at the world of ethics and how we can apply its principles in daily practice.

Ethics: What Are They, and Where Did They Come from?

The formal description of ethics includes the understanding that they are beliefs about behavior based on moral and value judgments that have been accepted by a group as the right way for members to conduct themselves. In our society, these beliefs begin with acknowledgment of the dignity and worth of individual human beings, which then provides guidelines for what a group considers to be acceptable rules of conduct. Beliefs and values also influence the extent to which individual rights are given priority over those of the group when there are contentious decisions that need to be made. While some principles are universal, such as the sacredness of human life, some are placed in order of relative importance according to social, religious, cultural, and ethnic custom. One example is the right of women to equal opportunities in education and employment; this is a principle accepted in fact, if not always in practice, in North America but not in place in many other countries. Ethics are often in harmony with the law but may at times depart from the law. That is why the common phrase in textbox 11.1 is often quoted.

> **Textbox 11.1. The Paradox of What Is Right**
> A maxim of ethics: You may have the right to do something, but that does not mean it is the right thing to do.

In human services there are several important areas where most of the common and difficult ethical issues are likely to come up. They involve the right of self-determination, due diligence in the performance of one's responsibilities, equal treatment for all, the avoidance of harm, the obligation to be truthful and respectful of the trusting (helping) relationship, the right of confidentiality, and, concomitantly, the respect for the helping relationship so that there is no abuse of power. The area of professional relationships can be among the most tricky on a daily basis because these relationships involve professional boundaries (the fine line between personal, social, and professional) as well as prohibitions against intimate or sexual relationships with clients. While many ethics conversations take place in academia with regard to conducting research, the most important fact to keep in mind is that, in the world of the homeless, people are part of a vulnerable population, often unable to protect themselves; they need to have their rights vigorously guarded. Before discussing specific ethical issues, we briefly look at the process of ethical decision making and the reasoning behind the principles used to make these determinations.

Health-care and social services professionals learn the code of ethics of their respective professions during their education and training. The values embedded in these codes, and the priority given to them, generally help to define how persons from different professions evaluate and react to dilemmas that arise in the course of trying to help people. For example, physicians "first do no harm" and nurses are taught that "patient safety is first." Social workers place respect for the dignity and worth of the individual and pursuit of social justice as first ethical principles that lead to empowerment of the individual. In contrast, psychologists place respect for the dignity of the individual as most important, followed by responsible caring, and police follow either a code of ethics or code of conduct, depending on the jurisdiction in which they work. The police code generally includes the responsibility to protect lives and property, preserve the peace, enforce the law, prevent crime, detect and apprehend offenders, and protect the rights and freedoms of all persons. On the other hand, lawyers have a code of conduct rather than a code of ethics, and this code places integrity of practice as primary and states that a lawyer should be above reproach. These examples show that some professions are more inclined to promote self-protection and self-interest while others are more concerned with care for others. As we explored in chapter 4, these values have a direct influence on how different professions make decisions when helping others.

All professional codes of conduct have some reference to preserving and respecting individual rights, including those of privacy and confidentiality. For workers who have not had the exposure to professional codes of ethics, the most common way to become aware of issues of confidentiality, client privilege, duty to warn, and other concerns is through daily work and, at times, in-service training. In this way, we increase our awareness of the need to protect individuals, especially vulnerable individuals.

BASIC ETHICAL PRINCIPLES

Ethical principles consist of a set of statements that guide decision making and involve issues of morals or values. These principles set the standards for discussions about how best to understand ethical problems and potentially offer answers. We have used the writings of some academics to guide this presentation about ethical principles and practices that face human services workers. As ethical issues have various nuances, they are best explored through case examples where the principles of practice can be illustrated and discussed. Following this discussion of basic principles, we will look at some of the numerous issues with ethical overtones that face homeless persons and their workers. The italicized English words in the following emphasize the essence of each principle. Basic ethical principles are as follows: nonmaleficence, beneficence, justice, autonomy, confidentiality, fidelity and veracity, utilitarianism, egoism, and formalism.

Nonmaleficence

The basic principle of medical and most other care of humans is to "do no harm." This principle is enshrined in the Hippocratic Oath taken by all physicians. It is recognized by all of the helping professions as a basic principle in caregiving. The primary principle is to do nothing that would ultimately hurt the patient or client. It is frequently applied in medical settings where the treatment options have varying degrees of risk and recovery potential. On the streets this principle may apply to simple acts that disrespect people.

For example, if a homeless family of two adult caregivers and two children, one of whom is an adolescent, requests shelter, do you send the adults to shelters and place the children in child welfare care? Or do you send the adolescent to a youth shelter? Or do you place them all together, even if this means two motel rooms because the adolescent is not allowed to sleep in the same bedroom as the parents? How important is family cohesions in this instance? What harms may there be to the adolescent or to the younger child if the family members are separated? What other ethical issues may be involved?

Beneficence

Beneficence addresses the attempt to do things that are *of benefit to another or will promote the good of others*. Situations that call on the principle of beneficence include those where the other person is incapacitated, cannot decide for himself, or is deemed incompetent. Homeless people are vulnerable and often at the mercy of others. It is tempting to want to be seen as "the doer of good deeds" for them. Many actions are done on behalf of others under this principle of beneficence. However, in many instances the good done is for the benefit of the doer and not the receiver.

For example, a town councilor who has been volunteering occasionally at the local soup kitchen is running for reelection. She wants to have the press take her picture while serving food, and wants to include some of those being served. In turn she promises to lobby for increased funding for the program. Whose interests are being served and what principles are in jeopardy?

Justice

Based on the principle of *fair and equal treatment for all people*, regardless of any distinguishing characteristics, justice refers to the distribution of goods and benefits. This distribution is not only for physical or tangible goods and benefits, but also for social, emotional, or relationship benefits. This principle is one of the thorniest that ethicists encounter; it often arises in situations where there are scarce resources. That is, when something is either very expensive or very scarce, who should receive it? The person most able to pay? Most able to return the benefit in future service? Likely to live the longest? Following are some troublesome examples:

- Should a premature baby born to a woman who is an active crack user have the same neonatal intensive care as a premature baby born to a woman who has no substance-abuse history? Does it make a difference if the care is paid under universal health care or if one woman has health-care coverage and the other's care is paid by government programs such as Medicaid or Medicare?

- Should undocumented people from other countries (that is, not in a country legally) be entitled to the same health-care benefits as citizens? How should their medical care be handled in an emergency when they can't afford the treatment?
- In a publicly funded treatment program, should a homeless cocaine-dependent person have the same access to residential treatment (publicly paid) as a business executive who must go to treatment or be fired from her job?
- Should a man who has custody of two children under the age of six be entitled to the same assistance as a woman with children of similar ages? Should he be given access to a homeless shelter for domestic abuse? Should he be offered alternatives?

Autonomy

We live in a democratic society, one that places a high value on *individual right to self-determination*. The freedom to choose, act on that choice, and live with the consequences are of premier importance; these freedoms are embodied in the Canadian Charter of Rights and Freedoms and in the US Constitution. As citizens of those countries we cherish our autonomy and relinquish it only reluctantly in critical situations involving health, life, and death.

For example, homeless people have had much of their autonomy stripped away. They have few choices about what, where, and when to eat; next to whom they will eat or sleep; what they will wear; and where they can keep their few possessions safe. Because of this major erosion in their autonomy, it is incumbent on workers to offer as much opportunity for choice as is feasible. In a small shelter, is it appropriate to require "lights out" so that staff can have free time?

Confidentiality

Confidentiality is a fundamental tenet in working with homeless persons. We all encounter issues of confidentiality, especially as this principle applies to our health, financial, and legal records. The *right to privacy* has led to the establishment of laws and regulations that affect all of us as individuals as well as the ways in which we work with vulnerable people. Workers should note that the attitudes and laws in Canada are different from those in the United States with regard to privacy and confidentiality. For example, in a client-worker relationship the duty to warn a person if they are in danger because of threats from another is different in the two countries and also in different jurisdictions in the United States (Felthous, O'Shaughnessay, Kuten, Francois-Purcel, & Medrano, 2007). Furthermore, laws regarding individual right to privacy also differ. Canada has adopted practices in line with stringent European Union requirements that focus on individual protections, whereas American laws favor business over individual concerns (Levin & Nicholson, 2005). We also need to distinguish between the statements of confidentiality in codes of ethics of individual professions, and the laws and regulations put forward by government and legal authorities that protect an individual's right to privacy.

In the real world of the streets, confidentiality can have some interesting implications. When a person seeks refuge in a homeless shelter, everyone who works and receives services there will know that this person is homeless—a fact with widespread ramifications. The example in textbox 11.2 provides a dramatic illustration of how far-reaching this knowledge can inadvertently become.

> **Textbox 11.2. Case Example**
> As a faculty advisor to social work students, the school's liaison was expected to meet regularly with students and their supervisors at the agency where their practicum occurred. On one such occasion the supervisor went to a secondary shelter for domestic violence. She encountered a student in the social work program on a temporary absence from her studies who was a resident of the shelter.
> The dilemma: Should the liaison acknowledge the fact that she knew this person to the woman herself? To others in the same room? Should she report this to the school?
> Alternative situation: If the location had been a psychiatric unit of the local general hospital, would the relevant issues be the same? Would there have been additional issues?
> What are the ethical principles underlying practice that are in conflict here?

Along with autonomy, confidentiality is one of the rights that often gets neglected or minimized when it is urgent to get a job done. All of us have a right to privacy about our personal lives and businesses. However, we cannot guarantee that we will not be recognized in a location where we would not want to be seen: in a preoperation waiting room, a cancer clinic, or perhaps at a food bank program or shelter. In small cities and towns, the probability that a person will be recognized by friends or acquaintances is much higher. For the totally homeless, there is no privacy in a shelter when you sleep thirty inches from the next person, stand in line for food with sixty others, or are seen in line at the local social services office.

Fidelity and Veracity

The importance of *promising only what you can deliver* has previously been mentioned as critical to establishing a working relationship with your (prospective) clients. Fidelity speaks to loyalty and commitment as essential to helping another. Veracity goes along with fidelity in that it addresses the need to *be truthful at all times*. This can be difficult, especially when we all have a tendency to shy away from difficult discussions, painful truths, and bad news. However, if another person cannot rely on your word as honest and truthful, then there cannot be any relationship that either of you can count on. We recognize that clients are also not comfortable with telling the truth at all times, as some information may make them more vulnerable to exploitation, legal action, and surveillance. It falls to the workers to set a standard of honesty and truth as nonnegotiable because without those fundamental elements there can be no trust, and trust glues relationships together.

Sometimes it is necessary to shelter a person from the complete truth—at least temporarily, to help the other to process information in stages rather than all at once. One example may be in the event of an unexpected and/or violent death of a family member, when news of the death may be sufficient and details left to another time. This does not mean that one avoids reality, but that the emotional processing should take place in stages and not all at once. Sometimes "found dead" may be the best place to stop, and to add later that the injury was self-inflicted. Veracity does mean that you do not tell the person that it was from "natural causes" or an accident when that was clearly not the case. You also need to decide when the answer "I don't know" is legitimate and when it is an avoidance of an unpleasant issue. People will find out if you have lied rather than revealing the truth when you knew it, and the repercussions will be hard to overcome for a long time.

Utilitarianism

Utilitarianism is a prime example where the importance of *what is best for the group* is more important than the rights and needs of the individual. That is, utilitarianism is "the greatest good for the greatest number." It is by itself not very helpful when a situation is relatively unique and does not affect the larger group except perhaps indirectly in monetary ways (such as a costly intervention that tax dollars have to pay for). For example, if a pandemic—a large-scale outbreak of a highly infectious disease—were to happen, public officials would be forced to make difficult decisions about who could be admitted to local shelters that had specialized quarantine areas, and who would have to be sent elsewhere. This may be an extra hardship for those shelter dwellers who need to live in a specific area where there are medical services they need. However, the decision would be made to accommodate the greatest good for the greatest number of people.

> **Textbox 11.3. Utilitarianism**
> Based on the philosophy expounded by John Stuart Mill (1806–73).

Individualism

Individualism, on the other hand, places *the rights of individuals over those of the group or society at large.* Individual rights and freedoms are closely aligned with the value of autonomy. These rights value independence and self-determination, but individualism faces challenges when the needs of one person are countered by opposing needs of a larger group of citizens. An example would be the provision of extremely expensive medical procedures, or very costly medicines, to save the life of a child when the cost is at public expense. When is this expense justified? Does it make a difference if the individual is an adult or has additional disabilities?

Egoism

Egoism, by contrast, refers to a situation where the needs and rights of the individual making a decision win out over what is in the best interests for the common good. It implies that "the self" is most important. This situation

> **Textbox 11.4. Individualism**
> Individualism, often associated with the existential school of thought that includes Sartre, Kant, and Nietzsche, is a twentieth-century development and is more espoused in Eurocentric countries than in societies with a communal value system such as China.

is likely to occur in instances where one person is the decision maker and that person is more interested in personal safety and financial gain than in the good of the group, program, or agency. This person also has the power and control to make the decision. Drug dealers and unscrupulous landlords are examples of egoism.

Formalism

Formalism, on the other hand, promotes *the even application of a rule across all situations,* as though equity (things being equal) is built on the equal treatment of all in all situations. This view comes from the words, "Do unto others as you would have them do unto you," attributed to Jesus in the Sermon on the Mount (Luke 6:31 and Matthew 7:12). It rarely takes into account unique or extenuating circumstances and instead uses a simple rule applied to everyone. Most people who work with people realize that life is filled with ambiguous situations where no single principle or rule can be applied to all people in all circumstances. Thus formalism has little relevance for the multiple times when there are fine shades of gray that nuance an ethical dilemma in people's lives. The formalism of government regulations often gets in the way of sensitive and appropriate services.

An example would be the custodial father of young girls whose mother is a substance abuser, but who cannot obtain help in parenting because he is a man and domestic violence programs serve only women.

WAYS OF APPLYING ETHICAL PRINCIPLES

Which of the above principles apply in any given situation is a source of considerable debate. This discussion has to also include consideration of times when the law may conflict with basic rights and principles, with professional ethics, and with your personal values and moral codes. This debate expands our views of human rights and needs to include the rights and

Ethics in Practice

needs of the individual as opposed to those of the group, those of the workers and agency, and those of society at large (figure 11.1). It also considers which rights and needs should take precedence. When working with the homeless there is a commitment to protect, care, and enhance the wellbeing of human beings. Thus we must

- understand their vulnerability;
- understand whether current practices "do no harm";

Figure 11.1. Multiple Contexts of Ethical Conduct

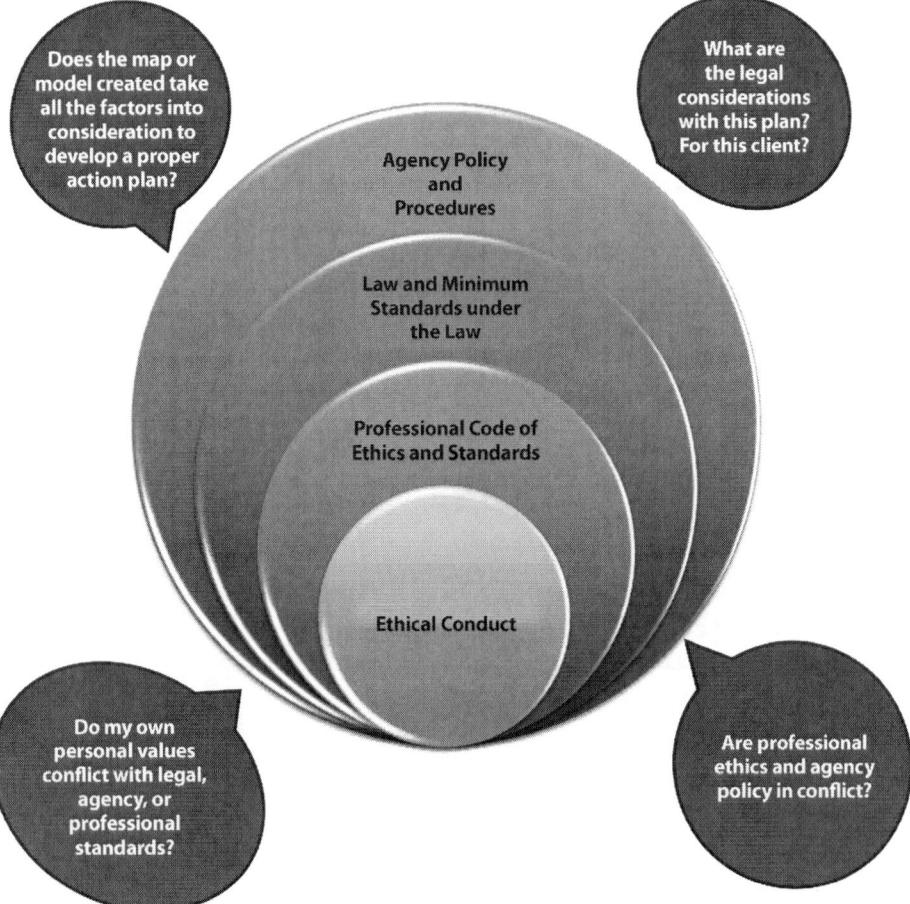

- understand the impact of staff attitudes and behavior, agency policy, and governmental policy and regulation; and
- understand challenging conflicts in the core values and standards of care.

A perfect example is the issue of panhandling. Should people be deprived of the opportunity to ask for money because they are not properly dressed, or may create a public nuisance, or be an embarrassment to the town as an example of need in an affluent society? On the other hand, does the scenario change if the panhandler is looking for money for drugs or alcohol? Is this panhandler any different from the well-heeled businessman who cheats his clients and then arranges for a cocaine supply for his next party?

What do these basic ethical principles have to do with the ethical issues that face workers and clients who are deprived of adequate housing? Where do you place your own values and attitudes using these theories? Table 11.1 gives a starting point to consider the implications of each school of thought on something as basic as shelter and housing.

Codes of Ethics

Professional codes of ethics delineate the standards by which members of a specific group should behave. While generally based on one or more of the decision-making principles described above, these codes are intended to ensure that all members of the group avoid practices that are considered illegal and/or immoral by the group. These codes classify the professional practice issues that may lead to abuse of power and harm to an individual or group. Each profession organizes the priorities of these values in somewhat different ways, although all follow a mandate to do no harm. A wide range of behaviors fall under this mandate and concern themselves with the range from physical harm and abuse; to psychological and sexual exploitation; and to conflict of interest, abuse of power, and influence. These issues are of particular importance for homeless persons who are most often vulnerable, without resources to adequately protect themselves, and without the ability to readily escape from problematic situations (McDermott, 2011). They risk further ostracism when they try to advocate for respectful and equal treatment for themselves and family and friends, as this assertiveness threatens their ability to obtain the food, shelter, and benefits that sustain them and

Table 11.1. Values and Ethics in Helping Homeless People

Theory	Argument to Support This Theory	Rebuttal
Utilitarianism	Give housing resources to all people needing housing, regardless of other issues, because doing so meets the greatest need.	What happens to those who have multiple and complex needs?
Individualism	We must meet the individualized needs of each person and household uniquely with whatever is required.	Who pays for this highly personalized service? Can government afford it?
Egoism	"My needs are taken care of and others should take care of themselves."	This leaves the disabled and unfortunate with no adequate means of survival.
Formalism	The government makes rules for the circumstances under which a person receives help.	Not everyone falls under these rules. There is no accounting for ethnicity or culture or individual disabilities.
Justice	All people should be treated equally, thus it is a human right for every person to have food, water, housing, and clothing, and the government needs to provide for those who can't provide this for themselves.	"The world is not fair" and "each person should look out for himself." "People will not want to work if they can get a handout."

may lift them out of homelessness. Following are some behaviors that are unethical because they are or can be interpreted as an abuse of power:

- Breaking client confidentiality without significant legal cause is an abuse of power.
- Wearing sexually provocative dress and displaying inappropriate sexual behavior (including that inappropriate to the client's cultural context) is an abuse of power.
- Any type of sexual contact is an abuse of power.
- Social interactions with a client that disadvantage the client are an abuse of power.

- Behavior that discriminates based on sex is an abuse of power.
- Actions that expect a reward or "payback" are an abuse of power.
- Engaging in legal or financial transactions with clients is an abuse of power.
- Threatened or actual legal action as a consequence for failure to follow demands that are not part of a court mandate is an abuse of power. This situation can be very subtle or very obvious, and is a frequent abuse of power among those connected with child welfare agencies and agencies serving those with mental illness. An example is if a worker says, "Do what I say [or want] or I will have the children removed . . . or make sure the children do not get returned to your care."
- Conflict of interest is using your knowledge, power, or influence to advantage one person or group of people over another and having yourself, friends, or family benefit from the result. Conflicts can be financial, psychological, or social, among others. An example of this would be the case worker who asks a client with landscaping skills to provide these services at his home at a major discount because he knows the homeless person has no income and few choices. This is also an abuse of power.
- An abuse of power is the act of threatening a person who has a mental disorder with hospitalization if he does not comply with worker demands that he take prescribed medication for his mental disorder.
- An abuse of power is threatening a newly housed person with eviction if she is seen in a local bar.
- Common situations that have ethical implications when working with homeless persons are
  - meeting with youths in nontraditional settings;
  - mistaking friendship for appropriate trust building;
  - not keeping confidentiality;
  - not reporting abuse and neglect;
  - not reporting runaways;
  - not addressing risky behaviors;
  - giving money, taking people home, leaving people in unsafe settings; and
  - failing to report or to act on information shared.

- Applying personal values and beliefs in decisions regarding clients. For example, a worker who values families staying together may encourage a runaway youth to return home, even though the parents are abusive, physically and emotionally.

ETHICAL BOUNDARIES

While there are certain universally accepted principles, such as the immorality of taking a life when self-protection is not involved, the territory between what is ethically right and ethically wrong can best be described by various shades of gray. War and acts of self-defense are a good example of where the sanctity of life is tempered by other circumstances. In this area there are often no clear-cut answers and what is right may be nuanced by the context of the situation. This leaves considerable judgment in the hands of the worker, which is one reason why we devote considerable space to this topic. Ethical boundaries are concrete—are easily described physically—and occur in the realm of feelings and relationships. Concrete boundaries take various shapes, such as the recognition of personal space, that distance from another that each of us treats as a comfort zone around ourselves. When we come too close to another for our comfort or that of the other person, we have entered someone's personal space without permission. In unavoidable places such as crowded elevators most people turn inwards and make little eye or body contact with surrounding strangers. Similarly, in an interview or other interaction with a homeless person, the signals about personal space are clear and indicate that the other person normally wants more rather than less space. Any move to reduce the space between you is often viewed as aggressive or confrontational behavior.

Boundaries also exist around social interactions. Clients do not become social friends who drop in at your home. You do not ask them out to dinner, but may share a couple of burgers. While having coffee together is common, sharing a bottle of wine is way outside of appropriate socializing regardless of the circumstances. Doing favors also violates professional or social boundaries, as does the lending of money—for any reason. The same applies to a worker providing a place to stay for a client or potential client who is suddenly left homeless. There may be unusual or extreme circumstances where a worker may provide shelter or go beyond customary boundaries, such as in extreme weather conditions, during a natural disaster, or in remote and rural areas when no other resources are accessible. But these are exceptions. The ethical principles for these rules come from the recognition that there is an inherent power imbalance between the worker and the homeless client. The power balance leads quickly to feelings of coercion or manipulation on the part of the client. Even when workers are not accustomed to the idea that they have some type of power over clients, they must recognize its existence and they should be vigilant to not misuse their power in any way.

Boundaries are also important in order to avoid situations where vulnerable clients may be subject to harm. Clients may confuse extra effort with romantic or personal interest, which may tap into latent dependency issues. Limits provide clients and workers with a sense of predictability and safety and thus define the extent to which a worker can and cannot do something. It allows the worker to avoid situations that encourage dependence of clients that leads to doing too much for clients. Sometimes doing too much can be as detrimental as doing too little. Thus, boundaries cannot always be absolute, but must be guidelines to appropriate roles and expectations.

These guidelines are not meant, however, to be so rigid that they stunt normal human interactions. There needs to be some flexibility in interpersonal boundaries, to include accepting and recognizing ambiguity. This flexibility acknowledges the changing needs of clients so that what is essential in one instance may not meet their requirements at another time. That is, a hug during a crisis situation may be permissible, but a hug at each meeting is not. This flexibility recognizes that each client is unique and has different needs for support. That means that the worker needs to be responsive and adaptive in finding informal solutions to pressing needs. Finally, boundaries are often set by paid work hours, but client needs may extend well beyond that. How does a worker balance client needs with personal needs?

For those working with homeless people, boundaries created by the workplace are usually not helpful or responsive to the behavior expected on the streets. Most references to boundaries imply that a person is interacting in an office environment that provides behavior guidelines and control over what is said and done. These guidelines do not exist in the open spaces of the street. Entering a person's place of sleep or rest, whether it is a tenting area or a shelter's sleeping hall, or coming close to the minimal structure that someone calls theirs, already touches the margins between public and private, and the boundaries that implies. Often, those who work on the streets find themselves exposed to inappropriate sexual language and behavior that would not be seen or tolerated in office settings. There are no rule books that explicitly guide a worker on what to do or not do (Fisk, Rakfeldt, Heffernan, & Rowe, 1999). Frequent discussions in groups and individually with managers and supervisors are important to being sensitive to and finding ways to respond to many of the boundary issues that workers confront on the streets. The opportunity to discuss daily events allows for examination of the details that are critical to determining ethical issues of boundaries, power, and control. This level of support is also helpful in preventing undue stress and burnout for workers.

ETHICAL DECISION-MAKING MAP

Ethical principles, as previously discussed, can be the basis for guidelines as to which principles should take priority. The following list, with items ordered in ethical priority, is one such approach (Dolgoff, Harrington, & Loewenberg, 2011). In prioritizing or ranking ethical principles, a higher-level principle is more compelling than one based on a lower-ranked principle:

1. The principle of protection of life
2. The principle of equality and inequality
3. The principle of autonomy and freedom
4. The principle of least harm
5. The principle of quality of life
6. The principle of privacy and confidentiality
7. The principle of truthfulness and full disclosure

While there are no fixed rules for what is right or wrong in the many ethical dilemmas that workers encounter, these principles can be applied in developing a decision map that can guide the worker. We suggest the following steps as an aid to identifying issues and determining a course of action.

Essential Steps for Ethical Problem Solving: A Frontline Worker's Toolbox

1. Evaluate the situation to determine if it may involve competing values and ways of acting.

2. Determine if there is a potential ethical issue and/or dilemma:
    a. Is there a conflict of values or rights or professional responsibilities?
    b. Are individual rights in conflict with agency or legal protocols or mandates?
    c. Are there boundary issues?
    d. Is confidentiality at risk?
    e. Is there an issue of self-determination of a woman versus the well-being of her child(ren)?
3. Identify the key values and principles involved:
    a. Should a homeless teen who has just given birth be allowed to keep her child or should it be placed in protective custody?
4. Rank the values or ethical principles that, in your professional judgment, are most relevant to the issue or dilemma. What reasons can you provide for prioritizing one competing value or principle over another? This process will allow the worker to step back from immediate and personal reactions and analyze the situation with some objectivity.
5. Develop an action plan that is consistent with the ethical priorities that you have determined are central to the situation.
6. Meet with colleagues and supervisors about potential risks and consequences of alternative courses of action. Be able to clearly describe the pros and cons of each alternative, and your reasoning for them. Can you support or justify your action plan with values or principles on which the plan is based?
7. Implement your plan, utilizing the most appropriate practice skills and competencies. How will you use core skills such as sensitive communication, skillful negotiation, and cultural competence? For example, skillful colleague or supervisory communication and negotiation may enable an impaired colleague to see his impact on clients and to take appropriate action.
8. Clearly document in case notes for each client any ethical issues that you have identified; current ethical practices, concerns, and conflicts; and any actions taken to address them, even if you were able to go no farther than supervisory consultation. In the event that there

is any future formal or legal action, you will have clearly indicated what you have done, which is important protection for you as the worker as well as for the client and the agency.

9. Reflect on the outcome of this ethical decision-making process. How would you evaluate the consequences of this process for those involved: clients, professionals, agencies?

For ongoing work with clients, it would be most helpful to develop with the program manager or supervisor an ethical decision map for specific issues with clients. This map should include and identify agency policies, practices, and procedures, as well as any relevant professional code of conduct.

BOUNDARY CROSSING OR VIOLATION

Some examples of boundaries can help to increase a worker's sensitivity and awareness of possible boundary crossing or violation. Boundaries recognize differences and the personal domains that exist between people. While a boundary crossing can be seen as an action or behavior that deviates from a recognized boundary such as not having physical contact with a client (i.e., hugging), if the deviation is by mutual consent it is not per se unethical. However, mutual consent does not negate the relationship differences and how any action could be perceived by either person or by onlookers. In other words, even a hug may be problematic under some circumstances. It is up to the worker to be aware of this possibility. In moments of extreme distress, calamity, and trauma, the comfort of human touch such as a hug is not in and of itself a boundary violation—in fact it may be the most therapeutic thing you can do. But in less-dramatic situations a hug could easily be misconstrued. Any action that abuses that personal space and takes advantage by force, intrusion, use of power, or intimidation, or that meets one's own needs at the expense of the client's needs (e.g., for emotional appreciation) can be viewed as a boundary violation. The same applies to emotional extortion or blackmail, which is often used when workers feel frustrated and out of their comfort zone. "If you don't move from this area I will throw you in jail." The previous examples do not refer to crossing major boundaries of social, financial, or sexual conduct. These boundary crossings are always unethical and may also be illegal in many circumstances.

Additional guidelines for workers include the following:

- Consider being friendly and real rather than being a friend.
- Do a weekly check-in with yourself and review if you have the right balance between being overinvolved and underinvolved with clients. It is normal to quickly get involved in situations of high need and high emotion.
- Include in the check-in reflective questions: Is this something that I would want others to know that I am doing? Is this an abuse of power or position? Am I looking for an ultimate reward?
- Form a work group or peer group or other professional relationship where you can do a quick review of troubling issues.
- Work in a team or in pairs whenever possible so that there is opportunity to share responsibility as well as deal with problematic situations.

There are additional basic guidelines that outreach workers should follow. They follow the premise that boundaries are necessary for both job performance and to reduce the possibilities of burnout from overinvolvement (Strike, O'Grady, Myers, & Millson, 2004).

- Do not give your home address or phone number to clients.
- Do not answer your work cell phone 24/7. It is best to have a personal cell for nonwork use.
- Do not involve yourself with client conflicts on the street.
- Do not engage with clients by talking, conducting home visits, and so on in off hours.
- Do not give or lend money to clients.
- Do not make decisions for clients.
- Do not drink, date, or socialize with clients.
- Do not involve yourself in activities that change your role and relationship such as that of employer or colleague.

If we look carefully at these guidelines it is quickly apparent that they speak primarily to role violations—crossing the line between being a helper and being a friend. They also include care around the use of the power inherent in any situation where the other person is disadvantaged, and where money and availability are equated with power.

BOUNDARIES IN RURAL AND REMOTE AREAS

Client confidentiality and client-worker interactions outside of formal service provision are more common in rural settings. In cities and suburban areas there is far less likelihood of meeting a client in another setting, whether on the street, in a shop, at a restaurant, or at a social event in someone's home. Small towns and rural areas do not provide as much opportunity to fade into the crowd, since places to go for anything are greatly reduced. The probability is also that you personally may wear several different hats or play several roles in the community. Most people know or know about those who live locally, and they are also privy to the people talk that fuels the local gossip mills. This challenges the guidelines around boundaries that usually guide the urban worker. Rural areas also have far fewer resources than cities, which means that any referral a worker makes could well be to someone the client knows, or is related to (Galambos, Watt, Anderson, & Danis, 2006). These issues are especially acute for native (Aboriginal) people living on reserves, and those in town who seek culturally aware services (staffed often by extended family and relatives of relatives). Family and friends make anonymity almost impossible in Native circles.

How does one handle boundaries in rural areas where your role is well known, and those you interact with are also known? Recognition and acceptance of your position and potential dilemmas paves the way for you to address this issue directly with clients and potential clients at the first meeting. As the issue of lack of anonymity faces both of you, it also addresses a concern that your client faces with you. In urban settings the decision to acknowledge a personal acquaintanceship in public should be mutual, but also should be based on the understanding that questions like, "Where do you know each other from?" or "How did you meet?" can be handled in general ways such as "I can't remember who introduced us" or by indicating the meeting was through church, school, bingo, and so on. The adage "to be forewarned is to be fore armed" is highly applicable in these instances. In rural settings such strategies may not be possible. You may already know or know of the individual. There may be family, church, or school ties. You may find yourself working on the same project through a local organization.

In that event, knowing nothing but the most obvious information—such as that a person is single or has children—should be the extent of any public recognition of each other. In public, let the client lead the way, but be careful not to step into personal areas as this may compromise your ability to help in your other role. As a worker, you need to be proactive and aware of the constant possibility that the next client could be someone you know that you will need to discuss the reality of your previous interactions/relationship at the onset of any work with that person. These are the situations where you need to have a direct and clear discussion with that person about the boundaries, and your varying roles should not cross over on each other. Your boundaries around them should be clear for the benefit of all concerned.

While the foregoing philosophies and values form the basis for making ethical decisions, the real challenge is in their recognition and application in real-life situations. Some examples from potential situations can be found in *Ragged Company* (Wagamese, 2008): a group of homeless persons tries to go to the movies to escape bitterly cold weather, and one of them finds a winning lottery ticket. In the process, they encounter a number of situations that challenge respectful and ethical treatment by Main Street movie attendants and lottery officials. They also become involved with a lawyer and a journalist, each of whom reminds them of the ethical issues of showing autonomy and respect for all the individuals in this situation.

ETHICS IN THE WORKPLACE

The application of ethical principles to individual situations is one of many in which workers find themselves and you will see in figure 11.2 some of the additional factors involved in ethical decision making. The workplace presents another wide range of booby traps that place individual and group needs in competition with those of the organization, its internal staff needs and demands, its overseers, and its funders. Workplace practices that are blatantly illegal—such as fraud, misrepresentation of services, illegal billing, misuse of agency property, charging the organization for personal expenses, and misappropriation of funds—are also clearly unethical. But in instances where there is no apparent violation of the law, ethical conflicts can still pose significant challenges.

Figure 11.2. Influences on Ethical Conduct

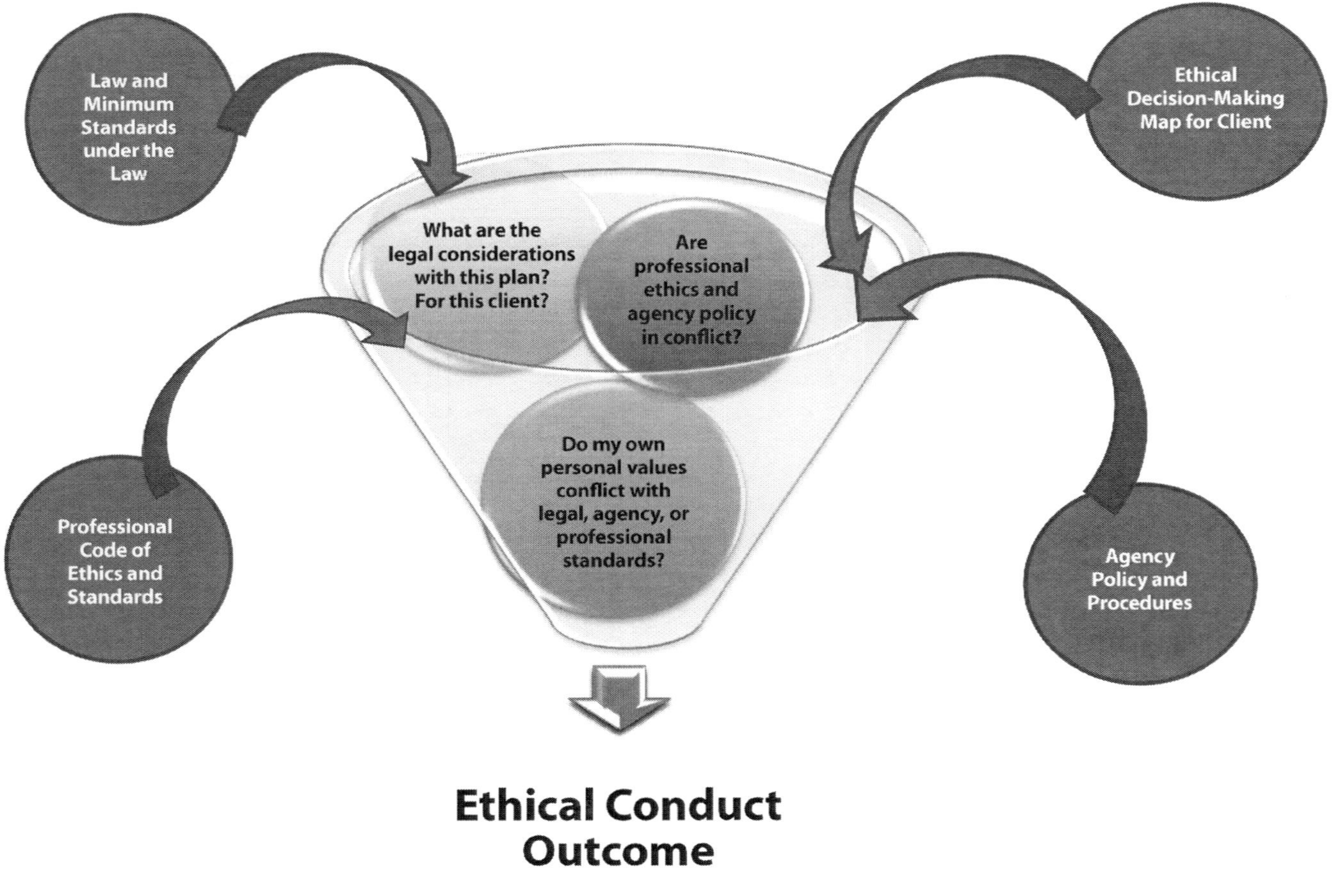

- Ethical Decision-Making Map for Client
- Agency Policy and Procedures
- Law and Minimum Standards under the Law
- Professional Code of Ethics and Standards

- Are professional ethics and agency policy in conflict?
- What are the legal considerations with this plan? For this client?
- Do my own personal values conflict with legal, agency, or professional standards?

Ethical Conduct Outcome

Boundary violations can as easily occur between a supervisor and staff member as they can between a worker and a client because the same problems of power imbalance and potential coercion can arise in both situations. This poses a dilemma for you, as a coworker, who becomes aware of the fact that a violation is occurring between two workers in your organization, or between a manager/supervisor and a coworker. For example, boundary violations may be inadvertent as in the case of coworkers who are both in substance-abuse recovery and meet at an AA meeting or attend the same meeting because there are no alternatives. If the issue of recovery is known by each person, then there may be no conflict, but if the issue is not known, then this personal information can become a source of power and could be used inappropriately. If one worker discloses a relapse in drug use at an AA meeting the other person is placed in an additional jeopardy—the confidentiality of AA meetings versus the need to protect clients in the workplace. It could also lead one or the other person to make compromising decisions in order for this information to remain hidden from employers.

The Unqualified or Impaired Worker

The competence and impairment of the worker are issues that have begun to receive more attention; they are serious issues that violate practice standards. While both issues are related, each has its own set of performance implications. Most professional codes of ethics expect that a person bound by that code will not undertake work or responsibilities that they are not competent to perform and that are outside of their training and experience (Corey, Corey, & Callanan, 2010). We do not accept a family physician as competent or qualified to perform neurosurgery, unless it is a circumstance involving life and death. Likewise, a substance-abuse counselor is usually not trained to provide intensive treatment for PTSD, and a domestic violence worker is usually not qualified to use specialized techniques such as Eye Movement Desensitization and Reprocessing approaches in clients (Davidson & Parker, 2001). Some recently trained individuals may attempt to practice outside their scope of training and experience. If you were to be working with someone who violates these boundaries, what would you do? Are there channels of complaint through your agency or a professional organization that can be used to alert authorities to persons unauthorized to practice in specific areas and interventions? If there is no national accreditation body to oversee competence with certain interventions, what recourse do you have? Is it ethical to remain silent in these situations?

How Do You Handle the Worker's Impairment?

The impaired worker poses many ethical difficulties in the office and in the community. Human service workers are not any more immune from the problems and difficulties of life than other people. Sometimes we may have a better understanding of how to respond—but not always. We have relationships that may be conflicted, children who act out, personal histories of maltreatment and abuse, mental health or addiction problems, psychosocial distress, or job burnout. Any and all of these can impact a person's ability to perform patiently, nonjudgmentally, and competently in helping others. Views and impressions of others' problems may be clouded and biased through how we are handling our own situations. In other words, we are impaired in the performance of our work. The extent of this impairment will affect job performance and may lead us to biased and unhealthy actions at work, violating the first rule of ethical conduct: "Do no harm."

The classic example of the impaired worker is one who has an addiction problem that has been under control until recently but now threatens the person's sobriety. Do you confront your impaired colleague? Do you present this matter to senior staff? What do you do if the senior staff or head of the organization is the person who has lost her sobriety? Do you wait to see if this will be harmful to the organization or to clients? What do you do if you hear of instances of public intoxication while the person is on professional business at a conference? To what extent do you risk becoming the whistle-blower at the potential expense of your own employment? In both Canada and the United States whistle-blower laws aim to protect public employees and not those in private and nonprofit organizations, thus your addressing the problematic behavior of a coworker may put you at risk. Does it make a difference if the agency is a substance treatment facility? These are questions that point to dilemmas between your own values and interests and those of the agency that employs you.

Impairment does not refer only to addictions. A person who is involved in a difficult and contentious marital breakup may be unable to put these concerns aside when attempting to deal with clients, especially if the clients are also persons involved in domestic disputes or child welfare supervision. A person who has recently lost a child or significant other may need extra time to grieve before being able to handle the caregiving involved in many social service jobs. A person who is the sole wage earner in the family may be working two or more jobs, and may consequently not be able to perform adequately in his primary job. The ethical concerns in these situations involve the ability to make decisions regarding the harm that may be done by not being able to fully and completely attend to the needs of a client and family, especially if there are competing emotional ties or reduced energy to deal with clients.

RECORD-KEEPING AND CONFIDENTIALITY

The relationship between ethical behavior and keeping records may not be obvious at first glance. Many workers assume that record-keeping is aimed only at documenting client and worker activities. It is also a testament to the delivery of appropriate, accountable, respectful services in a confidential and professional manner. Despite the fact that record-keeping may seem to be taking time away from direct service with clients, it is a vital component for delivering appropriate service. The documentation of what services are necessary, when and how they are to be delivered, and the result of service provision on client welfare are all important aspects of doing the best we can. Documentation addresses the accountability of workers for their job performance. The record provides evidence that the worker has competently assessed the situation, documented key facts, drawn appropriate conclusions, and acted accordingly. It also means that each item or progress note written into the record becomes an indication of whether or not the worker has done her job.

The burden of providing evidence to justify the need for specific services falls directly on the worker. Documentation is both a way of demonstrating competence and a means of accountability. The accountability may involve individual situations of client welfare, or organizational issues of proof of services provided for funders. It also has a legal aspect in that it provides evidence in the event that court action is required, such as child welfare custody situations as well as any potential lawsuits for malpractice. Service records should both be shared with and signed off by your supervisor, who remains ultimately responsible for their timely recording. This is a support and protection for workers; it signifies that you have not acted without supervisory knowledge and support.

Record-keeping involves writing skills and the ability to put information in logical and appropriate order. For many workers who have emerged as peer supporters from the ranks of the homeless, especially those for whom writing has been a challenge in the past, this can be a daunting task. Record-keeping taps immediately into fears about one's adequacy about being able to do the job, as reading and language skills come under scrutiny, especially if training and supervision have been light to nonexistent. Fortunately, present-day software can relieve some of the burden of grammatical and spelling errors, and typing hides poor writing skills. However, these advances are often not sufficient to overcome the fear of writing.

Some tips for record-keeping will be of help in providing structure. Three fundamental rules follow:

1. Separate fact from personal opinion, putting the facts first and leaving opinion, if stated at all, in a separate section.
2. Put information into logical, time-ordered facts. Short specific sentences suffice to convey the information that covers the *when* (day/time), *where* (the location of the interaction or service or incident), *what it was* (the issue or event), *what happened* (specific action), and *who* (was involved). Note that none of the above information includes the worker's observations or impressions. That belongs in a separate section, followed by *follow-up—next steps* (by who and when).
3. Clearly indicate the source of information—directly from clients, from a third party, or from other written material.

If the case notes or records state the facts, reported and observed, without personal commentary by the worker, a clear and focused report will be the result. While this may sound simple, most of us often intertwine fact and opinion; keeping these two apart will require a bit of practice. Some people are also accustomed to weaving related material into the account of an event in a way that shifts the logical and time sequence of what is being reported. As challenging as it may be, it is important, within mainstream service provision, to report information in a sequential manner as it is invaluable in situations where the record may be requested for legal action (criminal, child welfare, litigation, etc.).

Record-keeping also involves the ethical principle of nonmaleficence—do no harm. Potential harm in records stems from documenting information that you have acquired by hearsay, that is attributed to sources you cannot verify, or that is the opinion of yourself or another person, regardless of the authority or credentials that person may hold. Many examples come from the mental health and addictions fields, where labeling can be stigmatizing. Early in treatment a person may be given a preliminary diagnosis or a diagnostic impression. Unfortunately, when the label is transferred into the record as the diagnosis, a person may be labeled and thus stigmatized. When this diagnosis is an error the legacy may have long-lasting harmful effects. Such examples abound in the field of psychiatry where labels of schizophrenia and personality disorders, especially that of borderline personality disorder, are used when not accurately determined by a qualified professional. The result, in this instance, is that a person comes to be regarded as someone who is not amenable to treatment. When child welfare is involved, the consequences for parent and child may be irreparable if the parent is judged unfit for the responsibility of parenting.

The unintentional use of power can also occur in the handling of client records. Even if people have a right to see their records, clients who are homeless rarely make this request of an agency providing service as they are often fearful that any upset of the established order or questioning of authority may result in recriminations (denial of service, protracted waiting for services, being labeled as a troublemaker). They may not completely understand what is written, especially if there are literacy or English language problems. These situations can easily become coercive as service providers try to push realistic concerns aside for lack of time or fear of problems.

The provision of any help to others is always accompanied by ethical issues. These may be centered around decisions that workers and supervisors need to make or around the daily interactions that take place in the context of delivering services. They may involve using principles such as nonmaleficence (do no harm) or utilitarianism (the greatest good for the greatest number), or they may be concerned with issues of confidentiality, client empowerment, and the use of coercion in obtaining client cooperation. They may involve behaviors such as exploitation of clients, or written acts such as careless and inaccurate report writing. Whatever the situation, it is incumbent on the worker to be vigilant about the numerous ways in which ethical challenges present themselves. In the final section on exercises we have presented a number of examples to further your thinking on complex issues.

CODE OF ETHICS FOR FRONTLINE WORKERS

The following list presents a code of ethics for frontline workers. It borrows heavily from professional bodies such as social work, nursing, and psychology but recognizes and provides details on some of the specific ways workers can deal with ethical issues that arise in this field of work.

1. Respect the dignity and worth of all people.
   a. In all forms of communication, use language that is respectful of people.
   b. Avoid all derogatory comments, including jokes, sarcasm, or double meanings that are based on racial, ethnic, and cultural backgrounds; sex or gender preference; physical or mental disabilities; or other differences. Avoid any type of verbal harassment.
   c. Avoid activities that are disrespectful of others.
2. Have the highest regard for confidentiality.
   a. Treat all information and all interactions with the strictest of confidence.
   b. Share client names and identities only with client permission.
   c. Share client information only with those who have a need to know.
   d. Have discussions with and about clients only in private places.
   e. Keep written information in a secure place, not accessible to other clients or to the public, at all times.
   f. Inform clients about their rights to confidentiality when they first agree to participate in a service plan.
   g. Obtain written consents before releasing any information.
3. Recognize that the helping relationship is inherently an uneven one.
   a. Minimize all actions that emphasize this imbalance.
   b. Do not dictate days and times of meetings unless mandated by a legal authority to do so. Clients should determine where and when they will meet with or engage with a worker.

4. Respect cultural diversity.
   a. Workers should be trained in the recognition and respect for the values, attitudes, and expectations of different cultures and special interest groups.
   b. Be sure your helping expectations always consider the cultural context of the client.
   c. Respect the clients' cultural diversity in planning and intervention preferences: the customs, beliefs, rituals, and ceremonies that are fundamental to different groups of persons.
5. Respect the right to self-determination.
   a. Respect the right of individuals and families to make decisions about their own welfare and life circumstances.
   b. Do not use your status or power to directly or subtly coerce clients. This includes the ability to give or withhold services or other benefits that the client needs for successful independent living.
   c. Do not use guilt or other ways of influencing client behavior.
6. Respect the helping relationship.
   a. Accept that clients determine the extent to which they will accept interventions.
   b. Distinguish between helping and social relationships, and do not engage in social relationships or contact with clients.
   c. Do not seek any personal services or benefits from those who are clients. This includes providing employment that is below the acceptable wage for the specified activity.
7. Practice competence.
   a. Seek to obtain the knowledge and skills necessary for respectful practice.
   b. Seek regular opportunities to improve and expand your knowledge and experience through training and mentoring.
   c. Accept supervision of practice as an important aspect of responsible work.
   d. Be aware of your skills and their limitations. Do not provide services or practice interventions that you are not trained to perform.

      e. Maintain complete and accurate records of worker and client activities; this is a primary responsibility. Records should be factual and avoid negative value statements.
   8. Understand the implications of working in a helping organization.
      a. Understand the mission and aims of the organization in which you work.
      b. Respect and value collegial relationships.
      c. Do not exploit or use for personal gain any relationships with coworkers.
      d. Look for and advocate for ways that the organization can improve its work with clients.

EXERCISES

Case Examples

1. Marnie is a woman, age thirty-two, with two children, ages three and seven, who moved into a domestic violence shelter three weeks ago to escape from an abusive relationship with her common-law partner of eight years. She denies any history of alcohol abuse but admits to regular marijuana use, usually during the day, but never on the shelter premises. The children are in her care when she is using. They do not appear distressed or neglected.

   Do you report Marnie to child welfare authorities for child endangerment? Would you report a woman of Marnie's description who lives in her own home to child welfare? What would your response be if Marnie had a prescription for medical use of marijuana?

2. An older woman who has no family and who has some health issues but insists that she can function independently is adamant that she move from her shelter for the elderly into her own independent apartment. She cites the *housing first* philosophy as her right. The shelter staff are divided. As her continuing-care worker you would be responsible for monitoring her status and need for further care. It will be more difficult to get her placed into a retirement residence if she is living in her own apartment. What would you do? What would be in the client's best interest?

3. A program that helps victims of domestic violence has been forced to find a new office and program location. It has succeeded beyond its wildest dreams. The new location is central, in an office building, close to transportation and other services, and in a business neighborhood that caters to a large variety of people. Moreover, it is affordable and is in move-in condition, thus sparing the organization remodeling costs that it can ill afford. The only problem is that the landlord does not want program staff and participants using the main entrance, which is in an interior lobby, but instead wants them to use an outside doorway as the main program entrance. The landlord states that his position is nonnegotiable.

   What is the ethical issue? Is it a legal issue? What are the implications of resolution of this for each outcome?

4. Frank, a young man of about twenty-six, was referred by the local homeless shelter for men where he has been living for the past three months to a job skills training program for warehouse personnel. He has gradually struck up a good rapport with you, his primary counselor. He has confided that he has had several psychiatric hospitalizations for confused thinking and depression. Over the past few days he has become more silent and preoccupied. Today he arrived looking distressed and was speaking in a rambling way. Upon speaking with him you find out that he is very depressed, possibly thinking of suicide. He agrees to let you call the emergency mental health team who will come out to do an assessment.

   Do you tell the mental health team about Frank's past psychiatric history? What is the reason for your decision?

5. You are a contract supervisor in a small agency that provides substance-abuse programs. One program serves seniors. The program head recently went on a crash diet and has lost a sizable amount of weight in a few months. You learn that she is abusing alcohol every evening and is also deliberately starving herself to reduce her weight. Clients are concerned that she has a terminal illness and is not disclosing this. During supervision she has told you that she suffers from PTSD as a result of several traumatic experiences. She is depressed but continues to come to work daily. You advise her to take time off and she refuses. Her agency management supervisor will not deal with the problem.

What can you do? What may be the consequences? Ethically, what are the issues?

6. A local drop-in program that helps those with mental health and dual disorders is financed through health-care dollars on a per person basis. A recently enacted rule by the funder states that the person rate will be paid only for identified services users. This means that from now on people coming into the facility will be required to sign in with their health-card number (or Medicaid or Medicare card/number). Some people who have been attending regularly are reluctant to reveal their number and their use of medical services, claiming that this is confidential.

   What are the issues? What ethical principles are involved? How do you deal with the problem?

7. Tom is a young man, age twenty-two, who recently left home and came looking for work in an area booming with oil company projects. He didn't realize that the cost of hotels and food was as high as the local wages, and found himself with no money for a motel within three days of arriving. He went to seek help at a local drop-in program and was greeted by a young shelter worker whose winning smile had more nuances of a social welcome than he felt comfortable with. However, he had nowhere else to go and thus had to deal with the touch of her hands on his arms as she commiserated with him, her doe-like eyes, and her subtle glances.

   Is this provocative behavior unethical? How would you respond if you were her coworker?

8. A homeless American Indian/First Nations man, age thirty-eight, with a previous history of alcohol abuse and depression, has diabetes and is experiencing kidney failure. He is in recovery from his substance use, has a girlfriend, and is making many efforts at self-improvement. He will need a kidney transplant within the next two years if he is to live. Should he be placed on the transplant waiting list? Would there be a different decision if he has a history of a psychosis?

9. Max is a single senior who has been homeless since his landlord sold the SRO house where he was living three years ago. Fiercely independent, he has refused housing in a supportive living arrangement and continues to sleep at a local shelter. Occasionally he volunteers for an organization he has been involved with for the past

decade. On volunteer nights the shelter staff allow for his late return and keep his assigned bed for him. The rules that are relaxed for him provide some degree of individualism and autonomy and help Max keep his self-respect.

What do you do if a new supervisor decides to enforce strict rules about bed assignments and late entries into the shelter?

10. You work for an agency that provides street-level intervention for high-risk youths. Some of the youths are housed in your agency's emergency shelter. There have been a number of job changes in your agency and staff have had to adjust to new supervisors and new enforcement of agency rules. This has created stress for all staff. One of the staff you work with is especially anxious and jumpy. You learn that he has just broken up with his girlfriend whom he lived with. His mother, who lives alone in another city eight hundred miles away, has been diagnosed with breast cancer. He has started drinking excessively and is also smoking marijuana daily. He needs to work because he has no savings and has no earned sick leave from the job.

What do you do? What would you do if you were the supervisor? What would you do if you were the director of the agency? What ethical principles are involved in this situation?

11. A middle-aged professional woman who is in charge of a child-care program falls down a set of stairs, hits her head hard several times, and suffers an obvious broken nose. She refuses to have staff call an ambulance and insists on driving herself to the hospital. She is dressed casually because of the nature of her job. At the emergency room she registers and is asked to sit and wait. She notices people gradually moving away from her seat until she is all by herself. She looks disheveled, has blood on her face, and appears groggy from the fall. She is not seen until all others in the room have been attended to. She is eventually diagnosed with a broken nose, lacerations, and a severe concussion. Is this a situation of stigmatization? Is this an ethical problem?

12. Suzette, age about thirteen, is one of the street kids that regularly shows up at the only youth drop-in program in town, which you run. She lives at home—but barely, as she is on poor terms with her mother and stepfather. She has recently become sexually active and

has access to the condoms that are left out for the kids to use—no questions asked. She has asked for help in getting birth control pills. One issue, besides her age, is that her family belongs to an evangelical religious group and does not believe in any kind of birth control. What do you do? Would the issues be different if her parents were not devoutly religious with strong beliefs about sexual taboos?

The following are some additional exercises:

1. Illicit drug use is a reality of street life. Should workers adopt a harm reduction approach or demand total abstinence in order to receive help? What help would you withhold from someone who refuses to stop using? Respond in a class debate or reflective writing.
2. In *Ragged Company* Richard Wagamese (2008) presents a number of ethical dilemmas that the main characters face. They range from boundary recognition to harm reduction approaches. Can you identify at least five such instances?
3. Create a toolbox of forms and information that will guide your work. Include a copy of the "Essential Steps for Ethical Problem Solving: A Frontline Worker's Tool Box" that was presented in this chapter.

JOURNALING

1. Identify an ethical conflict at work in your agency. What issues are involved? How much is the argument clouded by moral judgments?
2. Identify a potential ethical conflict with a client. What issues are involved? How much is the argument clouded by moral judgments?

CHAPTER 12

Legal Issues in the Homeless Sector

KEY ISSUES	Victimization of the homeless
	Overview of the kinds of legal situations homeless persons encounter
	Legal processes in the event of criminal charge
	Accessing legal aid
	Boundaries with clients and avoiding legal pitfalls
	The child welfare systems
	Youth Justice Acts
	Legal guidelines related to mental health, addictions, and medical treatment
	Confidentiality and consent to treatment
	Legal implications for documentation and report writing
	Skills to write effective case notes, assessments, and discharge summaries

OVERVIEW

Being homeless inevitably means running into legal problems. They may have started before a person became homeless, such as with financial problems, landlord-tenant disputes, child welfare involvement, or criminal activity such as drug dealing and thievery. Once homeless, there are numerous additional legal problems that can surface. We know that homeless persons are frequently the target for arrest and harassment by police for vagrancy, loitering, and other normal behaviors for a person who has nowhere to go (Bellot, Raffestin, Royer, & Noël, 2005). Loss of ID and the process of trying to get social assistance can result in difficulties dealing with the legal system. In many encounters, homeless people may be the victims of crimes committed by others, and in other instances they may be the offender. Some encounters with the justice system occur more frequently because a person is homeless, such as when a person is charged with vagrancy or public intoxication because there was no place to go and "sleep it off," or because this was a way to provide safe shelter to an incapacitated person in extremely cold weather. Others, such as panhandling and squeegeeing, which are illegal in some jurisdictions, are ways to survive. As we look more closely it will become clear that there are numerous ways in which homeless persons become victims in legal struggles, and note that the violations of their civil rights are often flagrant. Beyond encounters with the law, issues that come up include violations of the rights to privacy and confidentiality that are often compromised in legal proceedings involving homeless people, especially those with a mental illness. Homeless people generally can't afford to hire a lawyer to defend their rights and are often unable to protect their civil rights. On a final note, we look at the worker context and examine the legal importance of documentation that protects both worker and client.

RIGHTS OF THE HOMELESS

Homelessness violates fundamental rights and freedoms accorded to the rest of society. The right to housing is embodied in both the United Nations Universal Declaration of Human Rights (United Nations, 1948) and the International Covenant on Economic, Social and Cultural Rights (United Nations, 1966).

> The right to adequate housing finds legal substance within more than a dozen international human-rights texts and has been re-affirmed in numerous international declarations, resolutions and policy-oriented instruments. More than fifty national Constitutions enshrine various formulations of housing rights and other housing-related state responsibilities, and a plethora of domestic laws in nearly all countries have a bearing upon one or more of the core elements of housing rights. Without exception, every government has explicitly recognized that adequate housing is a fundamental human right under international law. (United Nations Human Settlements Programme [UN-HABITAT], 2005, p. 79)

The United Nations (UN) statements on housing underscore the fact that lack of housing is a deprivation of individual rights. Violating a basic right to housing is just the tip of the iceberg of civil rights, entitlements, and encounters with the justice system for those who are homeless. Most people on Main Street believe that those who lack housing are inherently breaking the law, or have committed illegal acts that result in homelessness or that keep them homeless. In reality, although homeless people may commit minor infractions and break local bylaws, most are victims and not perpetrators of crime. Homeless advocates attest to the many times when those jumping the turnstiles to get a free ride on public transit and are convicted were sent to jail for their inability to pay the fine (Douglas, 2011). One fifty-year-old homeless man received 216 tickets in two years, 136 of them for being found asleep on a city transit bench. He owed the city $43,915 in fines and late fees. Yes, there is a group of individuals who commit serious offenses such as robbery, drug trafficking, and involvement in the sex trade, but these are not the majority of those who are homeless. In both Canada and the United States, most are victims more often than perpetrators (Fitzpatrick & Myrstol, 2011; Novac, Hermer, Paradis, & Kellen, 2006). Some of the ways that they are victims include illegalities such as questionable foreclosure of property, evictions, and quasi-questionable practices such as failure on the part of landlords and utility companies to work toward solutions to financial crises, and the failure of child welfare authorities to help homeless teens under eighteen because they are "too old" for their system of care. People are often fired from jobs without due notice, refused termination pay, or prevented from getting unemployment benefits because employers fail to truthfully report the reasons for termination. Other people fall victim to unscrupulous loan sharks who charge unlawfully high interest on short-term loans. Single parents, especially women with young children, do not receive their court-awarded child custody payments but can't afford a lawyer to take the non-paying husband to court. Other violations include those of human rights and civil liberties such as the right to vote and to receive government entitlements (Garland, Richards, & Cooney, 2010). These dilemmas are worsened by the inability of most poor persons to afford legal help to fight for their rights when they are in trouble: free legal help is generally only available to those charged with major criminal offenses.

VICTIMIZATION OF THE HOMELESS

The myriad problems stemming from the victimization of those who are homeless complicate the legal issues confronting social services providers

> **Textbox 12.1. Antidiscrimination**
>
> Both Canada and the United States have federal legislation that protects against discrimination, provides accessibility to housing rental and ownership, and acknowledges (some) government responsibility for social housing. In the United States these rights are embedded in the Civil Rights Code. In Canada some maintain that they implicitly belong in the Charter of Rights and Freedoms. However, the observance of these statutes is variable and has resulted in unequal distribution of resources, with some persons with disabilities, women, and children most likely to be beneficiaries of government programs and funding.

and their clients. People are evicted for failure to pay utilities and rent. They are then denied housing because of past debts. This is another form of victimization. Lack of stable housing leaves people vulnerable, without physical, emotional, and financial resources to fight for personal rights and civil liberties. Frequently the result is that homeless people become targets of criminal behavior and harsh police enforcement from local laws of conduct, and become victims of crimes of violence such as physical and sexual assaults. Homeless persons are less likely to be charged with violent offenses and more likely to be charged with property-related offenses, such as those they commit to meet their survival needs (Novac, Hermer, Paradis, & Kellen, 2009). They are frequently charged with violations of municipal bylaws, such as loitering, noise, and panhandling (Bellot et al., 2005). There are numerous examples of these situations, such as the targeting of homeless youths by transit police (Douglas, 2011) and police crackdowns of loitering- and vagrancy-related behaviors in high-profile urban areas such as downtown Los Angeles, New York, Ottawa, and Vancouver during high-profile public events such as the Olympics (Lenskyj, 2010).

Back-ending of charges is common (Eberle, Kraus, Serge, & Hulchanski, 2001). This occurs when youths, who may be defiant with police, are charged with obstruction of justice in addition to the original offense. It is also common for intoxicated offenders who become aggressive to be charged with resisting arrest or attempted assault on a police officer (Douglas, 2011). Finally, those with disabilities such as a mental disorder are more likely to be a target of crimes of opportunity than those without a mental disorder disability (Lenskyj, 2010). The mentally ill are often arrested not for posing a danger, but for violations of social norms such as jaywalking or for bizarre behavior (Novac et al., 2006). The common perception is that the mentally ill are at a greater risk of being arrested for minor infractions, and that police often have the misbelief that incarceration will provide access to medical and psychiatric services.

We are often reminded by advocates of rights for the homeless that current laws are not far removed from English Poor Laws of the sixteenth century that banned vagrancy and placed the poor, aged, and disabled in workhouses, and the laws of colonial America against vagrancy, loitering, and public intoxication (Stoner, 1995; Teplin, McClelland, Abram, & Weiner, 2005). In both those instances, poverty and the need for public assistance was seen as a moral failing and those requiring help should be given no more than what the lowest-paid worker in society could afford. Despite public efforts, these negative attitudes are continued in the ways in which police authorities target the public behavior of homeless persons. Panhandling, sleeping in automobiles, handing out free food, and establishing soup kitchens are banned in certain areas. Sometimes homeless persons deliberately break the law and are arrested in order to have a safe and warm place to sleep during cold weather. More often, police action is not intended to provide food and shelter, but to harass and target those with an undesirable appearance or behavior. Those who appear to be dishevelled are more likely to be targeted than those who are neatly dressed.

One of the troublesome problems for workers and clients is the criminalization of the victim: the treatment of those without a place to live as if they have in some way already broken the law. Those without a permanent place to stay often try to find alternatives that provide a bit of privacy and independence. Although sleeping rough in parks, beside railways, in tunnels, and under bridges is common for some of the homeless, abandoned buildings, nooks in alleyways not visible from the street, bushes, and wooded areas of suburban parks are also places where they search for a bit of privacy and shelter from public view. In most urban localities, illegal uses of public space can result in criminal charges; abandoned buildings are private property, and sleeping in them is trespassing. For those who have no means to pay fines and no eligibility for legal assistance, the result is a criminal record. A history of incarceration is higher among rough sleepers who sleep in places considered unfit for habitation. The reason for this higher rate is not clear in the research literature, however the reports are consistent (Belcher, 1988) and are supported by studies in Australia, Norway, and the United Kingdom (Bard, 2005). These studies indicate that rough sleepers are more likely than shelter users to have been arrested, held overnight, convicted, and to have served prison sentences.

Frequently, sleeping in one's own car, especially during the evening and nighttime hours, is also against the law. Ironically, this is not an issue for those who own a camping vehicle and who are allowed by property owners to (legally) park in parking lots of the local Walmart. Along with the restrictions on sleeping in personal vehicles are, for those without even that private space, the illegalities of loitering, being a public nuisance, public urination, and other behaviors of those who have no designated place to rest during the day and take care of bodily functions and hygiene. Public washrooms are scarce and those available are most often in stores that allow use by customers only. In other words, the lack of public toilets and washrooms in many cities and towns leaves the homeless with few choices. Jumping turnstiles or failing to pay bus fare adds to the list of infractions for those who are a distance from medical and social services help and have no means of transportation and no money to pay the fare. Law enforcement officials often harshly apply public nuisance and municipal infractions laws rather than looking for other solutions that do not place the burden of fines and jail time on already disadvantaged people. The mentally ill are most often targets of this police action (Bard, 2005).The additional stigma of a police record creates further obstacles to employment and makes rehousing increasingly difficult (Novac et al., 2006; Stoner, 1995). Novac also acknowledges the reciprocal risk factors of homelessness and incarceration: "Being homeless increases the odds of being jailed and being jailed increases the odds of being homeless" (Novac et al., 2006, p. 10). Many homeless persons are trapped in a revolving door between incarceration and the streets.

Certain subgroups are disproportionately vulnerable to postincarceration homelessness, including Aboriginal people in Canada and black males in the United States; people with a diagnosis of FASD; those with poor literacy skills, severe mental illness, TBI, or low intelligence; and those with prior criminal record, addictions, or heavy drug use. In Canada additional groups are racialized refugees (visible minorities), women (particularly those involved in the sex trade), youths who have been in foster care, and transgender persons whose gender issues are often misunderstood or ignored (Novac et al., 2006). In the United States these groups include Mexican Americans, and others of Spanish and Latino heritage.

Personal Identification (ID)

Lack of ID heads the list of legal difficulties that a homeless person faces. Without ID an individual is unable to access many resources for which he may be eligible. Included in ID are those listed in table 12.1.

Not all forms of ID are equal and some are necessary to get another. For example, a birth certificate is necessary for a passport and marriage license, in most jurisdictions. A social insurance (or social security) number and card are required for employment, as is proof of legal residency (that is, an immigrant or alien registration card or birth certificate). Some forms of ID are supplementary to primary ID, such as voter's cards and baptismal certificates, in some limited jurisdictions. One common denominator to all forms of ID is that they are essential to establish proof of who someone is, and of that person's eligibility to receive any form of public (government) entitlements and assistance.

How are ID loss and homelessness related, and what are the consequences of not being able to provide ID? Without a home one loses a secure place to keep valuables. As a result of a wandering, unstable life on the streets, with no place to keep valuable papers, the result is often loss of personal possessions, ID among them. A woman fleeing domestic violence may not realize the importance of taking these valuable documents with her,

Table 12.1. Forms of Personal ID

Primary Forms of ID	Supplementary Forms: Either Necessary or Secondary ID in Some Instances
Birth certificate	Utility bills
Alien registration card (or immigration certificate in Canada)	Baptismal certificate
	Certificate of citizenship
Social security or social insurance card	Voter's card (US)
Driver's license	Medicaid or Medicare (US) or health insurance card (Canada)
American Indian/Aboriginal Canadian status card	
Marriage license (certificate)	
Military discharge papers	
Passport	

and a youth leaving an abusive home may not even have access to a birth certificate. Anyone who has been the victim of a robbery where a wallet with their ID was stolen has a story to tell about the difficulties involved with replacing these items, not the least of which is proving one's right to these documents, and having the financial means to pay the replacement costs. For a homeless person, the lack of a mailing address is often an additional obstacle as most forms of ID will not be delivered to a post office box. Lack of a bank account means extra demands to use other forms to pay for replacement ID. Money orders and the like all come with additional costs. Without ID a person can't open a bank account, provide a credit check, obtain a credit card, get a driver's license, or enroll children in school. Getting health insurance (in Canada) requires proof of residency and legal status, and in the United States an application for Medicaid/Medicare requires a legal address. Speaking English (or French in Quebec) is not a requirement to establish legal residency in either country. Documentation of one's legal status as citizen or immigrant is essential in both countries in order to be employed and acquire other civil rights, privileges, and entitlements.

Debt

Financial difficulties, debt, and legal involvement are intertwined in complex and intractable ways. The inability to pay the rent is often the first, but rarely the last, foray into financial and legal difficulties for many people. Failure to pay utilities is often an additional stress. The legacy of nonpayment follows people into homelessness as the resulting debt, especially to utility companies and to the landlord if it is a government body such as municipal housing, is generally viewed as a debt to be repaid before subsidized housing is again provided. If there are irregularities in the process of accruing debt, such as the continual adding of interest and service charges to an unpaid balance, the victim has little recourse. There is double jeopardy for the persons involved; housing legalities are usually not handled by legal aid services, and fear of authority keeps many people from asserting their rights. In addition, many people who live on the margins lack the educational skills, abilities to advocate for self, and other abilities that would permit them to address irregularities and flagrant violations of rights. Many homeless persons rely on cell phones to provide vital connections with relatives and friends. However, failure to pay this bill may result in additional penalties for late payment.

These added penalties may go on indefinitely. Another inadvertent accumulation of debt occurs when there are insufficient funds to cover an automatic withdrawal from the bank at an ATM, and the added overdraft charges include interest that continues to increase the total owed as long as the debt is not paid. All of these possibilities result in increased difficulty in establishing solvency and paying for housing. The unpayable debt that accrues may lead to bankruptcy, but often even this recourse is not viable because the legal complexities of this course of action may be beyond the functional and financial capabilities of the affected persons. Finally, all of these events negatively impact a person's credit rating, which then makes it even more difficult for that person to acquire housing. Even when housing may become a possibility, many rental property owners and managers are now asking for references and credit checks. For many, it is an endless circle.

The Drug and Sex Trades

Most reports on criminal activity among homeless people focus on the public nuisance and social control factors of where they sleep, how they conduct their daily lives, and how they try to earn some spending money by activities such as squeegeeing and panhandling. However, the use of street drugs creates a more dangerous environment. While substance abuse is prevalent among homeless individuals, for many this abuse consists of alcohol abuse and is more often a result of homelessness than a cause (Dyb, 2009). Nonetheless, there is a cohort of drug abusers who lose housing because of their addictions and the lifestyle that this includes. While users are more likely to become homeless, the major dealers are rarely without housing. Usually it is the small local operators working at street level who are involved in both trafficking and housing loss, and it is these frontline dealers and users who are most often arrested, charged, and incarcerated. For adults this local dealing often supplies the resources for an addict to get the next fix.

For youths drug involvement may be among the survival tactics used to deal with homelessness. It provides communality with peers and a buffer against the alienation and depression that haunts many homeless youths. It also provides some anxiety relief and mind numbing for those who are self-medicating for untreated mental illnesses. Because youths are often victims of trauma and abuse before becoming homeless, and are also highly likely to be victims of trauma after hitting the streets, dealing with the effects of trauma is a major issue (Fitzpatrick & Myrstol, 2011). Their subsequent drug use, which is inordinately high in victims of trauma, is understandable. The most troubling concern is that the criminal activities involved in procuring and dealing in drugs also become the gateway to more serious offenses. Drug dealing is associated with additional crimes to get money to pay for drugs, as well as with violence, both on the part of users and on the part of dealers who are prone to use weapons to assert territorial control.

Involvement in the sex trade is the unfortunate result of those who seek shelter and/or drugs in exchange for a place to stay (Kushel, Hahn, Evans, Bangsberg, & Moss, 2005). Young women fleeing sexual abuse at home often find themselves abused and coerced into sex trade activities on the street (Didenko & Pankratz, 2007). Males, especially those who are gay, report similar coercive behavior. The net result is that those who are victimized before becoming homeless are again victimized while homeless, and seriously risk the possibility of being arrested for prostitution. The concern with the survival of young people is that trading sex for drugs and shelter can quickly lead to long-term abuse and other crimes (Coates & McKenzie-Mohr, 2010).

Prostitution in North America is most often the crime for which those seeking sexual services are ignored and those offering services are vigorously prosecuted, despite the fact that the sex trade worker is frequently a victim who has been forced into this lifestyle. Sex trade workers are also victims of their pimps who procure services for their women and who demand to be taken care of. While the women on the streets are pursued by police, the pimps are infrequently apprehended, despite their additional violence toward their women and their substance-abusing behavior. The serious problems this poses are especially poignant for victims who are homeless adolescents who are seduced or forced into prostitution and illegal aliens who have no legal supports to turn to.

INCARCERATION AND HOMELESSNESS

There is no evidence that homeless persons commit serious offenses such as murder, armed robbery, and other violent crimes more frequently than those who are housed. Indeed, the evidence points to the reverse: they are less likely to do so. However, drug-related offenses are prevalent, as are those related to the sex trade. Those who are homeless and/or have a mental disorder and/or substance abuse problems are much more likely to be jailed than sent for treatment (Weiser et al., 2006). Domestic violence and related offenses are also prevalent and often result in jail time for the perpetrator, as raising bail may be impossible. The same applies to less-serious offenses such as vagrancy, loitering, and other offenses targeted at the homeless for which one may spend time in jail awaiting disposition. Incarceration also raises the risk of becoming homeless for vulnerable people. Prior to a court hearing, an accused person may be held without bail on remand. In this case it is not possible to continue working, and it may be difficult to maintain the required income to make rent or mortgage payments on existing accommodations. An accused may be held for an undetermined length of time without knowledge of when he will be released, and usually lacks the resources to raise bail. In some cases they do not care about long-term consequences as their immediate human needs for shelter and food are paramount. The consequences of being homeless are that there is a much higher probability that one will also subsequently acquire a criminal record.

Lack of a place to stay is also a major concern for those who have been in jail or prison and have no place to live upon discharge. The prospect of going from a jail cell to a shelter bed is grim. Most shelters are near areas of increased crime and drug trafficking, which exposes newly released persons to the problems that often led to arrest. Lack of a secure place to go on discharge means that they now have an eleven-fold increase in the probability of being homeless and are identified as one group at serious risk of homelessness (Tyler, Gervais, & Davidson, 2013). An extensive report for the Urban Institute details the myriad difficulties and challenges facing those paroled from prisons and jails (Ferguson, Bender, Thompson, Xie, & Pollio, 2012).

The difficulties of release from prison or jail start with the reality that there is a lack of acceptable housing and appropriate reentry programs for former prisoners. For many there are no halfway houses available to help with reintegration, and employment supports may be ineffective in a depressed economy. For various reasons, many do not have a home or a job to go to when released. They may be alienated from family or relatives, or it may be that those who would take them in are living in housing that restricts the number of occupants or does not allow occupancy to those with a criminal record. Employers are reluctant to hire someone with a criminal record even when the offense has no bearing on a person's type of employment position. A driver's license may have expired and there may not be an easy way to have it restored, limiting where and how a person can find work. The result is that only too often those who are released have no option but to sleep in a public shelter. This unfortunately also paves the way for a rapid return to life on the streets. Statistics show that over half of those released are back in jail within three years, with most returning in less than a year. Lack of housing and supports have been shown to be chief contributors. Despite this grim picture, there are a number of cities that have introduced successful reentry programs (Roman, McBride, & Osborne, 2005; Sermons & Witte, 2011) that use employment strategies and supportive case management as fundamental aspects of success.

Diversion programs are another way in which the justice system has addressed the problems of incarceration of those with a history of mental health and/or substance-abuse problems. Several configurations of diversion exist, with some organized to provide intensive case management supports along with shelter in exchange for an agreement to remain in contact with support workers and clinical treatment providers. Another version of this approach offers a mandatory two-year drug treatment program along with a guilty plea to a felony charge in lieu of time in prison (Roman & Travis, 2004). Some question if this approach has placed the role of jailer in the hands of treatment personnel. Others criticize an approach that does nothing to avoid a criminal record. Diversion programs for women with dependents that mandate treatment have participants reporting on the stress of trying to meet treatment goals while dealing with caregiver responsibilities, lack of transportation, and child care (Roman et al., 2005; Solomon, 2006). A wider study of these diversion and reentry programs for persons with a mental illness concluded that they have mixed results and that the evaluation of their effectiveness has not been adequately studied (DeMatteo, LaDuke, Locklair, & Heilbrun, 2013; Sung, 2011). Thus workers need to use caution in advocating for diversion as the attendant consequences of diversion usually are not well understood.

CIVIL LAW AND CIVIL RIGHTS

Civil law refers to those matters involving relationships between people that do not concern criminal activity. Criminal law applies to those situations where there is a legal statute that has been violated (such as robbery, assault, homicide). The issues dealt with by civil law involve separation and divorce, child custody, property ownership, contracts, landlord and tenant disputes (e.g., eviction), bankruptcy, and damages to person and property such as in automobile accidents. In some instances there may be both criminal and civil law components to a situation, such as an accident that involves drinking and driving along with personal and property damage. While civil law intends to protect individual rights, homeless people often lack the emotional and experiential resources to deal with legal issues involving lawyers and courtroom proceedings. They may have no experience with the legal system, or they may have had negative encounters. The formalities of court may be intimidating, especially for women who have been oppressed. Legal documents may be written in ways that are incomprehensible to a layperson and that appear foreign to someone with limited education.

While legal assistance is available for those who commit a serious crime, lack of resources means that most people are not represented for minor offenses, and not at all for civil matters. This is a frequent problem for poor people whose rights may have been violated through unlawful eviction or firing from employment but who lack the money to obtain legal counsel and to pay for the court fees. They may be unaware of recourse through small claims court, not have the emotional willingness or ability to pursue legal violations through a court process, or be unwilling to confront their abuser. All of these factors continue experiences of disenfranchisement and oppression that poor people encounter.

The civil rights of homeless people have been widely debated in the United States and to some lesser extent in Australia, Canada, and the United Kingdom. In most instances a primary concern has been the denial of the rights of citizens such as voting, access to public entitlements, free education for children, family preservation, free access to public spaces, and the right to seek income through activities such as panhandling (Roman et al., 2005) in city areas where homeless persons are living. Many of these local ordinances are viewed as selectively targeting homeless persons, as they are the ones most likely to be sleeping in public or wandering in areas where food, shelter, and other amenities are available. Most common ordinances (local legislation in cities and towns) target behaviors of sleeping, camping, loitering, panhandling, peddling, and public bathing and toileting. Selective enforcement in areas known to have concentrations of homeless persons, often called "sweeps," result in the destruction of personal property, including important documents; personal property is thrown away and encampments are destroyed. Attempts by human rights groups such as the National Law Center on Homelessness and Poverty, the American Civil Liberties Union, and the Wellesley Institute in Toronto to seek policy and legal changes in the judicial system have met with some, but limited, success.

We encourage you to explore what efforts advocates have made, and what frontline workers can do, to deal with these inequalities.

> **Textbox 12.2. Mortgage Default**
>
> Assistance for those who are in danger of default on their mortgages is available through federal legislation in the United States through HUD (see http://portal.hud.gov/hudportal/HUD?src=/topics/avoiding_foreclosure).
> In Canada, because of more-stringent lending regulations, default on mortgages has not been a significant economic issue to date and thus there has not been government assistance for those facing foreclosure.

For many homeless persons, an encounter with civil law focuses on financial problems that lead to eviction and bankruptcy; domestic problems that lead to separation, divorce, and child custody; and involvement with child welfare in instances where the safety and protection of children is of concern. Since child welfare is in the realm of criminal law we will look at this separately. The major struggles encountered by those who face loss of housing due to eviction and bankruptcy include many persons living in poverty who generally do not have the resources (financial and other) to deal with the legal complexities involved. Even when there are assistance programs available to help avert housing loss due to mortgage default and failure to pay taxes, such as the HEARTH legislation (HUD, 2012), many people do not know the most expeditious ways to access these programs. Extensive use of these programs has depleted most of the allocated funding so that many homeowners are faced with current lack of availability of many aspects of the HUD programs intended to keep people housed. Those rendered homeless under these conditions fit a different profile as they are generally wage earners with a reasonable income who found themselves overcommitted by housing and personal debt. Their need for rehousing is high as many studies show that rapid rehousing will prevent a longer period of homelessness with its attendant social and legal problems.

Forced evictions have faced many persons recently rendered homeless. While legal protection is found under state and provincial landlord-tenant acts, many favor the landlord in rights of possession. Those that favor tenants usually have stipulations in lease and monthly tenancy agreements that spell out a detailed course of action for eviction that may take several months to execute. In these cases a rental tribunal may be available to deal with appeals and act as a mediator in landlord-tenant disputes. The role of the frontline worker can be invaluable in identifying this course of action and helping someone in danger of eviction to appeal for remediation. These actions can also buy time to find alternatives in case the appeal fails. However, in those legal jurisdictions where the tenancy acts favor the rights of landlords (as property owners with a right to protect their possessions), evictions may occur quickly and without much recourse to any appeal. Loss of housing can happen in as little as two weeks and those evicted usually do not have the financial means to challenge eviction in court.

The rights of low-income persons are often violated by unscrupulous landlords who take advantage of the reduced circumstances and helplessness of their tenants to ignore requests for repairs and cleaning in situations that violate health and safety codes. These opportunists will seek every means available to avoid repairs to heating and air conditioning equipment, plumbing, and safety of the building, thereby placing tenants at further health risk. Those who are living in these marginal circumstances usually do not have the money for a deposit on another rental and may find their current deposit withheld. Beyond rental deposit is the cost of actually moving personal and household furnishings. While there are some localities that have a volunteer moving service for those with low incomes, in most municipalities this service is not available. The cost of truck rental, even when there are friends and family to help, is not affordable and may not be available if the client has no credit card, or if the amount required as a security of the truck rental is over his credit limit.

CHILD WELFARE

Children's protective services, often referred to as child welfare, are mandated by law to provide supervision, monitoring, and alternative care for children who are experiencing or in danger of physical, mental, or emotional abuse and/or neglect. All states and provinces have legislation to this effect and also have legislation that requires providers of physical, psychological, and social services to report to child welfare authorities any instance where abuse or neglect is suspected. Child protective services, intended to ensure the safety of children, have a large cost as the disruption of the family is traumatic and children in foster care have poorer outcomes in terms of completing school and becoming self-sufficient than the rest of the population. These victims are also at higher risk of adult homelessness (HUD, 2012). The legal reporting requirements in instances of suspected or actual neglect and abuse often place frontline workers in an ethical conflict between the importance of family preservation and the need to protect vulnerable children.

> **Textbox 12.3. Child Welfare Quick Facts**
>
> **United States**
>
> 408,000 children in foster care in 2010 (out of a total population of 308,747,500)
>
> African American children represent 29 percent of the children in foster care but only 14 percent of the total child population (Annie E. Casey Foundation, 2013).
>
> **Canada**
>
> 67,000 children in foster care (out of a population of 34,000,000)
>
> Aboriginal children represent 26 percent of the children in foster care but only 6 percent of the total child population (Canadian Child Welfare Research Portal, 2014).

Child welfare services are very bureaucratic, highly legislated, and accorded powers of protective apprehension of children based on reports that may not be substantiated until presented in a court of law. This power of apprehension is a challenge for those who are self-righteous and claim to act in protection of children as there is a constant temptation to overprotect and apprehend when other actions may best serve children and parents. There are many times when apprehension is a form of abuse of power by those who lack the training and skills to seek alternatives that are more positive. While this can happen to people in all circumstances, the majority of child welfare apprehensions involve poor persons, and minority people are overrepresented in apprehensions. These are the very people who do not have the resources to obtain legal counsel and who lack other advocates. Once taken into custody, children may face an extended foster home placement before being returned to parental care. While this provides safety for the child, it also disrupts parent-child relationships and maternal bonding in the case of newborns. The process is traumatic for parents and children and is something many parents and all workers should seek to avoid if at all possible.

Some service providers consider the very situation of parental homelessness an indication that children are being neglected. Others watch with vigilance when families stay in shelters and temporary housing for indication of abuse and neglect of children or substance use or abuse on the part of parents. This places parents in an extremely stressful predicament where every

> **Textbox 12.4. Numbers of Homeless Children**
>
> In 2011 there were 1.6 million American children who were homeless (Annie E. Casey Foundation, 2013). As a result of the financial and housing crisis, between 2007 and 2010 there was a 38 percent rise in the number of children who were homeless. The variation across all fifty states is detailed in the report by Bassuk and colleagues (Bassuk, Murphy, Coupe, Kenney, & Beach, 2011). Statistics Canada collects data on numerous issues of importance to Canada but it does not collect information specifically on homeless children and youths, except for their type of dwelling, in the five-year census reports. Although total rates are lower than in the United States, homeless children and youths who have left home form a significant group and are of considerable concern.

move they make may be evaluated for their fitness as parental caregivers. Housed people do not receive such scrutiny, nor is there any evidence that homeless families are more or less likely to neglect or abuse their children than are housed parents. The fear of intrusion from child welfare representatives and the removal of children to foster homes results in other desperate situations. One alternative is that families remain doubled up despite the difficulties this creates, and parents are reluctant to seek help for fear of having their children removed. Children may be temporarily placed with relatives who are not under scrutiny but who may have their own set of coping difficulties. At times, some parents have children placed in foster care through the child welfare system in anticipation of becoming homeless and wanting to spare children the problems in the shelter system. This placement also complicates the return of children to parents when they are rehoused.

Drug and alcohol dependence are often contributing factors for child protective services involvement. However, when parents are clean and sober and want to have their children returned to their custody they encounter another set of obstacles as authorities impose stringent and not always realistic requirements for reunification. Return of children to their parents is usually dependent on their ability to demonstrate a clean and sober lifestyle, to live independently, and to have sufficient income and adequate housing for the children. A single person dependent on government assistance does not qualify for family housing unless the children are physically in the parent's custody. However, child protective services will not return a child unless accommodation is adequate (separate bedrooms for children and adults is one criterion). Parents also do not qualify for additional government income support and other subsidies for children unless they have custody. Alternatively, separation and divorce agreements regarding child-care payments may be effective only when the parent awarded custody actual has the child living with him or her. A third dilemma confronts the parent who is employed and now must have day care, but is unable to negotiate this and any attendant subsidies unless the child is in that person's custody. It is often the role of the frontline worker to try and negotiate with child-care workers and other support providers an acceptable plan to deal with these conflicting requirements.

ROLES FOR THE WORKER IN LEGAL ISSUES

There are a number of skills and attributes that contribute to the effectiveness of a good support worker. Advocacy is one of the most important. It may be worth considering whether advocacy and its related skills fit well with the proficiencies you already have and with those that you would like to develop:

- Become knowledgeable in social justice, local resources, and human rights legislation.
- Service users will often need an advocate, someone who will follow up on issues and/or legal rights in a strong voice. The advocate will be able to stand beside the service user, mentoring self-advocacy as an important life skill.
- You will have significant responsibility for managing the safety of your service users, and you will also need to deliver on what you offer service users in order to build a trusting relationship. An ability to work in a boundaried way, ensuring that your relationships with service users remain professional rather than crossing into friendship, is vital. You need to ensure that you act in the service user's best interests, recognizing the trust placed in you as a professional.
- It is important to have strong interpersonal skills, including being an empathetic good listener, and to be able to discuss difficult topics in a sensitive way, and to communicate equally well with service users and other professionals.

- An ability to work reflectively, challenging your own assumptions and thinking about the effectiveness of your work and possible ways forward, is key. This includes self-awareness about the impact the work has on you. Note: This is when self-care is of critical importance, and when check-ins with supervisors and a buddy system are worker self-protections that must be followed.
- As an advocate and support worker, you will need to have a nonjudgmental and empowering attitude, never imposing your own point of view, but instead supporting service users to achieve their own goals. You will need to demonstrate a genuine respect for the diversity, choice, and strengths of your service users.

> **Textbox 12.5. Sources of Legal Information**
> While legal matters can be complex, there are excellent reference books to guide practitioners through the criminal, legal, and child protective services. Legal issues are seen through different lenses in Canada and the United States, and within Canada they differ between Quebec and the rest of the country as the French heritage has a different basis than the British legal system that applies to the rest of the country. As laws vary from state to state and province to province, one needs to consult local and state sources for these details. Staff in the Office of the Public Defender, or in the local legal aid office, are often helpful in your quest to find the location of local and state legal references and resources.

CONFIDENTIALITY

Confidentiality, in addition to being an ethical concern, is a legal issue for those who work in health and human services. People who are recipients of a health or human service are entitled to have their identity protected. This expectation is embedded in many professional codes of ethics, but most importantly it is also woven into legislation in various forms. Some situations, such as the nondisclosure of medical, psychiatric, and information related to substance use, is guaranteed by laws that stipulate heavy penalties for violating those rights. Client-counselor privilege is also provided for lawyers who have a legal obligation to not disclose any client-related information.

To "confide" means literally to entrust with, to have full assurance that the recipient will respect that which has been shared. Confidentiality has

> **Textbox 12.6. The Identity of Victims of Crime and Violent Death**
> In Canada the disclosure of the identity of perpetrators and victims of crime and violent death is carefully controlled so as to not violate the right to privacy enshrined in the Canadian Charter of Rights and Freedoms. In the United States, privacy laws are more diffusely located in various legislative acts and local practices and are not as stringently controlled.

become increasingly important as modern technology has made the transmission of information almost instantaneous, and often not protected from violations of privacy (for example, social media and email offer little protection). Respect is essential for the privacy of those whose basic lives are exposed to the public because they have no private place to which to retreat. We are familiar with the codes of ethics that require confidentiality of medical and helping professionals: the maxim "do not tell without permission of the client." But confidentiality extends way beyond this because it is an essential building block of trust, and trust holds relationships together. Without trust there will be no effective partnership with another person, and without that partnership no real change can occur.

Confidentiality generally arises from three domains: (1) laws that enforce the privacy of specific information such as medical records, psychiatric, and substance-abuse treatment information; and the legal involvement of minors; (2) the codes of ethics of many professions that emphasize the privacy of client-practitioner relationships; and (3) the implicit or explicit agreements made between two persons about the sharing of specific information. An example of the latter is journalists who need to protect the confidentiality of their sources in certain situations. Organizations that serve a specific population may extend this code of confidentiality to employees, even when they are not explicitly covered by a specific professional code. Child welfare workers and workers in rehabilitation organizations fall under this application of confidentiality. It is common for employers of health and social service organizations to require employees to sign a statement of confidentiality. Members of boards of directors of these organizations are often required to sign similar statements.

The laws regarding confidentiality differ to some extent in Canada and the United States. Canadian confidentiality is legislated in two federal privacy laws: the Privacy Act of 1983 that limits government agencies in the information that can be collected and disseminated, and the Personal Information

Protection and Electronic Documents Act (PIPEDA; Office of the Privacy Commissioner of Canada, 2004) that stipulates how private organizations may collect, use, and disseminate or disclose personal information. In the United States a variety of laws are aimed at protecting privacy of information in specific sectors including the Health Insurance Portability and Accountability Act (HIPAA), the Children's Online Privacy Protection Act, the Electronic Communications Privacy Act, and the Right to Financial Privacy Act. However, this legislation does not have the wide-sweeping scope of personal protection legislated in Canada. One example of this difference is the differential use of the social security number (United States) and the social insurance number (Canada). The social security number is used extensively in areas such as credit applications, health insurance claims, and college and university applications, whereas the social insurance number is not used in these situations and is generally not necessary beyond employment documents (for tax-withholding purposes), filing taxes, and some government documents.

The code governing the PIPEDA provides a detailed proscription about the collection, storage, and dissemination of personal data that can be applied to the use of confidential information across all provinces and can be a guide in the states. This code readily forms a guide for those who routinely handle confidential information. The following list details major aspects of this code and provides guidance as to how you can put them into practice in the workplace.

1. Appoint an individual (or individuals) to be responsible for your organization's compliance; protect all personal information held by your organization or transferred to a third party for processing; and develop and implement personal information policies and practices.
2. Your organization must identify the reasons for collecting personal information before or at the time of collection. Before or when any personal information is collected, identify why it is needed and how it will be used; document why the information is collected; inform the individual from whom the information is collected why it is needed; identify any new purpose for the information; and obtain the individual's consent before using it.
3. Inform the individual in a meaningful way of the purposes for the collection, use, or disclosure of personal data; obtain the individual's consent before or at the time of collection, as well as when a new use is identified.

4. Do not collect personal information indiscriminately; collect only what is necessary and do not deceive or mislead individuals about the reasons for collecting personal information.

5. Use or disclose personal information only for the purpose for which it was collected, unless the individual consents, or the use or disclosure is authorized by PIPEDA; keep personal information only as long as necessary to satisfy the purposes; put guidelines and procedures in place for retaining and destroying personal information; keep personal information used to make a decision about a person for a reasonable time period to allow the person to obtain the information after the decision and pursue redress; destroy, erase, or render anonymous information that is no longer required for an identified purpose or a legal requirement. As part of a safety plan, journaling is an important tool. Have code names for particular clients during the street work to protect yourself and the client's identity.

6. Minimize the possibility of using incorrect information when making a decision about the individual or when disclosing information to third parties.

7. Protect personal information against loss or theft; safeguard the information from unauthorized access, disclosure, copying, use, or modification; protect personal information regardless of the format in which it is held.

8. Inform your customers, clients, and employees that you have policies and practices for the management of personal information; make these policies and practices understandable and easily available.

9. When requested, inform individuals if you have any personal information about them; explain how it is or has been used, and provide a list of any organizations to which it has been disclosed; give individuals access to their information; correct or amend any personal information if its accuracy and completeness is challenged and found to be deficient; provide a copy of the information requested, or reasons for not providing access, subject to exception set out in section 9 of PIPEDA; an organization should note any disagreement on the file and advise third parties where appropriate.

10. Develop simple and easily accessible complaint procedures; inform complainants of avenues of recourse. These include complaint procedures of your organization, of industry associations, of regulatory bodies, and of the Privacy Commissioner of Canada; investigate all complaints received; take appropriate measures to correct information handling practices and policies. (Tutty et al., 2009)

What Does Confidentiality Look Like in Practice?

Most workers are vigilant about the intentional disclosure of information, and the need to obtain informed consent from clients. There are, however, numerous ways in which disclosure may occur unintentionally and yet pose considerable risk for clients. Casual office behavior easily lends itself to unintentional violations of confidentiality. Some are common practices that may easily be assumed to be benign. In the office, privacy begins at the front door, where the receptionist should be placed at a distance from where others are waiting to be seen, so as not to be overheard. A person should not be greeted using their last name if there are others present. Within the office environment, files should be kept away from public view, and from coworkers where feasible. Clients should not be left in an office with any files that he could examine. When not in use, files should be in a locked cabinet. When it is imperative that a file has to leave the office, it should not leave the worker's possession for any reason.

Workplace conversations are another way in which confidentiality can inadvertently be compromised. Supervision is one place where workers can and should speak with candor and detail about the work they are doing and the clients they are trying to help. Coworkers may not have a need to know and thus should be brought into a conversation about a client only if they have additional information that may impact the situation. Here boundary violations are quite possible and the potential issues should be discussed with the supervisor who will need to be involved in this judgment call.

In team settings confidentiality has different boundaries. For many workers, talking about work challenges offers a chance to release pent-up emotional energy, to get some peer support, and to recharge one's batteries. The extent to which a group of peer workers acts as a team will determine the degree to which information can be shared, and peer support offered. In team settings it is important to inform the client that the worker belongs to a team, that this team acts together to provide an array of services, and that information needs to be shared in order to work to the best of everyone's ability. This sharing should not extend to the lunchroom or a public location where conversations can be overheard. Even in team settings care should be taken in mentioning names, especially last names. One of the real challenges for a worker is the discretion that must be used at home, with friends and family, in not sharing information that may identify a client. Confidentiality does not extend to one's inner circle; that is, you are not permitted to share client information with people with whom you have close personal relationships. The challenge of this is apparent when there is a critical incident or extreme situation that evokes a marked response in the worker. Debriefing should be done with supervisors and coworkers.

Technology and electronic communication are also fraught with potential violations of confidentiality. Cell phones, answering machines, and fax and copy machines that are not password protected can easily be intercepted. Lost mobile devices that also receive email are full of potential violations as people also store phone numbers and other incidental information on them. Laptops also require a secure password, especially if any client- or organization-related material is stored on them. The same applies to memory sticks that store and transmit information. Any Internet-based form of communication, email, blogs, Twitter, and so on can easily be intercepted by hackers. Even government-based communications have been compromised. The utmost caution should be used in conveying information that identifies clients or is otherwise highly confidential.

What Does Confidentiality Not Include?

By law, some information cannot be kept confidential and must be reported to authorities. These laws exist in various forms in all states, provinces, and territories in the United States and Canada. They include

- child abuse and neglect, including physical, sexual, and emotional abuse;
- client threats to harm themselves or others;
- elder abuse and neglect (specific legal requirements for reporting); and
- assault by or to a client in any organizational setting.

Confidentiality and Release of Information

The rules and boundaries of confidentiality are challenged in situations requiring rapid sharing of information about mutual clients between workers of different organizations. The need to obtain required release of information from clients is a frequent issue and potential obstacle when time is of the essence. It is imperative that the worker be able to access appropriate help and/or resources as quickly as possible. In these situations, privacy laws may complicate this process. In other situations, the worker may have information that is needed by another agency or government organization, but that also cannot be shared without informed consent. The issues around privacy may be complicated in those instances where a person with acute psychotic symptoms needs to be rapidly assessed and treated.

Laws and regulations dealing with confidentiality and privacy of information may make this a challenge since no information—including acknowledgment of whether the individual is a client of the organization—is permitted without that person's authorization. What does this entail? No information should be released without the client's written consent (that of a parent or guardian in the case of a minor). In the United States the most stringent requirements target those presently or formerly in substance-abuse treatment and those with HIV/AIDS. In Canada the requirements follow federal privacy laws. The consent should always address the following items:

1. The consent must name the organization *providing the information*.
2. The consent must name the organization *to which the information is to be provided*.
3. The consent must indicate *specific information* to be released. Note: Words such as "all clinical records" or "all assessments" is too broad. The information should be specific about the period to be covered, e.g., "in the past six months."
4. The consent must *give the reason* for the release of information.
5. The consent must give *the length of time that the release is valid*. In general, a release should be valid for no longer than six months and should be renewed periodically if there is an ongoing need to exchange information. If this is a long-term plan of coordinated care, it should be renewed with an annual review of the care plan.

6. The consent must include a statement that the *consent can be revoked* at any time to the extent that it has not already been acted on by the organization.
7. The consent must be *dated, signed, and witnessed*.
8. The consent should be *on organization letterhead*.

Documentation

Workers have a legal, professional, and ethical responsibility to document their work with clients. The paperwork of documentation often seems like the most unrewarding aspect of a worker's job. Over time, however, it becomes an excellent indication of client progress and those interventions that have been helpful as well as those that have not. Record-keeping for most frontline workers involves noting events, conversations, and interventions; when they occurred; what the immediate response was (if applicable); worker assessment of the situation/incident; plan of action; and planned follow-up. This information needs to be factual, with events and conversations separated from worker impressions (which should be in a separate section). Technical wording is not as important as clear direct factual information. Most information can be captured with simple, direct, unambiguous language. As it is both legally and professionally responsible, this approach will help avoid pitfalls where a worker unintentionally communicates opinions or biases about a client or client's situation.

Access to information is but one of the numerous issues confronting the worker. Criminal and civil law come to mind for the many situations where a homeless person may be in violation of minor infractions or major offenses. But those who have children will also be faced with the complex legislation of the child welfare laws, more complicated still if the children are in custody in a different jurisdiction from the parents.

EXERCISES

1. Identify local efforts that are in place to help persons who have lost their ID documents to replace them.

2. If a local business allows campers to stay overnight in its parking lot, without charge, should the same courtesy be extended to those who are sleeping in their cars? Discuss both sides of this issue.
3. Is there a local organization that helps homeless individuals deal with human rights violations where they are victims? With other legal difficulties apart from major crimes?

JOURNALING

1. Have you worked with a person who panhandles for income? How do you feel about this behavior? Do you see all panhandling as a means to pay for alcohol and drugs?
2. How do you react to a person who is busking (playing some instruments, juggling, or performing on the street or sidewalk in some other way) for income? Do you believe this is different from panhandling? Is this activity legally sanctioned (allowed) locally? Explore some common and divergent themes.

APPENDIX 1

Canadian Definition and Topology of Homelessness (Canadian Homelessness Research Network, 2012)

Below is a full definition and description of what we mean by homelessness. It was developed by the Canadian Homelessness Research Network and is reproduced here with its permission.

CANADIAN DEFINITION OF HOMELESSNESS

Canadian Homelessness Research Network

DEFINITION

Homelessness describes the situation of an individual or family without stable, permanent, appropriate housing, or the immediate prospect, means and ability of acquiring it. It is the result of systemic or societal barriers, a lack of affordable and appropriate housing, the individual/household's financial, mental, cognitive, behavioural or physical challenges, and/or racism and discrimination. Most people do not choose to be homeless, and the experience is generally negative, unpleasant, stressful and distressing.

Homelessness describes a range of housing and shelter circumstances, with people being without any shelter at one end, and being insecurely housed at the other. That is, homelessness encompasses a range of physical living situations, organized here in a ***typology*** that includes 1) **Unsheltered**, or absolutely homeless and living on the streets or in places not intended for human habitation; 2) **Emergency Sheltered**, including those staying in overnight shelters for people who are homeless, as well as shelters for those impacted by family violence;

3) **Provisionally Accommodated**, referring to those whose accommodation is temporary or lacks security of tenure, and finally, 4) **At Risk of Homelessness**, referring to people who are not homeless, but whose current economic and/or housing situation is precarious or does not meet public health and safety standards. It should be noted that for many people homelessness is not a static state but rather a fluid experience, where one's shelter circumstances and options may shift and change quite dramatically and with frequency.

The *problem* of homelessness and housing exclusion refers to the failure of society to ensure that adequate systems, funding and support are in place so that all people, even in crisis situations, have access to housing. The goal of ending homelessness is to ensure housing stability, which means people have a fixed address and housing that is appropriate (affordable, safe, adequately maintained, accessible and suitable in size), and includes required services as needed (supportive), in addition to income and supports.

Numerous populations, such as youth, individuals from different ethnocultural backgrounds, families, newcomers to Canada, people impacted by family violence, the elderly, etc., experience homelessness due to a unique constellation of circumstances and as such the appropriateness of community responses has to take into account such diversity. The over-representation of Aboriginal peoples (including First Nations, Métis, and Inuit peoples), for instance, amongst Canadian homeless populations, necessitates the inclusion of their historical, experiential and cultural differences, as well as experiences with colonization and racism, in their consideration of homelessness.

TYPOLOGY

The typology describes the range of accommodations that people without appropriate, stable, and permanent housing may experience. Those without acceptable housing experience a range of different types of homelessness, from being unsheltered to having housing that is insecure or inappropriate. As homelessness is not one single event or state of being, it is important to recognize that at different points in time people may find themselves experiencing different types of homelessness.

1) Unsheltered

This includes people who lack housing and are not accessing emergency shelters or accommodation, except during extreme weather conditions. In most cases, people are staying in places that are not designed for or fit for human habitation.

1.1 PEOPLE LIVING IN PUBLIC OR PRIVATE SPACES WITHOUT CONSENT OR CONTRACT
- *Public space, such as sidewalks, squares, parks, forests, etc.*
- **Private space and vacant buildings (squatting)**

1.2 PEOPLE LIVING IN PLACES NOT INTENDED FOR PERMANENT HUMAN HABITATION
- *Living in cars or other vehicles*
- **Living in garages, attics, closets or buildings not designed for habitation**
- **People in makeshift shelters, shacks or tents**

2) Emergency Sheltered

This refers to people who, because they cannot secure permanent housing, are accessing emergency shelter and system supports, generally provided at no cost or minimal cost to the user. Such accommodation represents a stop-gap institutional response to homelessness provided by government, non-profit, faith based organizations and / or volunteers.

2.1 EMERGENCY OVERNIGHT SHELTERS FOR PEOPLE WHO ARE HOMELESS

These facilities are designed to meet the immediate needs of people who are homeless. Such short-term emergency shelters may target specific sub-populations, including women, families, youth or Aboriginal persons, for instance. These shelters typically have minimal eligibility criteria, offer shared sleeping facilities and amenities, and often expect clients to leave in the morning. They may or may not offer food, clothing or other services. Some emergency shelters allow people to stay on an ongoing basis while others are short term and are set up to respond to special circumstances, such as extreme weather.

2.2 SHELTERS FOR INDIVIDUALS/FAMILIES IMPACTED BY FAMILY VIOLENCE

These shelters provide basic emergency and crisis services including safe accommodation, meals, information, and referral. They provide a high security environment for women (and sometimes men) and children fleeing family violence or other crisis situations. Residents are not required to leave during the day. These facilities offer private rooms for families and a range of supports to help residents rebuild their lives.

2.3 EMERGENCY SHELTER FOR PEOPLE FLEEING A NATURAL DISASTER OR DESTRUCTION OF ACCOMMODATION DUE TO FIRES, FLOODS, ETC.

3) Provisionally Accommodated

This describes situations in which people, who are technically homeless and without permanent shelter, access accommodation that offers no prospect of permanence. Those who are provisionally accommodated may be accessing temporary housing provided by government or the non-profit sector, or may have independently made arrangements for short-term accommodation.

3.1 INTERIM HOUSING FOR PEOPLE WHO ARE HOMELESS

Interim housing is a systems-supported form of housing that is meant to bridge the gap between unsheltered homelessness or emergency accommodation and permanent housing. In some cases referred to as 'transitional housing', this form of accommodation typically provides services beyond basic needs, offers residents more privacy, and places greater emphasis on participation and social engagement. Interim housing targets those who would benefit from structure, support and skill-building prior to moving to long term housing stability, with the ultimate goal of preventing a return to homelessness. In the case of second-stage housing for those impacted by family violence, the key characteristics of this housing are the safety and security it provides, trauma recovery supports, along with the ultimate goal of preventing re-victimization. Interim housing has time limitations on residency, but generally allows for a longer stay (in some cases up to three years) compared to emergency shelters.

3.2 PEOPLE LIVING TEMPORARILY WITH OTHERS, BUT WITHOUT GUARANTEE OF CONTINUED RESIDENCY OR IMMEDIATE PROSPECTS FOR ACCESSING PERMANENT HOUSING

Often referred to as 'couch surfers' or the 'hidden homeless', this describes people who stay with friends, family, or even strangers. They are typically not paying rent, their duration of stay is unsustainable in the long term, and they do not have the means to secure their own permanent housing in the future. They differ from those who are staying with friends or family out of choice in anticipation of prearranged accommodation, whether in their current hometown or an altogether new community. This living situation is understood by both parties to be temporary, and the assumption is that it will not become permanent.

3.3 PEOPLE ACCESSING SHORT TERM, TEMPORARY RENTAL ACCOMMODATIONS WITHOUT SECURITY OF TENURE

In some cases people who are homeless make temporary rental arrangements, such as staying in motels, hostels, rooming houses, etc. Although occupants pay rent, the accommodation does not offer the possibility of permanency. People living in these situations are often considered to be part of the 'hidden homeless' population.

3.4 PEOPLE IN INSTITUTIONAL CARE WHO LACK PERMANENT HOUSING ARRANGEMENTS

Individuals are considered to be provisionally accommodated and 'at risk' of homelessness if there are no arrangements in place to ensure they move into safe, permanent housing upon release from institutional care. This includes individuals who:

a) were homeless prior to admittance (where their stay may be short-term or long-term) and who have no plan for permanent accommodation after release; or

b) had housing prior to admittance, but lost their housing while in institutional care

c) had housing prior to admittance, but cannot go back due to changes in their needs.

In either case, without adequate discharge planning and support, which includes arrangements for safe and reliable housing (and necessary aftercare or community-based services), there is a likelihood that these individuals may transition into homelessness following their release. Institutional care includes:

- Penal institutions
- Medical / mental health institutions
- Residential treatment programs or withdrawal management centers
- Children's institutions / group homes

3.5 ACCOMMODATION / RECEPTION CENTERS FOR RECENTLY ARRIVED IMMIGRANTS AND REFUGEES

Prior to securing their own housing, recently arrived immigrants and refugees may be temporarily housed while receiving settlement support and orientation to life in Canada. They are considered to be homeless if they have no means or prospects of securing permanent housing.

4) At Risk of Homelessness

Although not technically homeless, this includes individuals or families whose current housing situations are dangerously lacking security or stability, and so are considered *to be at risk of homelessness*. They are living in housing that is intended for permanent human habitation, and could potentially be permanent (as opposed to those who are provisionally accommodated). However, as a result of external hardship, poverty, personal crisis, discrimination, a lack of other available and affordable housing, insecurity of tenure and / or the inappropriateness of their current housing (which may be overcrowded or does not meet public health and safety standards) residents may be "at risk" of homelessness.

An important distinction to make is between those who are at "imminent risk" of becoming homeless and those who are "precariously housed".

No matter the level of probability, all who can be categorized as being "at risk" of homelessness possess a shared vulnerability; for them, a single event, unexpected expense, crisis, or trigger is all it may take for them to lose their housing. As the risk factors mount and compound, so too does the possibility of becoming homeless.

4.1 PEOPLE AT IMMINENT RISK OF HOMELESSNESS

Many factors can contribute to individuals and families being at imminent risk of homelessness. Though in some cases individual factors (such as those listed below) may be most significant, in most cases it is the interaction of structural and individual risk that, in the context of a crisis, influence pathways into homelessness. In other words, what separates those who are at risk of homelessness due to *precarious housing* from those who are at *imminent risk*, is the onset of a crisis, a turn in events, or the increase in acuity of one or more underlying risk factors. Factors that may contribute (as singular or co-occurring factors) include:

- **Precarious employment.** Many people have unstable employment and live pay cheque to pay cheque. Precarious employment describes non-standard employment that does not meet basic needs, is poorly paid, part time (when full time work is desired), temporary, and/or insecure and unprotected. An unanticipated expense, increases in cost of living or a change in employment status may undermine their ability to maintain housing.
- **Sudden unemployment** with few prospects and little to no financial savings or assets, or social supports to turn to for assistance.
- **Supported housing with supports that are about to be discontinued.** Some Housing First models provide supports, but on a time-limited basis. If such resources (aftercare, services) are withdrawn but are still needed, individuals and families may be at imminent risk of re-entering homelessness.
- **Households facing eviction**, lacking the resources needed to afford other housing including social supports, or living in areas with low availability of affordable housing.
- *Severe and persistent mental illness, active addictions, substance use and/or behavioural issues.*
- **Division of Household** – caused by situations (such as separation, divorce, conflicts between caregivers and children, or roommates moving out) where the affected do not have the resources to keep the existing housing or secure other stable housing.
- *Violence / abuse (or direct fear of) in current housing situations, including:*
  - People facing family/gender violence and abuse
  - Children and youth experiencing neglect, physical, sexual, and emotional abuse
  - Seniors facing abuse
  - People facing abuse or discrimination caused by racism or homophobia or misogyny
- **Institutional care that is inadequate or unsuited** to the needs of the individual or family.

4.2 INDIVIDUALS AND FAMILIES WHO ARE PRECARIOUSLY HOUSED

Many individuals and families experience severe housing affordability problems, due to their income, the local economy and / or the lack of availability of affordable housing that meets their needs in the local market. The income of these households is not sufficient to cover the household's basic shelter and non-shelter costs. This includes people who are on government benefits but who do not have sufficient funds to pay for basic needs.

The greater the shortfall of income in covering basic costs, the more at risk of homelessness the household is. Those classified as "precariously housed" face challenges that may or may not leave them homeless in the immediate or near future (in the absence of an intervention). Those who manage to retain their housing in such circumstances often do so at the expense of meeting their nutritional needs, heating their homes, providing proper child care and other expenses that contribute to health and well-being.

Precarious and inadequate housing not only relate to household income and the physical structure of the dwelling, but also to lack of access to necessary supports and opportunities, including employment, health care services, clean water and sanitation, schools, child care centres and other social supports and facilities. Housing that is not culturally appropriate in the way it is constructed, the building materials used, and the policies that support it is also considered inadequate.

CMHC defines a household as being in core housing need if its housing: "falls below at least one of the adequacy, affordability or suitability standards and would have to spend 30% or more of its total before-tax income to pay the median rent of alternative local housing that is acceptable (meets all three housing standards)." (CMHC, 2012)

- **Adequate** housing is reported by residents as not requiring any major repairs. Housing that is inadequate may have excessive mold, inadequate heating or water supply, significant damage, etc.
- **Affordable** dwelling costs less than 30% of total before-tax household income. Those in extreme core housing need pay 50% or more of their income on housing. It should be noted that the lower the household income, the more onerous this expense becomes.
- **Suitable** housing has enough bedrooms for the size and composition of the resident household, according to National occupancy Standard (NoS) requirements."

Source: Canadian Homelessness Research Network (2012). Reprinted with permission.

APPENDIX 2

Professional Quality of Life Scale (ProQOL)

COMPASSION SATISFACTION AND COMPASSION FATIGUE (ProQOL) V. 5 (Stamm, 2009)

When you help people you have direct contact with their lives. As you may have found, your compassion for those you help can affect you in positive and negative ways. Below are some questions about your experiences, both positive and negative, as a helper. Consider each of the following questions about your current work situation. Select the number (on the scale from 1 to 5) that honestly reflects how frequently you experienced these things in the past thirty days.

1 = Never	2 = Rarely	3 = Sometimes	4 = Often	5 = Very Often

____ 1. I am happy.

____ 2. I am preoccupied with more than one person I help.

____ 3. I get satisfaction from being able to help people.

____ 4. I feel connected to others.

____ 5. I jump or I am startled by unexpected sounds.

____ 6. I feel invigorated after working with those I help.

____ 7. I find it difficult to separate my personal life from my life as a helper.

____ 8. I am not as productive at work because I am losing sleep over traumatic experiences of a person I help.

____ 9. I think that I might have been affected by the traumatic stress of those I help.

____ 10. I feel trapped by my job as a helper.

____ 11. Because of my helping, I have felt "on edge" about various things.

___ 12. I like my work as a helper.
___ 13. I feel depressed because of the traumatic experiences of the people I help.
___ 14. I feel as though I am experiencing the trauma of someone I have helped.
___ 15. I have beliefs that sustain me.
___ 16. I am pleased with how I am able to keep up with helping techniques and protocols.
___ 17. I am the person I always wanted to be.
___ 18. My work makes me feel satisfied.
___ 19. I feel worn out because of my work as a helper.
___ 20. I have happy thoughts and feelings about those I help and how I could help them.
___ 21. I feel overwhelmed because my case (work) load seems endless.
___ 22. I believe I can make a difference through my work.
___ 23. I avoid certain activities or situations because they remind me of frightening experiences of the people I help.
___ 24. I am proud of what I can do to help.
___ 25. As a result of my helping, I have intrusive, frightening thoughts.
___ 26. I feel "bogged down" by the system.
___ 27. I have thoughts that I am a "success" as a helper.
___ 28. I can't recall important parts of my work with trauma victims.
___ 29. I am a very caring person.
___ 30. I am happy that I chose to do this work.

What Is My Score and What Does It Mean?

In this section you will score your test so you can understand the interpretation for you. To find your score *on each section*, total the questions listed on the left and then find your score on the right of the section.

Compassion Satisfaction Scale

Copy your score for each of the following questions and add them up. Look up your total score on the table to the right.

3. ____

6. ____

12. ____

16. ____

18. ____

20. ____

22. ____

24. ____

27. ____

30. ____

Total ____

The sum of my Compassion Satisfaction questions is	My score equals	My compassion satisfaction level is
22 or less	43 or less	Low
Between 23 and 41	Around 50	Average
42 or more	57 or more	High

Compassion satisfaction is about the pleasure you derive from being able to do your work well. For example, you may feel it is a pleasure to help others through your work. You may feel positively about your colleagues or your ability to contribute to the work setting or even the greater good of society. Higher scores on this scale represent a greater satisfaction related to your ability to be an effective caregiver in your job.

The average score is 50. (SD 10, alpha scale reliability .88). About 25 percent of people score higher than 57 and about 25 percent of people score lower than 43. If you are in the higher range, you probably derive a good deal of satisfaction from your position. If your scores are below 40, you may either find problems with your job, or there may be some other reason—for example you may derive your satisfaction from activities other than your job.

Burnout Scale

For this scale you will need to take an extra step. Starred items are "reverse scored." If you scored the item as a 1, write 5 beside it. The reason we ask you to do this is because scientifically the measure works better when these questions are asked in a positive way but they can tell us more about their negative form. For example, the question "I am happy" tells us more about the effects of helping when you are not happy when you reverse the score.

You wrote	Change to
1	5
2	4
3	3
4	2
5	1

1. ____ *
4. ____ *
8. ____
10. ____
15. ____ *
17. ____ *
19. ____
21. ____
26. ____
29. ____ *

Total ____

The sum of my Burnout questions is	My score equals	My burnout level is
22 or less	43 or less	Low
Between 23 and 41	Around 50	Average
42 or more	57 or more	High

Most people have an intuitive idea of what burnout is. From the research perspective, burnout is one of the elements of Compassion Fatigue (CF). It is associated with feelings of hopelessness and difficulties dealing with work or in doing your job effectively. These negative feelings usually have a gradual onset. They can reflect the feeling that your efforts make no difference, or they can be associated with a very high workload or a non-supportive work environment. Higher scores on this scale mean that you are at higher risk for burnout.

The average score is 50 (SD 10, alpha scale reliability .75). About 25 percent of people score higher than 57 and about 25 percent of people score lower than 43. If your score is below 43, this probably reflects positive feelings about your ability to be effective in your work. If you score above 57 you may wish to think about what at work makes you feel like you are not effective in your position. Your score may reflect your mood; perhaps you were having a "bad day" or are in need of some time off. If the high score persists, or if it is reflective of other worries, it may be cause for concern.

Secondary Traumatic Stress Scale

Copy your score for each of the following questions and add them up. Look up your total score on the table to the right.

2. ____
5. ____
7. ____
9. ____
11. ____
13. ____
14. ____
23. ____
25. ____
28. ____
Total ____

The sum of my Secondary Traumatic Stress questions is	My score equals	My secondary traumatic level is
22 or less	43 or less	Low
Between 23 and 41	Around 50	Average
42 or more	57 or more	High

The second component of Compassion Fatigue (CF) is secondary traumatic stress (STS). It is about your work related, secondary exposure to extremely traumatic or stressful events. Developing problems due to exposure to other's trauma is somewhat rare but does happen to many people who care for those who have experienced extremely or traumatically stressful events. For example, you may hear stories about the traumatic things that happen to other people, commonly called Vicarious Traumatization. If your work puts you directly in the path of danger, for example, field work in a war or area of civil violence, this is not secondary exposure, your exposure is primary. However, if you are exposed to others' traumatic events as a result of your work, for example as a therapist or an emergency worker, this is secondary exposure. The symptoms of STS are usually rapid in onset and associated with a particular event. They may include being afraid, having difficulty sleeping, having images of the upsetting event pop into your mind, or avoiding things that remind you of the event.

The average score on this scale is 50 (SD 10; alpha scale reliability .81). About 25 percent of people score below 43 and about 25 percent of people score above 57. If your score is above 57, you may want to take some time to think about what at work may be frightening to you or if there is some other reason for the elevated score. While higher scores do not mean that you do have a problem, they are an indication that you may want to examine how you feel about your work and your work environment. You may want to discuss this with your supervisor, a colleague, or a health care professional.

APPENDIX 3

Addiction Abstinence Self-Efficacy Scale

The following scale is a modified version of the one developed by McKiernan and colleagues. These questions look at your temptation to use alcohol and drugs and how confident you feel in resisting the opportunities and urges to use. The higher your score, the more susceptible you are to relapse.

Rate yourself on the following items using the scale: 1 = not at all to 5 = extremely

A. How *tempted would you be* to drink or use drugs when:

1. you are emotionally upset (feeling down, angry, afraid or guilty)? 1 2 3 4 5
2. you are around others or seeing others who are using—such as during social gatherings, celebrations or on vacation? 1 2 3 4 5
3. you experience physical pain, such as headache, injury, or are physically tired? 1 2 3 4 5
4. you have thoughts of using—either when awake or dreaming? 1 2 3 4 5
5. you are feeling a physical need or craving for drugs or alcohol? 1 2 3 4 5
6. you have the urge to drink or use drugs just once to see what happens? 1 2 3 4 5

B. How *confident would you be not to* drink or use drugs when:

7. you are emotionally upset (feeling down, angry, afraid or guilty)? 1 2 3 4 5

8. you are around others or seeing others who are using—such as during social gatherings, celebrations or on vacation?   1   2   3   4   5

9. you experience physical pain, such as headache, injury, or are physically tired?   1   2   3   4   5

10. you have thoughts of using—either when awake or dreaming?   1   2   3   4   5

11. you are feeling a physical need or craving for drugs or alcohol?   1   2   3   4   5

12. you have the urge to drink or use drugs just once to see what happens?   1   2   3   4   5

Source: McKiernan et al. (2011). Used with permission.

APPENDIX 4

Trauma Self-Assessment

The Trauma Self-Assessment scale is a self-administered tool that helps an individual determine if he or she has trauma-related feelings and behaviors that may warrant clinical attention. This is a public document and can be freely used. It is *not* recommended that you give this to clients as its use in this context should be determined by a trained trauma therapist. This tool will help workers to identify if they have trauma-related issues that may impact their work, provide emotional triggers, and thus warrant further attention.

PTSD Checklist—Civilian Version (PCL-C)

Not at all (1)　　A little bit (2)　　Moderately (3)　　Quite a bit (4)　　Extremely (5)

To what extent do you experience:

____ 1. Repeated, disturbing memories, thoughts, or images of a stressful experience from the past?

____ 2. Repeated, disturbing dreams of a stressful experience from the past?

____ 3. Suddenly acting or feeling as if a stressful experience were happening again (as if you were reliving it)?

____ 4. Feeling very upset when something reminded you of a stressful experience from the past?

____ 5. Having physical reactions (e.g., heart pounding, trouble breathing, or sweating) when something reminded you of a stressful experience from the past?

____ 6. Avoiding thinking about or talking about a stressful experience from the past or avoid having feelings related to it?

____ 7. Avoiding activities or situations because they remind you of a stressful experience from the past?

_____ 8. Trouble remembering important parts of a stressful experience from the past?
_____ 9. Loss of interest in things that you used to enjoy?
_____ 10. Feeling distant or cut off from other people?
_____ 11. Feeling emotionally numb or being unable to have loving feelings for those close to you?
_____ 12. Feeling as if your future will somehow be cut short?
_____ 13. Trouble falling or staying asleep?
_____ 14. Feeling irritable or having angry outbursts?
_____ 15. Having difficulty concentrating?
_____ 16. Being "super alert" or watchful, on guard?
_____ 17. Feeling jumpy or easily startled?

Scoring: Add your scores for all items. If the total is fifty or greater you are urged to seek professional help. If your score is under fifty you may still elect to seek help if you have answered a four or five to specific questions that continue to trouble you.

Source: Weathers, Litz, Huska, & Keane (1994).

Note: This is a government document in the public domain.

APPENDIX 5

Alcohol and Other Drugs: Intoxication and Withdrawal

SIGNS OF ALCOHOL INTOXICATION

- Odor of alcohol on the breath
- Difficulty focusing; glazed appearance of the eyes
- Irritability
- Slowed or slurred speech
- Slowed reaction times such as while driving
- Loss of sense of balance
- Uncharacteristically passive behavior; or combative and argumentative behavior

SIGNS OF MARIJUANA INTOXICATION

Many signs are subtle and may go unrecognized except to the trained/experienced observer.

- Early stages: often rapid, loud talking, and bursts of laughter
- Later stages: sleepy or stuporous
- Forgetfulness and/or slow in conversation
- Slowed reaction times
- Slow while driving
- Misperceived sense of time—time intervals overestimated
- Inflammation in whites of eyes; pupils likely dilated

SIGNS OF DEPRESSANT INTOXICATION (CAN BE PRESCRIPTION DRUGS)

- Symptoms of alcohol intoxication with no odor on breath (depressants frequently used with alcohol)
- Lack of facial expression or animation
- Flat affect
- Flaccid appearance
- Slurred speech
- Slow reactivity
- Lethargy, drowsiness
- Pupils that fail to respond (constrict) to light

Narcotic and cocaine intoxication may have these additional signs (in addition to the depressant signs):

- Redness and raw nostrils from inhaling heroin or cocaine in powder form
- Scars (tracks) on inner arms or other parts of the body from needle injections (can also be from cocaine, which is a stimulant)
- Presence of paraphernalia for smoking or injecting drugs, including syringes, bent spoons, bottle caps, eye droppers, rubber tubing, cotton and needles, little bottles of white powder, and straws (plastic, glass, or metal)

SIGNS OF STIMULANT INTOXICATION

- Dilated pupils
- Dry mouth and nose, bad breath, frequent lip licking
- Agitation, excessive activity, difficulty sitting still, lack of interest in food or sleep
- Irritable, argumentative, nervous
- Talkative, but conversation often lacks continuity; changes subjects rapidly

- May appear suspicious or paranoid
- Runny nose, cold or chronic sinus/nasal problems, nose bleeds
- Possession of paraphernalia including small spoons, razor blades, mirror

SIGNS OF INHALANT ABUSE

- Substance odor on breath and clothes
- Runny nose
- Watering eyes
- Poor muscle control
- Drowsiness or unconsciousness
- Prefers group activity to being alone
- Presence of bags or rags containing dry plastic cement or other solvent
- Discarded cans of whipped cream, spray paint, or similar chargers (users of nitrous oxide)
- Small bottles labeled "incense" or "head cleaner" (users of butyl nitrate)

SIGNS OF HALLUCINOGEN ABUSE

- Extremely dilated pupils
- Warm skin, excessive perspiration, and body odor
- Distorted sense of sight, hearing, touch; distorted image of self and perception of time
- Mood and behavior changes, the extent depending on emotional state of the user and environmental conditions
- Unpredictable flashback episodes even long after withdrawal (although these are rare)

SIGNS OF PCP ABUSE

- Unpredictable behavior; mood may swing from passive to violent for no apparent reason

- Symptoms of intoxication
- Pupils may appear dilated
- Floating pupils, appear to be following a moving object
- Mask-like facial appearance
- Disorientation; agitation and violence if exposed to excessive sensory stimulation
- Fear; terror
- Rigid muscles
- Strange gait
- Deadened sensory perception (may experience severe injuries while appearing not to notice)
- Comatose (unresponsive) if large amount consumed: eyes may be opened or closed

REFERENCES

Al-Krenawi, A., & Graham, J. R. (2000). Culturally sensitive social work practice with Arab clients in mental health settings. *Health and Social Work, 25*(1), 9-22.

American Psychiatric Association. (2013). *Diagnostic and Statistical Manual of Mental Disorders* (DSM-5) (5th ed.). Washington, DC: Author.

Annie E. Casey Foundation. (2013). Kids Count Data Center: Children in poverty. Retrieved from http://datacenter.kidscount.org/data/across states/Rankings.aspx?i nd=43

Bachrach, L. L. (1987). Homeless women: A context for health planning. *Milbank Quarterly*, 371-396.

Bandura, A. (1993). Perceived self-efficacy in cognitive development and functioning. *Educational Psychologist, 28*(2), 117-148.

Bard, J. (2005). Rearranging deck chairs on the Titanic: Why the incarceration of individuals with serious mental illness violates public health, ethical, and constitutional principles and therefore cannot be made right by piecemeal changes to the insanity defense. *Houston Journal of Health Law and Policy, 5*(1), 1.

Barrow, S., & Zimmer, R. (1998). Transitional housing and services: A synthesis. Paper presented at the Practical Lessons: The 1998 National Symposium on Homelessness Research, Arlington, VA, October 29-30.

Bassuk, E. L., Murphy, C., Coupe, N. T., Kenney, R. R., & Beach, C. A. (2011). America's youngest outcasts 2010: State report card on child homelessness. The National Center on Family Homelessness. Retrieved from http://www.homelesschildrenamerica.org/reportcard.php

Belcher, J. R. (1988). Are jails replacing the mental health system for the homeless mentally ill? *Community Mental Health Journal, 24*(3), 185-195.

Bellot, C., Raffestin, I., Royer, M.-N., & Noël, V. (2005). *Judiciarisation et criminalisation des populations itinérantes à Montréal.* Montreal, QC: Rapport de recherché pour le Secretariat National des Sans-Abri.

REFERENCES

Berry, J. W. (2010). Immigrant acculturation. In A. E. Azzi, X. Chryssochoou, B. Klandermans, & B. Simon (Eds.), *Identity and participation in culturally diverse societies*. Oxford, UK: Wiley-Blackwell.

Berry, J. W., Phinney, J. S., Sam, D. L., & Vedder, P. (2006). Immigrant youth: Acculturation, identity, and adaptation. *Applied Psychology, 55*(3), 303-332.

Bouchard, T. J., & McGue, M. (2003). Genetic and environmental influences on human psychological differences. *Journal of Neurobiology, 54*(1), 4-45.

Braveman, P., Egerter, S., & Williams, D. R. (2011). The social determinants of health: Coming of age. *Annual Review of Public Health, 32*, 381-398.

Briere, J., & Scott, C. (2006). *Principles of trauma therapy: A guide to symptoms, evaluation, and treatment*. Thousand Oaks, CA: Sage Publications.

Brown, S. A. (2008). Factors and measurement of mental illness stigma: A psychometric examination of the Attribution Questionnaire. *Psychiatric Rehabilitation Journal, 32*(2), 89.

Brown, S. A., Vik, P. W., Patterson, T. L., Grant, I., & Schuckit, M. A. (1995). Stress, vulnerability and adult alcohol relapse. *Journal of Studies on Alcohol and Drugs, 56*(5), 538.

Brown, S. L. (2005). *The history of housing and treatment services for people with serious psychiatric disabilities: Models of residential service delivery*. University of Hartford, CT. Retrieved from http://proquest.umi.com/pqdweb?did=1014322451&Fmt=7&clientId=20829&RQT=309&VName=PQD

Burg, M. A. (1994). Health problems of sheltered homeless women and their dependent children. *Health & Social Work, 19*(2), 125-131.

Burt, M. (2001). Homeless families, singles, and others: Findings from the 1996 National Survey of Homeless Assistance Providers and Clients. *Housing Policy Debate, 12*(4), 737-780.

Calgary Homeless Foundation. (2009). Calgary Homeless Foundation facts and figures. Retrieved from http://www.calgaryhomeless.com

Canadian Child Welfare Research Portal. (2014). Statistics. Retrieved from http://cwrp.ca/statistics1zn

Canadian Homelessness Research Network. (2012). Canadian Definition of Homelessness. Toronto: Homeless HUB, York University. Retrieved from www.homelesshub.ca/CHRNhomelessdefinition/

Canning, I., Sherman, E., & Unwin, G. (Producer), & Hooper, T. (Director). (2010). The king's speech [Motion picture]. United Kingdom: Momentum Pictures.

Centers for Disease Control and Prevention (CDC). (2013). *Integrated Disease Surveillance and Response (IDSR)*. Atlanta, GA: Author. Retrieved from http://www.cdc.gov/globalhealth/healthprotection/ghsb/idsr/default.htm

Chang, J. (2003). *Wild swans: Three daughters of China*. New York: Touchstone.

Chiu, L., Emblen, J. D., Van Hofwegen, L., Sawatzky, R., & Meyerhoff, H. (2004). An integrative review of the concept of spirituality in the health sciences. *Western Journal of Nursing Research, 26*(4), 405–428.

Christensen, R. C., Hodgkins, C. C., Garces, L., Estlund, K. L., Miller, M. D., & Touchton, R. (2005). Homeless, mentally ill and addicted: The need for abuse and trauma services. *Journal of Health Care for the Poor and Underserved, 16*(4), 615–622.

Chudley, A. E., Kilgour, A. R., Cranston, M., & Edwards, M. (2007). Challenges of diagnosis in fetal alcohol syndrome and fetal alcohol spectrum disorder in the adult. *American Journal of Medical Genetics* Part C, Seminar in Medical Genetics 145C: 261–272.

Clarren, S., Weinberg, J., & Jonsson, E. (2010). Incidence, prevalence, and economic aspects of FASD. In E. P. Riley, S. Clarren, J. Weinberg, & E. Jonsson (Eds.), *Fetal alcohol spectrum disorder: Management and policy perspectives of FASD* (vol. 14). Edmonton, AB: Wiley-Blackwell.

Coates, J., & McKenzie-Mohr, S. (2010). Out of the frying pan, into the fire: Trauma in the lives of homeless youth prior to and during homelessness. *Journal of Sociology and Social Welfare, 37*, 65.

Cochran, B. N., Stewart, A. J., Ginzler, J. A., & Cauce, A. M. (2002). Challenges faced by homeless sexual minorities: Comparison of gay, lesbian, bisexual, and transgender homeless adolescents with their heterosexual counterparts. *American Journal of Public Health, 92*(5), 773–777.

Cohen, K. (1998). Native American medicine. *Alternative Therapies in Health and Medicine, 4*(6), 45–57.

Commission for Case Management Certification. (2013). Case Management Certification. Retrieved from http://ccmcertification.org/case-managers/board-certified-case-manager

Corey, G., Corey, M. S., & Callanan, P. (2010). *Issues & ethics in the helping professions* (8th ed.). Pacific Grove, CA: Brooks/Cole.

Corrigan, J. D., Selassie, A. W., & Orman, J. A. L. (2010). The epidemiology of traumatic brain injury. *Journal of Head Trauma Rehabilitation, 25*(2), 72-80.

Corrigan, P., Markowitz, F.E., Watson, A., Rowan, D. &, Kubiak, M.A. (2003). An attribution model of public discrimination towards persons with mental illness. *Journal of Health and Social Behavior,* (44), 162-179.

Currie, J. (2004). *Women offenders: Characteristics, needs and impacts of transitional housing.* Ottawa, ON: Canada Mortgage and Housing Corporation.

D'Amour, D., Ferrada-Videla, M., San Martin Rodriguez, L., & Beaulieu, M.-D. (2005). The conceptual basis for interprofessional collaboration: Core concepts and theoretical frameworks. *Journal of Interprofessional Care, 19*(S1), 116-131.

D'Andrea, W., Ford, J., Stolbach, B., Joseph Spinazzola, J., & van der Kolk, B. A. (2012). Understanding interpersonal trauma in children: Why we need a developmentally appropriate trauma diagnosis. *American Journal of Orthopsychiatry, 82*(2), 187-200.

Damron-Rodriguez, J. (2008). Developing competence for nurses and social workers. *Journal of Social Work Education, 44*(3), 27-37.

Davidson, P. R., & Parker, K. C. H. (2001). Eye movement desensitization and reprocessing (EMDR): A meta-analysis. *Journal of Consulting and Clinical Psychology, 69*(2), 305-316.

DeMatteo, D., LaDuke, C., Locklair, B. R., & Heilbrun, K. (2013). Community-based alternatives for justice-involved individuals with severe mental illness: Diversion, problem-solving courts, and reentry. *Journal of Criminal Justice, 41*(2), 64-71.

DiClemente, C. O., Carbonari, J. P., Montgomery, R. P., & Hughes, S. O. (1994). The alcohol abstinence self-efficacy scale. *Journal of Studies on Alcohol, 55*(2), 141-148.

DiClemente, R. J., Hansen, W. B., & Ponton, L. E. (1996). *Handbook of adolescent health risk behavior.* New York: Springer.

Didenko, E., & Pankratz, N. (2007). Substance use: Pathways to homelessness? Or a way of adapting to street life. *Visions: British Columbia's Mental Health and Addictions Journal, 4*(1), 9-10.

Dolgoff, R., Harrington, D., & Loewenberg, F. (2011). *Brooks/Cole empowerment series: Ethical decisions for social work practice.* Belmont, CA: Brooks/Cole.

Dombovy, M. L. (2011). Traumatic brain injury. *CONTINUUM: Lifelong Learning in Neurology, 17*(3), 584-605.
Donovan, D. M., & O'Leary, M. R. (1978). The drinking-related locus of control scale: Reliability, factor structure and validity. *Journal of Studies on Alcohol and Drugs, 39*(05), 759.
Donovan, V. (2009). Houses for homeless, no strings attached. Retrieved from http://ezproxy.lib.ucalgary.ca:2048/login?url=http://search.ebs cohost.com/login.aspx?direct=true&db=rch&AN=6FP3719330243& site=ehost-live
Douglas, J. (2011). The criminalization of poverty: Montreal's policy of ticketing homeless youth for municipal and transportation by-law infractions. *Appeal: Review of Current Law and Law Reform, 16,* 49.
Drake, R. E., & Mueser, K. T. (2000). Psychosocial approaches to dual diagnosis. *Schizophrenia Bulletin, 26*(1), 105-118.
Drake, R., Yovetich, N., Bebout, R., Harris, M., & McHugo, G. (1997). Integrated treatment for dually diagnosed homeless adults. *Journal of Nervous & Mental Disease, 185*(5), 298-305.
Drake, R. E., & Wallach, M. A. (2000). Dual diagnosis: 15 years of progress. *Psychiatric Services, 51*(9), 1126-1129.
Dyb, E. (2009). Imprisonment: A major gateway to homelessness. *Housing Studies, 24*(6), 809-824.
Eberle, M., Kraus, D., Serge, L., & Hulchanski, D. (2001). *Homelessness: Causes and effects, vol. 1: The relationship between homelessness and the health, social services and criminal justice system; a literature review.* Prepared for the BC Ministry of Social Development and Economic Security, and BC Housing.
Elliott, D. E., Bjelajac, P., Fallot, R. D., Markoff, L. S., & Reed, B. G. (2005). Trauma-informed or trauma-denied: Principles and implementation of trauma-informed services for women. *Journal of Community Psychology, 33*(4), 461-477.
Evans-Campbell, T. (2008). Historical trauma in American Indian/Native Alaska communities: A multilevel framework for exploring impacts on individuals, families, and communities. *Journal of Interpersonal Violence, 23*(3), 316-338.
Felthous, A., O'Shaughnessay, R., Kuten, J., Francois-Purcel, I., & Medrano, J. (2007). The clinician's duty to warn in the United States, England, Canada, New Zealand, France and Spain. In A. Felthous & H. Sass (Eds.),

International handbook of psychopathic disorders and the law (vol. 2, pp. 57-94). Chichester, UK: John Wiley & Sons.

Ferguson, K. M., Bender, K., Thompson, S. J., Xie, B., & Pollio, D. (2012). Exploration of arrest activity among homeless young adults in four US cities. *Social Work Research,* doi: 10.1093/swr/svs023.

Figueiredo, R. L. F., Hwang, S. W., & Quiñonez, C. (2012). Dental health of homeless adults in Toronto, Canada. *Journal of Public Health Dentistry, 73*(1), 74-78.

Fisk, D., Rakfeldt, J., Heffernan, K., & Rowe, M. (1999). Outreach workers' experiences in a homeless outreach project: Issues of boundaries, ethics and staff safety. *Psychiatric Quarterly, 70*(3), 231-246.

Fitzpatrick, K. M., & Myrstol, B. (2011). The jailing of America's homeless: Evaluating the rabble management thesis. *Crime & Delinquency, 57*(2), 271-297.

Folman, A., Lalou, S., Meixner, G., Nahlieli, Y., & Roman, P. (Producers), & Folman, A. (Director). (2008). *Waltz with Bashir* [Motion picture]. Israel: Sony Pictures Classics.

Folsom, D., Hawthorne, W., Lindamer, L., Gilmer, T., Bailey, A., Golshan, S. . . . & Jeste, D. (2005). Prevalence and risk factors for homelessness and utilization of mental health services among 10,340 patients with serious mental illness in a large public mental health system. *American Journal of Psychiatry, 162*(2), 370-376.

Foster, G., & R. Krasnoff (Producer), & Wright, J. (Director). (2009). *The soloist* [Motion picture]. United States: Paramount Pictures.

Foucault, M. (1988). *Madness and civilization: A history of insanity in the age of reason.* New York: Random House Digital.

Frankish, C. J., Hwang, S. W., & Quantz, D. (2005). Homelessness and health in Canada: Research lessons and priorities (Commentary). *Canadian Journal of Public Health, 96*(Suppl. 2).

Frost, R. B., Farrer, T. J., Primosch, M., & Hedges, D. W. (2012). Prevalence of traumatic brain injury in the general adult population: A meta-analysis. *Neuroepidemiology, 40*(3), 154-159.

Gaetz, S. (2010). The struggle to end homelessness in Canada: How we created the crisis, and how we can end it. *Open Health Services and Policy Journal, 3,* 21-26.

Galambos, C., Watt, J. W., Anderson, K., & Danis, F. (2006). Ethics forum: Rural social work practice: Maintaining confidentiality in the face of dual relationships. *Journal of Social Work Values & Ethics*. Retrieved from http://www.socialworker.com/jswve/content/view/23/

Garland, T. S., Richards, T., & Cooney, M. (2010). Victims hidden in plain sight: The reality of victimization among the homeless. *Criminal Justice Studies, 23*(4), 285-301.

Gately, I. (2008). *Drink: A cultural history of alcohol.* New York: Penguin.

Gibelman, M., & Furman, R. (2008). *Navigating human service organizations* (2nd ed.). Chicago: Lyceum.

Goering, P., Veldhuizen, S., Watson, A., Adair, C., Kopp, B., Latimer, E. . . . & Aubry, T. (2014). National at home/chez soi final report. Mental Health Commission of Canada, Calgary, AB.

Grob, G. N. (1994). Mad, homeless, and unwanted. A history of the care of the chronic mentally ill in America. *Psychiatric Clinics of North America, 17*(3), 541-558.

Hanselmann, C. (2001). *Urban Aboriginal people in western Canada*. Calgary: CanadaWest Foundation.

Harper, G. W., Davidson, J., & Hosek, S. G. (2008). Influence of gang membership on negative affect, substance use, and antisocial behavior among homeless African American male youth. *American Journal of Men's Health, 2*(3), 229-243.

Hartman, A. (1995). Diagrammatic assessment of family relationships. *Families in Society, 76,* 111-122. (Original work published 1978).

Hawkins, E. H., Cummins, L. H., & Marlatt, G. A. (2004). Preventing substance abuse in American Indian and Alaska Native youth: Promising strategies for healthier communities. *Psychological Bulletin, 130*(2), 304.

Health Canada. (2012). Canadian Alcohol and Drug Use Monitoring Survey, Table 8: Prevalence of alcohol use and exceeding LRDG, total population, CAS 2004, CADUMS 2008-2011. Government of Canada, Ottawa. Retrieved from http://www.hc-sc.gc.ca/hc-ps/drugs-drogues/stat/_2011/tables-tableaux-eng.php#t8

Health Canada. (2013). Health concerns. Retrieved from http://www.hc-sc.gc.ca/hc-ps/index-eng.php

Hecht, L., & Coyle, B. (2001). Elderly homeless: A comparison of older and younger adult emergency shelter seekers in Bakersfield, California. *American Behavioral Scientist, 45*(1), 66-79.

Hepworth, D., Rooney, R., Dewberry-Rooney, G., Strom-Gottfried, K., & Larsen, J. (2010). *Direct social work practice* (8th ed.). Belmont, CA: Brooks/Cole.

Herman, J. L. (1992). *Trauma and recovery*. New York: Basic Books.

Herrman, H., Saxena, S., & Moodie, R. (2005). Promoting mental health: Concepts, emerging evidence, practice: A report of the World Health Organization, Department of Mental Health and Substance Abuse, in collaboration with the Victorian Health Promotion Foundation and the University of Melbourne. World Health Organization, Geneva.

Hill, D., & Obst, L. (Producer), & Gilliam, T. (Director). (1991). *Fisher king* [Motion picture]. United States: TriStar Pictures.

Hollingshead, A. B., & Redlich, F. C. (1953). Social stratification and psychiatric disorders. *American Sociological Review, 18*(2), 163–169.

Holmes, T., & Rahe, R. (1967). Holmes-Rahe social readjustment rating scale. *Journal of Psychosomatic Research, 11*(2), 213–218.

Hooker, S. D., Freeman, L. H., & Stewart, P. (2002). Pet therapy research: A historical review. *Holistic Nursing Practice, 17*(1), 17–23.

Hopper, E. K., Bassuk, E. L., & Olivet, J. (2010). Shelter from the storm: Trauma-informed care in homelessness services settings. *Open Health Services and Policy Journal, 3*, 80–100.

Hudson, C. G. (2005). Socioeconomic status and mental illness: Tests of the social causation and selection hypotheses. *American Journal of Orthopsychiatry, 75*(1), 3–18.

Hwang, S. W. (2001). Homelessness and health. *Canadian Medical Association Journal, 164*(2), 229–233.

Hwang, S. W., Colantonio, A., Chiu, S., Tolomiczenko, G., Kiss, A., Cowan, L. . . . & Levinson, W. (2008). The effect of traumatic brain injury on the health of homeless people. *Canadian Medical Association Journal, 179*(8), 779–784.

Hwang, S. W., Lueng, J., M., Chiu, S., Kiss, A., Tolomiczenko, G., Cowan, L. . . . & Redelmeier, D. A. (2010). Universal health insurance and health care access for homeless persons. *Journal Information, 100*(8).

Hwang, S. W., Tolomiczenko, G., Kouyoumdjian, F. G., & Garner, R. E. (2005). Interventions to improve the health of the homeless: A systematic review. *American Journal of Preventive Medicine, 29*(4), 311, e75. Retrieved from http://www.ajpmonline.org/article/S0749-3797%2805%2900295-3/abstract

Interprofessional Education Collaborative Expert Panel. (2011). *Core competencies for interprofessional collaborative practice: Report of an expert panel*. Washington, DC: Author.

Jack, T., & Robert, A. R. (2012). Consumer choice over living environment, case management, and mental health treatment in supported housing and its relation to outcomes. *Journal of Health Care for the Poor and Underserved, 23*(4), 1671-1677.

Jellinek, E. M. (1960). *The disease concept of alcoholism.* New Haven, CT: College and University Press.

Jencks, C. (1995). *The homeless.* Cambridge, MA: Harvard University Press.

Kahn, A. (1979). *Social policy & social services* (2nd ed.). New York: Random House.

Keeshin, B. R., & Campbell, K. (2011). Screening homeless youth for histories of abuse: Prevalence, enduring effects, and interest in treatment. *Child Abuse & Neglect, 35*(6), 401-407.

Kidd, A. H., & Kidd, R. M. (1994). Benefits and liabilities of pets for the homeless. *Psychological Reports, 74*(3), 715-722.

Kloos, B., Zimmerman, S. O., Scrimenti, K., & Crusto, C. (2002). Landlords as partners for promoting success in supported housing: "It takes more than a lease and a key." *Psychiatric Rehabilitation Journal, 25*(3), 235-244.

Kohls, R. (1984). *The values Americans live by.* Washington, DC: Meridian House International.

Kortrijk, H., Mulder, C., van Vliet, D., van Leeuwen, C., Jochems, E., & Staring, A. (2013). Changes in motivation for treatment in precontemplating dually diagnosed patients receiving assertive community treatment. *Community Mental Health Journal, 49*(6), 733-741.

Kraus, D. (2001). *Housing for people with alcohol and drug addictions: An annotated bibliography.* Vancouver, BC: City of Vancouver.

Kryda, A. D., & Compton, M. T. (2009). Mistrust of outreach workers and lack of confidence in available services among individuals who are chronically street homeless. *Community Mental Health Journal, 45*(2), 144-150.

Kushel, M. B., Hahn, J. A., Evans, J. L., Bangsberg, D. R., & Moss, A. R. (2005). Revolving doors: Imprisonment among the homeless and marginally housed population. *American Journal of Public Health, 95*(10), 1747.

Kushel, M. B., & Miaskowski, C. (2006). End-of-life care for homeless patients. *JAMA: Journal of the American Medical Association, 296*(24), 2959-2966.

Langlois, J. A., Rutland-Brown, W., & Wald, M. M. (2006). The epidemiology and impact of traumatic brain injury: A brief overview. *Journal of Head Trauma Rehabilitation, 21*(5), 375-378.

Lenskyj, H. J. (2010). Women and the Olympics: Research, activism, and an alternative view. *Thirdspace: A Journal of Feminist Theory & Culture, 9*(2).

Leung, C. S., Ho, M. M., Kiss, A., Gundlapalli, A. V., & Hwang, S. W. (2008). Homelessness and the response to emerging infectious disease outbreaks: Lessons from SARS. *Journal of Urban Health, 85*(3), 402-410.

Levin, A., & Nicholson, M. J. (2005). Privacy law in the United States, the EU and Canada: The allure of the middle ground. *University of Ottawa Law and Technology Journal, 2*(2), 357-395.

Lieberman, S. (1973). The genogram. The family tree as a tool. *Transgenerational family therapy*. London: Croom Helm, 23-32.

Link, B. G., Struening, E. L., Neese-Todd, S., Asmussen, S., & Phelan, J. C. (2001). Stigma as a barrier to recovery: The consequences of stigma for the self-esteem of people with mental illnesses. *Psychiatric Services, 52*(12), 1621-1626.

Link, B. G., Yang, L. H., Phelan, J. C., & Collins, P. Y. (2004). Measuring mental illness stigma. *Schizophrenia Bulletin, 30*(3), 511-541.

Littlechild, B., Smith, R., & Work, S. (2012). *A handbook for interprofessional practice in the human services: Learning to work together*. New York, Routledge.

Lowinson, J., Ruiz, P., Millman, R., & Langrod, J. (2004). *Substance abuse: A comprehensive textbook* (4th ed.). Philidelphia: Lippincott, Williams & Wilkins.

Lozoff, B., Jimenez, E., Hagen, J., Mollen, E., & Wolf, A. W. (2000). Poorer behavioral and developmental outcome more than 10 years after treatment for iron deficiency in infancy. *Pediatrics, 105*(4).

Marlatt, G. A., Larimer, M. E., & Witkiewitz, K. (2011). *Harm reduction: Pragmatic strategies for managing high-risk behaviors*. New York: Guilford Press.

Maslach, C., Schaufeli, W. B., & Leiter, M. P. (2001). Job burnout. *Annual Review of Psychology, 52*, 379-422.

Maslow, A. H. (1954). *Motivation and personality*. New York: Harper & Bros.

Mathieu, F. (2012). *The compassion fatigue workbook*. New York: Routledge.

Matsumoto, D., & Juang, L. (2012). *Culture and psychology*. Belmont, CA: Wadsworth.

May, P. A., Gossage, J. P., Kalberg, W. O., Robinson, L. K., Buckley, D., Manning, M., & Hoyme, H. E. (2009). Prevalence and epidemiologic characteristics of FASD from various research methods with an emphais on recent in-school studies. *Developmental Disabilities Research Reviews, 15*(3), 176-192.
McCormarck, D., Johnston, C., Boivin, J.-F., & Thompson, C. (2010). Naming health determinants that influence the health status of homeless persons. *Social Development Issues, 32*(3), 92-108.
McDermott, S. (2011). Ethical decision making in situations of self-neglect and squalor among older people. *Ethics and Social Welfare, 5*(1), 52-71.
McKiernan, P., Cloud, R., Patterson, D. A., Golder, S., & Besel, K. (2011). Development of a brief abstinence self-efficacy measure. *Journal of Social Work Practice in the Addictions, 11*(3), 245-253.
Mechanic, D. (2007). Mental health services then and now. *Health Affairs (Millwood), 26*(6), 1548-1550.
Mental Health Commission of Canada. (2012). *At home/chez soi early findings report* (vol. 2, 22). Calgary, AB: Author.
Miley, K. K., O'Melia, M. W., & DuBois, B. L. (2012). *Generalist social work practice: An empowering approach* (7th ed.). Old Tappan, NJ: Pearson Education.
Mojtabai, R. (2011). National Trends in Mental Health Disability, 1997-2009. *American Journal of Public Health, 101*(11), 2156-2163.
Montgomery, A. E., Metraux, S., & Culhane, D. (2013). Rethinking homelessness prevention among persons with serious mental illness. *Social Issues and Policy Review, 7*(1), 58-82.
Morse, G., Salyers, M. P., Rollins, A. L., Monroe-DeVita, M., & Pfahler, C. (2011). Burnout in mental health services: A review of the problem and its remediation. *Administrative Policy in Mental Health, 39*, 341-352.
Munson, C. (2001). *The mental health diagnostic desk reference.* New York: The Haworth Press.
Musto, D. F. (1991). Opium, cocaine and marijuana in American history. *Scientific American, 265*(1), 40-47.
Musto, D. F. (2002). *Drugs in America: A documentary history.* New York: NYU Press.
National Alliance to End Homelessness. (2011). Housing First. Retrieved from http://www.endhomelessness.org/content/article/detail/1424
National Alliance to End Homelessness. (2012). Ending family homelessness: National trends and local system response. Retrieved from http://

www.endhomelessness.org/library/entry/ending-family-homelessness-national-trends-and-local-system-responses

National Alliance to End Homelessness. (2013). *The state of homelessness in America*. Washington, DC: Author.

National Case Management Network. (2009). Canadian Standards of Practice for Case Management. Retrieved from http://www.ncmn.ca/resources/documents/english%20standards%20for%20web.pdf

National Coalition for the Homeless. (2009). Minorities and homelessness. Retrieved from http://www.nationalhomeless.org/factsheets/minorities.html

National Institute on Drug Abuse (NIDA). (2013). *National survey of drug use and health*. Washington, DC: US Government Printing Office. Retrieved from http://www.drugabuse.gov/national-survey-drug-use-health

Norris, F. H., & Slone, L. B. (2007). The epidemiology of trauma and PTSD. In M. J. Friedman, T. M. Keane, & P. M. Ressick (Eds.), *Handbook of PTSD: Science and practice* (pp. 78–98). New York: Guilford Press.

Novac, S., Hermer, J., Paradis, E., & Kellen, A. (2006). *Justice and injustice: Homelessness, crime, victimization, and the criminal justice system* (Research Paper 207). Toronto: Centre for Urban and Community Studies, University of Toronto and The John Howard Society of Toronto.

Novac, S., Hermer, J., Paradis, E., & Kellen, A. (2009). A revolving door? Homeless people and the justice system in Toronto. *Centre for Urban and Community Studies Research Bulletin, 36*, 3. Toronto: University of Toronto.

Noyce, P., Olsen, C., & Winter, J. (Producer), & Noyce, P. (Director). (2002). *Rabbit proof fence*. Australia: Miramax.

O'Connell, D. F. (1998). *Dual disorders: Essentials for assessment and treatment*. New York: Routledge.

O'Connell, J. J. (2005). *Premature mortality in homeless populations: A review of the literature*. Nashville, TN: National Health Care for the Homeless Council.

Office of the Privacy Commissioner of Canada. (2004). The Personal Information Protection and Electronic Documents Act (PIPEDA). Ottawa: Government of Canada. Retrieved from http://www.priv.gc.ca/leg_c/leg_c_p_e.asp

Office of the United Nations High Commissioner for Human Rights. (2009). *Human rights fact sheet 21*. Geneva: Author.

Olivet, J., McGraw, S., Grandin, M., & Bassuk, E. (2010). Staffing challenges and strategies for organizations serving individuals who have experienced chronic homelessness. *Journal of Behavioral Health Services and Research, 37*(2), 226-238.

Olson-Madden, J. H., Forster, J. E., Huggins, J., & Schneider, A. (2012). Psychiatric diagnoses, mental health utilization, high-risk behaviors, and self-directed violence among veterans with comorbid history of traumatic brain injury and substance use disorders. *Journal of Head Trauma Rehabilitation, 27*(5), 370-378.

O'Toole, T. P., Conde-Martel, A., Gibbon, J. L., Hanusa, B. H., & Fine, M. J. (2003). Health care of homeless veterans. *Journal of General Internal Medicine, 18*(11), 929-933.

Palepu, A., Gadermann, A., Hubley, A. M., Farrell, S., Gogosis, E., Aubry, T., & Hwang, S. W. (2013). Substance use and access to health care and addiction treatment among homeless and vulnerably housed persons in three Canadian cities. *PloS ONE, 8*(10), e75133.

Paris, M., & Hoge, M. A. (2010). Burnout in the mental health workforce: A review. *Journal of Behavioral Health Services Research,* (37), 519-528.

Perlman, H. H. (1957). *Social casework: A problem-solving process.* Chicago: University of Chicago Press.

Perlman, J., & Parvensky, J. (2006). *Denver housing first collaborative cost benefit analysis and program outcomes report.* Colorado Commission for the Homeless. Retrieved from http://mdhi.org/download/files/Final%20DHFC%20Cost%20Study.pdf

Podymow, T., Turnbull, J., & Coyle, D. (2006). Shelter-based palliative care for the homeless terminally ill. *Palliative Medicine, 20*(2), 81-86.

Prochaska, J. O., & DiClemente, C.C. (1986). Toward a comprehensive model of change. In W. R. Miller & N. Heather (Eds.), *Treating addictive behaviors: Processes of change.* (pp. 3-27). New York: Plenum Press.

Prochaska, J. O., & Norcross, J. C. (2003). *Systems of psychotherapy: A transtheoretical analysis.* Pacific Grove, CA: Brooks/Cole.

Rew, L. (2000). Friends and pets as companions: Strategies for coping with loneliness among homeless youth. *Journal of Child and Adolescent Psychiatric Nursing, 13*(3), 125-132.

Rog, D., McCombs-Thornton, K., Gilbert-Mongelli, A., Brito, M., & Holupka, C. (1995). Implementation of the Homeless Families Program: 2. Characteristics, strengths, and needs of participant families. *American Journal of Orthopsychiatry, 65*(4), 514-528.

Rogers, C. R. (1966). Client-centered therapy. *American Handbook of Psychiatry, 3*, 183-200.

Rohnke, C., & Buttler, S. (1995). *QuickSilver: Adventure games, initiative problems, trust activities, and a guide to effective leadership.* Dubuque, IA: Kendall/Hunt.

Rollnick, S., & Miller, W. R. (1995). What is motivational interviewing? *Behavioural and Cognitive Psychotherapy, 23*, 325-334.

Roman, C. G. (2009). *Moving toward evidence-based housing programs for persons with mental illness in contact with the justice system.* Center for Mental Health Services, National GAINS Center. http://gainscenter.samhsa.gov/pdfs/ebp/MovingTowardEvidence-BasedHousing.pdf

Roman, C. G., McBride, E., & Osborne, J. W. (2005). Principles and practice in housing for persons with mental illness who have had contact with the justice system. *Housing Expert Panel Meeting: The National GAINS Center for Systemic Change for Justice-Involved Persons through the Center for Mental Health Services, SAMHSA* (p. 44). Bethesda, MD: Center for Mental Health Services (CMHS).

Roman, C. G., & Travis, J. (2004). *Taking stock: Housing, homelessness, and prisoner reentry.* Urban Institute, Washington, DC.

Rosenthal, R. N., Hellerstein, D. J., & Miner, C. R. (1992). Integrated services for treatment of schizophrenic substance abusers: Demographics, symptoms, and substance abuse patterns. *Psychiatric Quarterly, 63*(1), 3-26.

Roy, É., Haley, N., Leclerc, P., Sochanski, B., Boudreau, J.-F., & Boivin, J.-F. (2004). Mortality in a cohort of street youth in Montreal. *JAMA: Journal of the American Medical Association, 292*(5), 569-574.

Schein, E. H. (2006). *Organizational culture and leadership* (vol. 356). San Francisco, CA: John Wiley and Sons.

Schiff, R., & Waegemakers Schiff, J. (2010). Housing needs and preferences of relatively homeless Aboriginal women with addiction. *Social Development Issues, 32*(3), 65-76.

Schutt, R. K. (2011). At home on the street: People, poverty & a hidden culture of homelessness. *Contemporary Sociology: A Journal of Reviews, 40*(1), 100-101.

Sermons, M. W., & Henry, M. (2010). *Demographics of homelessness series: The rising elderly population.* Washington, DC: National Alliance to End Homelessness.

Sermons, M. W., & Witte, P. (2011). *State of homelessness in America: A research report on homelessness.* National Alliance to End Homelessness, Washington, DC.

Shapcott, M. (2008). *Wellesley Institute national housing report card*. Toronto: Wellesley Institute.

Shelley, B. M., Sussman, A. L., Williams, R. L., Segal, A. R., & Crabtree, B. F. (2009). "They don't ask me so I don't tell them": Patient-clinician communication about traditional, complementary, and alternative medicine. *Annals of Family Medicine, 7*(2), 139–147.

Smith, J. (2010). Capabilities and resilience among people using homeless services. *Housing, Care and Support, 13*(1), 9–18.

Solomon, A. L. (2006). *Understanding the challenges of prisoner reentry: Research findings from the urban institute's prisoner reentry portfolio*. Washington, DC: Urban Institute.

Song, J., Bartels, D. M., Ratner, E. R., Alderton, L., Hudson, B., & Ahluwalia, J. S. (2007). Dying on the streets: Homeless persons' concerns and desires about end of life care. *Journal of General Internal Medicine, 22*(4), 435–441.

Stamm, B. H. (1995). *The ProQOL manual: The professional quality of life scale compassion satisfaction, burnout & compassion fatigue/secondary trauma scales*. Baltimore: Sidaren Press.

Stamm, B. H. (2009). Professional quality of life: Compassion satisfaction and fatigue version 5 (ProQOL). Retrieved from www.isu.edu/~bhstamm or www.proqol.org

Statistics Canada. (2007). Population density by dissemination area (DA) in Canada, 2006. Retrieved from http://www.statcan.gc.ca/pub/91-003-x/2007001/figures/4129885-eng.htm

Stefancic, A., Larissa, H., Colleen, G., John, J., Sam, T., & Heather, J. (2012). Reconciling alternative to incarceration and treatment mandates with a consumer choice Housing First model: A qualitative study of individuals with psychiatric disabilities. *Journal of Forensic Psychology Practice, 12*(4), 382–408.

Stoner, M., R. (1995). *The civil rights of homeless people: Law, social policy, and social work practice*. Hawthorne, NY: Walter deGruyter.

Streissguth, A. P., Barr, H. M., Kogan, J., & Bookstein, F. L. (1996, August). Understanding the occurrence of secondary disabilities in clients with fetal alcohol syndrome (FAS) and fetal alcohol effects (FAE). Final Report to the Centers for Disease Control and Prevention (CDC, Tech. Rep. No. 96–06). Seattle: University of Washington, Fetal Alcohol and Drug Unit.

Strike, C., O'Grady, C., Myers, T., & Millson, M. (2004). Pushing the boundaries of outreach work: The case of needle exchange outreach programs in Canada. *Social Science & Medicine., 59*(1), 209–219.

Sundin, E. (2011). Homelessness and experiences of psychological trauma in the Western world: A research review and a qualitative study. *European Psychiatry, 26.* Retrieved from http://www.europsy-journal.com/article/S0924-9338%2811%2973515-5/abstract

Sung, H.-E. (2011). From diversion to reentry: Recidivism risks among graduates of an alternative to incarceration program. *Criminal Justice Policy Review, 22*(2), 219–234.

Sylvestre, M.E. (2010). Policing the homeless in Montreal: Is this really what the population wants? *Policing & Society, 20*(4), 432–458.

Tanzman, B. (1993). An overview of surveys of mental health consumers' preferences for housing and support services. *Hospital and Community Psychiatry, 44,* 450–455.

Tashiro, J., Byrne, C., Kitchen, L., Vogel, E., & Bianco, C. (2011). The development of competencies in interprofessional health care for use in health science educational programs. *Journal of Research in Interprofessional Practice and Education, 2*(1).

Teplin, L. A., McClelland, G. M., Abram, K. M., & Weiner, D. A. (2005). Crime victimization in adults with severe mental illness: Comparison with the national crime victimization survey. *Archives of General Psychiatry, 62*(8), 911–921.

Test, M. A., & Stein, L. I. (1976). Practical guidelines for the community treatment of markedly impaired patients. *Community Mental Health Journal, 12*(1), 72–82.

Topolovec-Vranic, J., Ennis, N., Colantonio, A., Cusimano, M. D., Hwang, S. W., Kontos, P. . . . & Stergiopoulos, V. (2012). Traumatic brain injury among people who are homeless: A systematic review. *BMC Public Health, 12*(1), 1059.

Torrey, E. F. (1988). *Nowhere to go: The tragic odyssey of the homeless mentally ill.* New York: Harper & Row.

Totten, S., & Bartrop, P. (2008). *Dictionary of genocide* (vol. 1). Westport, CT: Greenwood Press.

Trattner, W. I. (2007). *From poor law to welfare state: A history of social welfare in America.* New York: Simon and Schuster.

Truss, L. (2005). *Eats, Shoots & Leaves.* New York: Gotham Books.

Tsemberis, S. (1999). From streets to homes: An innovative approach to supported housing for homeless adults with psychiatric disabilities. *Journal of Community Psychology, 27*(2), 225–241.

Tsemberis, S. (2010). *Housing First: The Pathways model to end homelessness for people with mental illness and addiction*. Center City, MI: Hazelden.

Tsemberis, S., Gulcur, L., & Nakae, M. (2004). Housing first, consumer choice, and harm reduction for homeless individuals with a dual diagnosis. *American Journal of Public Health, 94*(4), 651-656.

Tutty, L., Bradshaw, C., Waegemakers Schiff, J., Worthington, C., McLaurin, B., Hewson, J., & McLeod, H. (2009). *Risks and assets for homelessness prevention: A literature review for The Calgary Homeless Foundation*. Calgary, AB: Calgary Homeless Foundation.

Tyler, K. A., Gervais, S. J., & Davidson, M. M. (2013). The relationship between victimization and substance use among homeless and runaway female adolescents. *Journal of Interpersonal Violence, 28*(3), 474-493.

Ulloa, E. W., Marx, B. P., Vanderploeg, R. D., & Vasterling, J. J. (2012). Assessment. In J. Vasterling, R. Bryant, & T. Keane (Eds.), *PTSD and mild traumatic brain injury* (pp. 149-173). New York: Guilford Press.

United Nations. (1948). Universal declaration of human rights. Author, New York. Retrieved from http://www.un.org/en/documents/udhr/

United Nations. (1966). International Covenant on Economic, Social and Cultural Rights. June 30, 2014. Retrieved from https://treaties.un.org/pages/Result.aspx?searchText = International%20Covenan t%20on%20 Economic,%20Social%20and%20Cultural%20Rights&dir = Publication\MTDSG&file = &query = All&tab = UN.

United Nations Human Settlements Programme (UN-HABITAT). (2005). Compilation of selected United Nations documents on housing rights (2nd ed.). Nairobi, Kenya. Retrieved from http://www.unrol.org/files/3672_81984_1.pdf

US Census Bureau. (2011). Population density for counties and Puerto Rico municipios: July 1, 2011. Retrieved from http://www.census.gov/popest/data/maps/2011/County-Density-11.html

US Department of Housing and Urban Development (HUD). (2012). Homeless emergency assistance and rapid transition to housing: Defining "homeless." US Government Printing Office, Washington, DC. Retrieved from http://portal.hud.gov/hudportal/HUD?src = /program_offices/comm _planning/homeless

US Department of Housing and Urban Development (HUD). (2013). 24 CFR Part 579.Homeless Emergency Assistance and Rapid Transition to Housing: Rural Housing Stability Assistance Program and Revisions to the

Definition of "Chronically Homeless"; Proposed Rule. Federal Register, Washington, DC. Retrieved from http://www.gpo.gov/fdsys/pkg/FR-2013-03-27/html/2013-06521.htm

US Department of Housing and Urban Development (HUD). (2014). Homelessness assistance. Retrieved from http://portal.hud.gov/hudportal/HUD?src=/program_offices/comm_planning/homeless

van der Kolk, B. A., Roth, S., Pelcovitz, D., Sunday, S., & Spinazzola, J. (2005). Disorders of extreme stress: The empirical foundation of a complex adaptation to trauma. *Journal of Traumatic Stress, 18*(5), 389–399.

Wadsworth, M., & Kuh, D. (1997). Childhood influences on adult health: A review of recent work from the British 1946 national birth cohort study, the MRC National Survey of Health and Development. *Paediatric and Perinatal Epidemiology, 11*(1), 2–20.

Waegemakers Schiff, J. (2009). Development of a measure of organizational culture in mental health. *Best Practices in Mental Health: An International Journal, 5*(2), 89–111.

Waegemakers Schiff, J., & Schiff, R. (2014). Housing First: Paradigm or program? *Journal of Social Distress and the Homeless.* Accessed at http://www.maneyonline.com/doi/full/10.1179/1573658X14Y.0000000007

Waegemakers Schiff, J., & Turner, A. (2014). *Housing First in rural Canada: Rural homelessness and Housing First feasibility across 22 Canadian communities.* Report prepared for Human Resources and Development Canada.

Waegemakers Schiff, J., & Turner, A. (2014). *Rural homelessness in Canada & Alberta: A review of the literature.* Calgary, AB: Alberta Centre for Child, Family and Community Research.

Wagamese, R. (2008). *Ragged company* (1st ed.). Toronto: Anchor Canada.

Weathers, F. W., Litz, B., Huska, J., & Keane, T. (1994). *PCL-C for DSM-IV.* Boston: National Center for PTSD-Behavioral Sciences Division.

Weaver, T., Renton, A., Stimson, G., & Tyrer, P. (1999). Severe mental illness and substance misuse: Research is needed to underpin policy and services for patients with comorbidity. *BMJ: British Medical Journal, 318*(7177), 137.

Weinstock, M. (2005). The potential influence of maternal stress hormones on development and 1znmental health of the offspring. *Brain, Behavior, and Immunity, 19*(4), 296–308.

Weiser, S., Dilworth, S., Neilands, T., Cohen, J., Bangsberg, D., & Riley, E. (2006). Gender-specific correlates of sex trade among homeless and marginally housed individuals in San Francisco. *Journal of Urban Health, 83*(4), 736-740.

Winick, C. (1992). Epidemiology of alcohol and drug abuse. In J. H. Lowinson, P. Ruiz, & R. B. Millman (Eds.), *Substance abuse: A comprehensive textbook*, 2nd ed. (pp. 15-29). Baltimore: Williams and Wilkins.

Witte, P. (2012). *The state of homelessness in America, 2012.* Washington, DC: National Alliance to End Homelessness, Homeless Research Institute.

World Health Organization (WHO). (2007). Mental health. Retrieved from http://www.who.int/features/qa/62/en/

World Health Organization (WHO). (n.d.). Mental disorders. Retrieved from http://www.who.int/topics/mental_disorders/en/

Yoder, K. A., Whitbeck, L. B., & Hoyt, D. R. (2003). Gang involvement and membership among homeless and runaway youth. *Youth & Society, 34*(4), 441-467.

Zeidner, M., Hadar, D., Matthews, G., & Roberts, R. D. (2013). Personal factors related to compassion fatigue in health professionals. *Anxiety, Stress & Coping, 26*(6), 595-609.

Ziskin, L. (Producer), & Brooks, J. (Director). (1997). *As good as it gets* [Motion picture]. United States: TriStar Pictures.

Zorzi, R., Scott, S., Doherty, D., Engman, A., Lauzon, C., McGuire, M., & Ward, J. (2006). *Housing options upon discharge from correctional facilities.* Ottawa, ON: Canada Mortgage and Housing Corporation.

Index

Aboriginal people
  boundaries and, 347
  child welfare and, 377
  colonization and, 285-286, 319-320
  communication and, 315
  family and, 145, 187
  fetal alcohol spectrum disorder (FASD) and, 223, 297
  genocide and, 319
  medicine and, 320
  rates of homelessness for, 10*t*
  studies of, 185
  trauma and, 285-286
abuse of power, 339-341
accountability, 110
acculturation, 308, 318
action plan, developing, xxiii, 30, 45, 100-102, 194
active listening, 43-44
addiction abstinence self-efficacy scale, 403-404
addictions
  abstinence self-efficacy scale for, 403-404
  diagnostic labels for, 220
  exercises on, 270
  factors leading to, 256*fig*
  history of homelessness and, 5-6
  housing first philosophy and, 175
  Jellinek Curve and, 255, 257*fig*, 258-259
  mechanisms and pathways for, 255
  overview of, 235-236
  stages of, 260*fig*
  stages of change model and, 259-260, 261*fig*
  statistics on, 236*t*
addictive disorders, 202-203, 211, 218, 261, 268

advocacy, 156, 379-380
affect regulation, 282, 284
affordability, 161-164
affordable housing, disappearance of, 4-5
after-care, 261
agencies, definition of, 124-125
agency resource books, 126
alcohol
  effects and appeal of, 253*t*
  history of, 240-243
  internal/external locus of control and, 268*t*
  intoxication signs for, 407
  major effects of, 248-249
  traumatic brain injury (TBI) and, 295, 296
  widespread use of, 242, 248
  withdrawal from, 248-252
  See also fetal alcohol spectrum disorder (FASD)
alcohol abuse/addiction
  effects of, 250*t*
  history of homelessness and, 5-6
  Jellinek Curve and, 255, 257*fig*, 258-259
  mental illness/mental health disorders and, 204, 224
  statistics on, 236*t*, 237
  See also addictions; fetal alcohol spectrum disorder (FASD)
alcohol withdrawal syndrome, 249-252
alcoholic hallucinosis, 250
Alcoholics Anonymous (AA), 244, 266
American Civil Liberties Union, 374
American Psychiatric Association, 281
American Society of Addiction Medicine, 264-265
animals, 73-74

antidiscrimination, 365
anxiety/anxiety disorders, 209, 214-215, 220, 263, 273, 283
appearance, mental health disorders and, 212-213
apprehensions, 377
As Good As It Gets, 221
assertive community treatment (ACT), 183-184, 279
assertiveness, 107-108, 156
assessments, 31, 97, 100, 124, 138, 141, 142-143, 144-145
assets, included in an action plan, 100, 127*t*, 143, 194
asylums, 160, 171, 172. *See also* deinstitutionalization
attentive listening, 34
attitudes
  practitioner, 26
  valid and invalid, 26-28, 27*t*
Attribution Questionnaire (AQ-27), 208, 231-234
autonomy, 108, 332
avoidance, 16, 208, 281, 282-283, 286, 292

Bandura, A., 280
barbiturates, 252, 255
basic premises, xv-xvi
Bassuk, E. L., 378
behavioral compliance, 173-174, 178
beneficence, 331
bioavailability, 276, 278
biological factors, 203
birth certificates, 20, 130, 137, 368. *See also* identification
blood, 60
bodily fluids, 60, 61, 62
body reactions to drugs, 247-252
boundaries, 28, 32, 341-343
brain injuries. *See* traumatic brain injury (TBI)
burnout, 28, 77-86, 400-401

Canada Pension Plan, 129*t*
cannabinols, 254*t*
case management
  certification in, 140
  continuing support services and, 143-150
  description of, 139-140
  exercises on, 157
  overview of, 123-125
  process of, 146*fig*
  responsibilities of, 141-142
  service coordination and, 139-143
case studies, 118-120, 121-122
casing, 32
Centre for Addiction and Mental Health, 281
change
  ambivalence toward, 43
  looking for, 44-45
Charter of Rights and Freedoms (Canada), xvi, 365, 381
Charter of Rights (United Nations), 186
child welfare, 376-379, 385
children
  custody of, 136
  education for, 136-137
  trauma and, 281-282, 287
Children's Online Privacy Protection Act, 382
choice
  importance of, 179, 181
  lack of, 200
civil law, 373-376
civil rights, 373-376
Civil Rights Code, 365
civil rights legislation (US), xvi
client, meaning of, xxii-xxiii
client-centered approach, 34, 42
client-centered services, 96-97, 98*fig*, 100, 106-107, 116, 145
Clostridium Difficile (C. diff.), 62
clothing
  as a right, xv-xvi, 76, 339
  as a sign of homelessness, 11-12, 15, 19-20, 24, 212, 321
  appropriate for frontline workers, 29, 38, 64-65
  and cultural awareness, 304*t*, 306*t*
  team dynamics and, 109-110
code of ethics, 111
cognitive difficulties, 213-215
cognitive disorders, 209, 220

Index

cognitive/developmental disorders, 220
cold water flats, 161
colonization, 319-320
Commission for Case Management Certification, 139-140
communicable diseases, 58, 59-67, 60*t*
communication, 108-110, 117, 315
companion pets, 73-74
compassion fatigue, 78-82, 401-402
compassion satisfaction scale, 399-400
confidentiality, 29, 332-334, 352-354, 355, 380-387
conflict of interest, 340
conflict tolerance and resolution, 110-116
consent for release of information, 386-387
continuing support services, 143-150
continuum of care (COC), 173, 175*fig*, 177, 178*fig*, 185, 264-265
co-occurring disorders (dual diagnosis)
    deinstitutionalization and, 227
    description of, 272-278
    exercises on, 298-299
    harm reduction approach and, 174
    terminology for, 236, 271-272
    treatment of, 278-279
    See also traumatic brain injury (TBI)
cooperation, 25, 27, 106, 108, 110, 354
coordination of care, 56, 108. *See also* interprofessional practice
couch surfing, 20-22
Coyle, B., 51
cross-cultural awareness, 305
cultural awareness
    definition of, 303
    levels of, 306*t*
    personal, 308-311
    stages of, 304-305*t*
cultural competence
    cultural sensitivity and, 303, 305, 307-308
    differences and, 314-318
    exercises on, 323-324
    overview of, 301-302
cultural diversity, 356
cultural lens, 313
cultural misconceptions, 312*t*
cultural norms, variations in, 314-316

cultural sensitivity, 303, 305, 307-308, 310*t*
cultural suppression, 319-320
culture
    description of, 302-303, 309
    family and, 145
    mental illness diagnosis and, 218, 219
    organizational, 322-323

daily living, needs for, xvi
death/death rates, 51, 70-71. *See also* life expectancy
debt, 369-370, 375
Declaration of Human Rights (United Nations), xvi
deinstitutionalization, 160, 171-173, 225-227. *See also* institutionalization
delirium tremens (DTs), 250
dental care, 19-20, 56, 58
depressants, 253*t*, 408
depression, 209, 214-215, 263, 273
11depressive disorders, 220
detoxification, 261, 265
developmental disorders, 211
Diagnostic and Statistical Manual of Mental Disorders (APA), 218-219, 281
DiClemente, C. C., 259, 269
direct service roles, 94*t*
directories, 126
disability benefits, 162-163, 164
disability income, 129*t*
disability insurance, 127*t*, 129*t*
discrimination, 207, 365, 389, 394-395
disinfectant, 62, 63
dissociation, 283, 286-287
diversion programs, 373
diversity, xiv
domestic violence, xiii, xv, 2, 31. *See also* family violence
    behavioral compliance and, 174
    as cause of homelessness, 19, 21
    housing first philosophy and, 174, 178, 183, 186
    trauma and, 222, 282, 284, 288
Donovan, D. M., 267
doubling up, 20-22

INDEX

Drink, A Cultural History of Alcohol (Gately), 240
drug abuse, 204, 224, 236t. *See also* addictions; co-occurring disorders (dual diagnosis); substance abuse
drug availability, 246
drug pathways, 247
drug trade, 370-371
drugs
  body reactions to, 247-252
  co-occurring disorders and, 273-277, 275*fig*
  effects and appeal of, 253-254t
dual diagnosis. *See* co-occurring disorders (dual diagnosis)
dysfunctional responses, 34-35, 37

early developmental influences, 203-204, 224
Eats, Shoots & Leaves (Truss), 108
ecomaps, 147*fig*, 152
education, 314-315
egoism, 335-336, 339t
elderly, 128t
  health issues and, 50-51, 295
Electronic Communications Privacy Act, 382
eligibility requirements, 138, 142
emergency medical kit, 61
emotional attachment, 31
emotional contagion, 79
employment insurance, 129t
empowerment, 21, 30, 37, 41, 73, 95, 124, 139, 143, 179, 182, 280, 292, 326
end of life, 70-71
engagement
  goals of, 29-34
  overview of, 24-26
  steps for, 41-45
entitlements, 41, 126, 131t, 137, 140, 145, 174, 364, 369, 374
environmental influences, 204, 224
epidemics, 59-67
epigenetics, 203
equality, 313-314
ethical decision-making map, 343-345
ethics
  basic principles of, 330-338

  boundaries and, 341-343, 345-348
  code of, 111, 329, 338-341, 354-357
  decision-making and, 343-345
  description of, 328-330
  exercises on, 357-361
  influences on ethical conduct, 349*fig*
  multiple contexts of, 337*fig*
  overview of, 325-328
  record-keeping and, 352-354
  violations of, 345-347
  in workplace, 348, 350-352
evictions/eviction laws, 167-168, 188-189, 375-376
exercises
  on addictions, 270
  on budgets, 195
  on case management, 157
  on co-occurring disorders, 298-299
  on cultural competence, 323-324
  on ethics, 357-361
  on health, 88-89
  on interprofessional practice, 116-122
  on legal issues, 387-388
  on mental illness/mental health disorders, 230-234
  on outreach and engagement, 45-47
  on self-care, 89
eye contact, 31, 34

family
  cultural differences in, 145
  extended, 187
family violence, 119, 389, 390-392. *See also* domestic violence
fetal alcohol spectrum disorder (FASD), 59, 223, 296-298, 298-299
fidelity, 330, 334
financial assistance programs, 125-126
financial challenges, 193-194
Fisher King, The, 221
flexibility
  ethics and, 342
  importance of, 25
  in services, 153, 342
foot care, 57-58
foreclosure, 375
formalism, 336, 339t
fragilely housed, meaning of, xxii, 49, 51, 72

Index

frontline workers
  challenges for, 28-29
  code of ethics for, 354-357
  roles of, 94*t*
  stress and, 76
  trust and, 27-28
  See also workers
frostbite, 56, 57
functional organizations, characteristics of, 86-88*t*

Gately, Iain, 240
gender constructions, 313-314
genetics, 203, 224
genocide, 318-319
genograms, 149-150, 150*fig*, 151*fig*, 152
guarded people, working with, 37, 39-41

Habitat for Humanity, 164
Hadar, D., 78
hallucinogens, 254*t*, 409
harm reduction approach, 174, 180, 182, 244, 269-270
Hartman, A., 152
health, mental. *See* mental health; mental illness/mental health disorders
health, oral, 19-20, 58
health, physical
  common medical conditions, 56-67
  exercises on, 88-89
  immediate needs when ill, 66*t*
  journaling on, 90
  needs related to, 67-74
  overview of, 49-51, 54-55
  primary care and, 71-72
  psychosocial determinants, 52-54
Health Insurance Portability and Accountability Act (HIPAA), 382
health of provider
  burnout and, 77-86
  overview of, 74-76
  See also burnout; compassion fatigue; self-care
HEARTH legislation, 375
Hecht, L., 51
hereditary factors, 203, 224
homelessness
  areas of concern and, 131-135*t*
  in Canada, 6-8, 9*t*, 10*t*, 11*t*
  causes of, 12
  culture of, 320-322
  definition of, 389-390
  description of, xiii-xiv, 3-4, 12
  emotional burden of, 8
  experience of, 16-18
  history of, 4-6, 159-161
  rural, 7, 9, 11*t*, 21, 55
  scenarios of, 13-15
  statistics on, 6-8
  typology of, 390-396
  in United States, 6-8, 9*t*, 10*t*, 11*t*
homeostasis, 249, 263
hope, 1, 21, 73, 79, 195
hopelessness, 73, 210*t*, 212, 215, 228, 401
Hopper, E. K., 289
hospice care, 70-71
hospitalizations, 55, 72, 170-171, 274, 340
hostile people, working with, 37, 39-41
House Link, 174-175
housing
  affordability of, 161-164
  getting and keeping, 186-187, 189, 194-195
  right to, 363
  subsidized, 164, 168-169
  vulnerability, 164-165
Housing and Community Development Act, 128*t*
housing assistance, Canadian vs. US, 165, 166-167*t*
Housing First
  culture of, 181-183
  description of, 175-179
  development of, 177
  essential values of, 182-183
  guidelines for, 183
  organizational culture and, 182
  program components, 179-181
  studies of, 184
  variations in, 178
housing first philosophy
  appropriateness of, 184-186
  continuum of, 178*fig*
  description of, 176-177
  effectiveness of, 185
  elements of, 176*t*

436 INDEX

housing first philosophy (*continued*)
  engagement and, 41
  importance of, xix
  overview of, 158-159
  support services and, 181
  variations in, 176
Housing for the Elderly (Section 202), 128*t*
housing loss
  needs assessment for, 192-193*fig*
  steps before, 189, 190-191*fig*
Housing Opportunities for People with AIDS (HOPW), 128*t*
housing readiness programs, 185
Hwang, S. W., 49
hypothermia, 56

identification, 15, 55, 130, 136, 368-369, 368*t*
immersion foot, 57
immigrants, 10*t*, 185, 313, 315-316. *See also* refugees
incarceration, 6, 366-367, 371-373
income standard, 162
individualism, 335, 339*t*
influenza, 59-67
inhalants, 254*t*, 255, 409
institutionalization, 170-171. *See also* deinstitutionalization
intake process, 100, 102, 153-156, 202
intensive treatment, 169, 260-261, 264-266, 350
International Classification of Diseases (ICD; World Health Organization), 218
International Covenant on Economic, Social and Cultural Rights, 363
interpretation services, 322
interprofessional practice
  case example for, 103
  conflict and, 110-115
  description of, xiv, 92-96
  disciplines involved in, 93*t*
  diverse settings and, 94
  domains of, 98*fig*
  elements of teamwork for, 105-110
  exercises on, 116-122
  housing first philosophy and, 101*fig*
  importance of, xix

  importance of teamwork for, 102-104, 104-106
  key components of, 97, 99, 114*t*
  overview of, 91-92
  practice principles for, 97, 99, 115-116
  services team and, 99-106
  structure of, 95*fig*
intervention skills/strategies, 34-37, 35*t*, 36*t*, 38*t*, 40, 44*t*, 227-229
intoxication, 246, 251*t*, 407-410

jargon, 99, 109, 117
Jellinek Curve, 255, 257*fig*, 258-259, 261
journaling
  prompts for, 47, 90, 122, 157, 197, 234, 270, 299-300, 324, 361, 388
  role of, xx-xxi
justice, 331-332, 339*t*
  criminal, 93, 185
  social, 12, 329, 379
justice system, 12, 134*t*, 138, 193, 363-364, 373

King's Speech, The, 221
Kushel, M. B., 70

landlords, 187-189. *See also* evictions/eviction laws
language differences, 316
legal issues
  child welfare, 376-379
  civil law, 373-376
  debt, 369-370
  drug and sex trades, 370-371
  exercises on, 387-388
  lack of identification, 368-369
  mortgage default, 375
  overview of, 362-363
  rights, 363-364
  victimization, 364-367
  worker roles in, 379-380
  See also confidentiality
Lieberman, S., 149
life balance, 83, 84*fig*
life expectancy, 54, 55. *See also* death/death rates
limit testing, 32-33
living rough, meaning of, xxii

low-income persons, vulnerability of, 164-165

mania (bipolar disorder), 215-217
marginally housed, meaning of, xxii
marijuana intoxication, 407
Maslow's hierarchy of needs, xvi, xvii*fig*, 19, 30
Matthews, G., 78
McKiernan, P., 269
medical care, 49, 58, 144, 265, 332
  as a basic right, xvi, 181
  difficulties in getting, 19, 73
medical kit, 61
medicine, traditional, 317, 320
mental disorders, definition of, 198-199. *See also* mental illness/mental health disorders
mental health
  definition of, 198-199
  housing and, 200
  terminology and, 72-73
Mental Health Commission of Canada, 175, 177, 184
mental health disability, 129*t*, 201
mental illness/mental health disorders
  causes of, 203-205, 223-227
  common signs and symptoms of, 209, 210*t*, 211-212
  diagnostic labels for, 211, 217-220
  diagnostic manuals for, 218-219
  exercises on, 230-234
  housing first philosophy and, 186
  housing programs for people with, 169-175
  identifying, 208-223
  intervention strategies and, 227-229
  legal issues and, 365-366, 367
  misunderstandings regarding, 202-203
  statistics on, 201
  stereotypes regarding, 208
  stigma and, 205-208
  treatment of, 225-227
Methicillin Resistant Staphylococcus Aureus (MRSA), 62
Miller, W. R., 42
minimum wage, 5, 162, 163*t*
minorities, overrepresentation of, xiv

misdiagnosis, 286-290
mixed-feature disorders, 211, 220
Model Residential Landlord-Tenant Code, 168
mood- and mind-altering drugs
  history of, 239-246
  types of, 252-255, 253-254*t*
mood lability, 216, 252
moral treatment, 225-226
mortality rates. *See* death/death rates
motivational interviewing, 42-45, 266-268
multigenerational trauma, 285-286, 320

narcotics, 244, 253*t*
Narcotics Anonymous, 204, 244
National Health Care for the Homeless Council, 54
National Law Center on Homelessness and Poverty, 374
National Standards of Practice, 139-140
Native American Housing Assistance and Self-Determination Act (NAHASDA), 128*t*
navigation, 153
need-based programs, 126
needs assessment, 192-193*fig*
negative mood and cognitions, 283
networking, 155
nonmaleficence, 330-331, 353-354
nonverbal behaviors/communication, 37, 39-41, 109-110
Norcross, J. C., 279
Novac, S., 367
Nowhere to Go (Torrey), 172
nutrition, 67-68

O'Connell, J. J., 49
Old Age Security Pension (OAS), 129*t*
Old-Age and Survivors Insurance (OASI), 127*t*
O'Leary, M. R., 267
One Flew Over the Cuckoo's Nest, 172
one-third rule, 162
opioids, 253*t*
oppression, 318-320
oral health, 19-20, 56, 58
organic disorders, 209
organizational culture, 182, 322-323

organizational factors, burnout and, 85-86, 86-88*t*
organizations
　definition of, 124-125
　responsibilities of, 131-135*t*
outreach, overview of, 24-26

Pathways to Housing, 175, 177
peer influences, 204
peer support programs, 266
Personal Information Protection and Electronic Documents Act (PIPEDA; 2004), 381-383
personal space, 32-33
personality disorders, 221-222
personality influences, 224
pets, 73-74
phencyclidine (PCP), 254*t*, 409-410
Poor Laws, 174, 366
poorhouses, 159-160, 161
post-traumatic stress disorder (PTSD), 222
poverty, xiv, xvi, 2, 4, 7, 9-11, 13, 49, 52, 165, 170, 366, 375
practitioner attitudes and values, 26
pregnancy, 59
prenatal influences, 203, 224
preventative health care, 71-72
primary health care, 71-72
prisons. *See* incarceration
privacy, right to, 332-333, 381. *See also* confidentiality
Privacy Act (1983), 381
Prochaska, J. O., 259, 279
professional degree requirements, 113*t*
Professional Quality of Life Scale (ProQOL), 82, 397-402
programs
　definition of, 125
　income support, 126-127*t*, 128*t*
　publicly administered, 125-126, 130
Prohibition era, 243
prostitution, 371
psychedelics, 254*t*
psychiatric hospitals, 5. *See also* asylums; deinstitutionalization
psychoeducation, 184
psychological health, 72-73. *See also* mental health; mental illness/mental health disorders

psychosis, 209, 214
public housing, 128*t*, 164, 168-169

Quebec Pension Plan, 129*t*

Rabbit Proof Fence (Noyce, Olsen, Winter, & Noyce), 319
Ragged Company (Wagamese), 8, 37, 260, 297, 321, 348
rape vs. sexual assault, 285
reactivity/arousal, 283
rebound effect, 249, 273
record-keeping, 352-354, 387. *See also* confidentiality
reentry programs, 373
refugees, 10*t*, 15, 131-132*t*, 313. *See also* immigrants
rehousing, first steps toward, 189
relapse and relapse prevention, 268-269
relationships
　ecomaps for, 152
　genograms for, 149-150, 150*fig*, 151*fig*, 152
　influences of, 204
rental assistance, 165
rental tribunals, 168, 375
Residential Tenancy Act, 167-168
residential treatment programs, 169
resource depletion, in workers 79
resources, locating, 126
responsibility, 110
Right to Financial Privacy Act, 382
rights
　civil, xvi, 365, 373-376
　legal, 363-364
Roberts, R. D., 78
Rogers, C., 34, 42
role assumption, 112, 121
role clarification, 116-117
role confusions, 95-96
Rollnick, S., 42
Roy, É., 59
rule enforcement, 27
rural areas and communities, 2, 5, 21, 126, 133*t*, 168, 196, 252
rural and remote settings, boundaries and, 347-348

Index

Rural Housing Stability Assistance programs, 166*t*
Rush, B., 243

SAMHSA, 281
screening, 142
secondary traumatic stress scale, 401-402
Section 8, 128*t*
sedative-hypnotics, 252, 253*t*, 255
seizures, 251
self-assessments
 addictions and, 403-404
 for trauma, 405-406
self-care, 81, 83-85, 89, 90, 212-213
self-determination, 332, 335, 356
self-efficacy, 267, 268, 280, 293
self-esteem, 289
self-stigma, 205, 206
service brokers and service coordination, 138-143, 153-157
service fairs, 20
service system, 131-135*t*
services
 array of, 148*fig*
 for client and family, 147*fig*
Severe Acute Respiratory Syndrome (SARS), 65-66
sex trade, 370-371
sexual assault vs. rape, 285
sexual comments, 32
sexual health, 58-59
shelters, 25-26, 124, 139, 176
shoes, 29, 64, 65
silence, engagement and, 31-32
single room occupancy hotels (SROs), 160, 169, 225-226
skill deficiencies, assumptions of, 174
sleep, providers and, 77
sleeping place, secure, 18-19
Smith, B., 244
social housing, 169
Social Insurance/Social Security, 130, 131*t*, 368, 382
social services
 description of, 125-126
 responsible organizations and, 131-135*t*
social welfare programs, 125-126
socioeconomic influences, 204-205, 224
Soloist, The, 220-221

solvents, 254*t*
stages of change model, 259-260, 261*fig*
STDs, 59
Stein, L. I., 183
stigma, 13, 199, 203, 205-208, 230, 316
stimulants, 253*t*, 408-409
street skills, for frontline workers, 29
strength-based approach, 31
stress, 52-54, 74-75, 80, 82, 224
stressful life events, 52, 53-54*t*, 54-55
subcultures, 302, 312-313
subsidized housing, 168-169
substance abuse
 description of, 247
 levels and locations of care for, 262*t*, 263-266
 overview of, 237-238
 programs/treatment for, 169, 260-266
 statistics on, 201
 See also addictions; co-occurring disorders (dual diagnosis)
substance dependency, 247
supervision
 burnout and, 86
 confidentiality and, 384
 shadowing and, 39
 stress and, 75
supplemental security income (SSI), 127*t*, 163
support services, *housing first* philosophy and, 181
swearing, 32
systems navigation, 153

takeovers, 188
team building, 107
teamwork
 elements of, 105-110
 exercises on, 117-120
 importance of, xv, 102-104, 104-106
temperance movement, 243, 244
Temporary Assistance to Needy Families (TANF), 127*t*
terminology, xxi-xxiii, 24
Test, M. A., 183
therapeutic treatment communities, 169
therapeutic window, 276-277, 276*fig*
thinking and cognition, 213-215

thought and emotional processing disorders, 209
Tipping Act (1751), 242
tobacco use, 243. *See also* substance abuse
toolkits, 154–156
transitional housing models, 185–186
translation services, 322
trauma
  children and, 281–282, 287
  common reactions and, 281, 290–291*t*
  complex, 285
  current care-related information on, 280
  definition of, 279–280, 281–282
  drug abuse and, 370–371
  homelessness and, 281–286
  impact of, 68–69
  mental illness/mental health disorders and, 204, 222, 224
  multigenerational, 285–286
  secondary, 401–402
  self-assessment scale for, 405–406
  terminology and, 280–281
  vicarious, 68, 78–82
trauma-induced cognitive distortions, 288–290
trauma-informed care, 279–281, 293–294
traumatic brain injury (TBI), 69–70, 222–223, 294–296
traumatic reactions, 281, 282–285, 290–291*t*
treatment-resistant pathogens, 62
trust
  building, 27
  confidentiality and, 381
  teamwork and, 106–107
  trauma and, 288–289
tuberculosis, 59–60
turnover, 75

unemployment insurance, 127*t*
unethical behavior, 339–341. *See also* ethics
Uniform Residential Landlord and Tenant Residency Act, 168. *See also* evictions/eviction laws; landlords
United Nations, xvi, 186, 363
United Way, 126

Universal Declaration of Human Rights, 363
universal health-care coverage, 55
universality of feelings, 209
Urban Institute, 372
utilitarianism, 335, 339*t*
utilities, 165, 167, 168

vaccinations, 62
values, practitioner, 26
Vancomycin Resistant Enterococcus (VRE), 62
veracity, 334
veterans, traumatic brain injury (TBI) and, 295
vicarious trauma, 68, 78–82
victimization, 364–367, 370–371
voting, 16, 136

Wagamese, R., 37
Waltz with Bashir, 221
war on drugs, 244
Wellesley Institute, 374
Wild Swans, 316
Wilson, B., 244
withdrawal, from substance use, 246–252, 261–265, 262*t*, 276, 407–410
women
  cultural differences and, 313–314, 315
  gender constructions and, 313–314
  health issues and, 50
  housing first philosophy and, 186
  pregnant, 59
worker reactions and interventions, 289, 292–294
workers
  health issues and, 51
  impaired, 350–352
  unqualified, 350
  See also frontline workers
workers' compensation, 127*t*, 129*t*
World Health Organization (WHO), 73, 198–199, 218

youths
  health issues and, 50–51
  housing first philosophy and, 186
  See also children

Zeidner, M., 78